Pancreatic Cancer

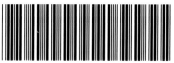

369 0246707

This book is due for return on or before the last date shown below.

Pancreatic Cancer

Pathogenesis, Diagnosis, and Treatment

Edited by

Howard A. Reber, MD

UCLA School of Medicine,
Los Angeles, CA

Springer Science+Business Media, LLC

ISBN 978-1-4612-7294-6   ISBN 978-1-4612-1810-4 (eBook)
DOI 10.1007/978-1-4612-1810-4

© 1998 Springer Science+Business Media New York
Originally published by Humana Press Inc. in 1998
Softcover reprint of the hardcover 1st edition 1998

This publication is printed on acid-free paper. ∞
ANSI Z39.48-1984 (American Standards Institute) Permanence of Paper for Printed Library Materials.

Cover design by Patricia F. Cleary.

Photocopy Authorization Policy:
Authorization to photocopy items for internal or personal use, or the internal or personal use of specific clients, is granted by Springer Science+Business Media, LLC,
provided that the base fee of US $8.00 per copy, plus US $00.25 per page, is paid directly to the
Copyright Clearance Center at 222 Rosewood Drive, Danvers, MA 01923. For those organizations that have been granted a photocopy license from the CCC, a separate system of payment has been arranged and is acceptable to Springer Science+Business Media, LLC,
The fee code for users of the Transactional Reporting Service is: [0-89603-466-6/98 $8.00 + $00.25].

Library of Congress Cataloging-in-Publication Data

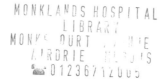

Preface

In spite of the fact that pancreatic cancer continues to be a devastating disease in which few patients are cured, the last decade has seen a number of truly significant advances in the field. Enormous strides have been made in our understanding of the basic cellular and molecular processes that influence the development of this malignancy, and the characterization of the genetic abnormalities that are associated with it. These advances in basic science represent the most likely area from which significant improvements in the management of pancreatic cancer are likely to come. Thus, a number of the contributions to this book are concerned with these issues, as well as their potential clinical relevance.

Advances have been made as well in the areas of the diagnosis and staging of pancreatic cancer, as well as its nonoperative management. They have resulted in fewer patients undergoing surgery for the disease, increased the likelihood of resection in those who are operated on, and generally improved the quality of life. These are reviewed in chapters that discuss the latest techniques for genetic screening for pancreatic cancer, the value of tumor antigens, advances in diagnostic radiology, and the roles of laparoscopy (diagnostic and therapeutic) and palliative endoscopic stenting.

The section on treatment of pancreatic cancer includes contributions from surgeons in the United States and Japan, who review their experiences with standard forms of pancreatic resections and the so-called radical or extended pancreatic resection, which some have viewed as an improvement over the standard Whipple pancreaticoduodenectomy. Up-to-date information is also provided about the efficacy and roles of chemotherapy and radiotherapy in this disease, as well as the theoretical basis and potential for gene therapy. The final chapter is devoted to a consideration of the quality of life of pancreatic cancer patients, an area that is assuming increasing importance in the discussion of cancer treatment in general.

Pancreatic Cancer: Pathogenesis, Diagnosis, and Treatment was created in an effort to reflect the current state of both the art and the science in the field of pancreatic cancer, with contributions from renowned experts in Asia, Europe, and the United States. It should be of interest to basic scientists as well as all clinicians who are working in this challenging area.

Howard A. Reber, MD

Contents

Preface .... *v*

List of Contributors .... *ix*

PART I.   ETIOLOGY AND PATHOGENESIS 1

1   Molecular Genetics of Pancreatic Carcinoma
    Christopher A. Moskaluk and Scott E. Kern................................... 3

2   Role of Polypeptide Growth Factors and Their Receptors
    in Human Pancreatic Cancer
    Murray Korc 21

3   Growth Factors and Growth Factor Receptors in Chronic Pancreatitis,
    and the Relation to Pancreatic Cancer
    Helmut Friess, Pascal Berberat, and Markus W. Büchler 33

4   Clues from Experimental Models
    Daniel S. Longnecker 53

5   Role for Transforming Growth Factor-β: *Clues from Other Cancers*
    Leslie I. Gold and Trilok Parekh 71

PART II.   DIAGNOSIS AND STAGING 111

6   Screening for Pancreatic Cancer Using Techniques to Detect Altered
    Gene Products
    Robb E. Wilentz, Robbert J. C. Slebos, and Ralph H. Hruban 113

7   Tumor Antigens in Pancreatic Cancer
    Carlos Rollhauser and William Steinberg 137

8   Radiologic Techniques for Diagnosis and Staging of Pancreatic
    Carcinoma
    Mark E. Baker 157

9   Diagnosis and Staging of Pancreatic Cancer: *The Role of Laparoscopy*
    Margaret Schwarze and David W. Rattner 171

PART III.   TREATMENT 179

10   Standard Forms of Pancreatic Resection
    Peter W. T. Pisters, Jeffrey E. Lee, and Douglas B. Evans 181

11   Extended Radical Whipple Resection for Cancer of the Head
    of the Pancreas: *Operative Procedure and Results in Our Institution*
    F. Hanyu, T. Imaizumi, M. Suzuki, N. Harada, T. Hatori,
       and A. Fukuda... 201

12　Extended Pancreatic Resection for Carcinoma of the Pancreas
　　Tatsushi Naganuma and Yoshifumi Kawarada......................................213

13　Endoscopic Stents for Palliation in Patients with Pancreatic Cancer
　　Richard C. K. Wong and David L. Carr-Locke.................................235

14　Laparoscopic Biliary and Gastric Bypass
　　Kevin C. Conlon and Stanley W. Ashley...253

15　Chemotherapy of Pancreatic Cancer
　　Margaret Tempero...265

16　Radiation Therapy for Pancreatic Cancer
　　Tyvin A. Rich...281

17　Gene Therapy for Pancreatic Cancer
　　Nicholas R. Lemoine...295

18　Quality of Life in Pancreatic Cancer
　　D. Fitzsimmons and C. D. Johnson...319

　　Index...339

Contributors

STANLEY W. ASHLEY • *Department of Surgery, Brigham and Women's Hospital, Boston, MA*

MARK E. BAKER • *Department of Radiology, Cleveland Clinic, Cleveland, OH*

PASCAL BERBERAT • *Department of Visceral and Transplantation Surgery, University of Bern, Switzerland*

MARKUS W. BÜCHLER • *Department of Visceral and Transplantation Surgery, University of Bern, Switzerland*

DAVID L. CARR-LOCKE • *Gastroenterology Division, Brigham and Women's Hospital, Boston, MA*

KEVIN C. P. CONLON • *Department of Surgery, Memorial Sloan-Kettering Cancer Center, New York, NY*

DOUGLAS B. EVANS • *Department of Surgery, M. D. Anderson Cancer Center, University of Texas, Houston, TX*

HELMUT FRIESS • *Department of Visceral and Transplantation Surgery, University of Bern, Switzerland*

A. FUKUDA • *Department of Gastroenterological Surgery, Tokyo Women's Medical College, Tokyo, Japan*

D. FITZSIMMONS • *Southampton General Hospital, University of Southampton, UK*

LESLIE I. GOLD • *Department of Pathology, The Stanley Kaplan Cancer Center, New York University Medical Center, New York, NY*

F. HANYU • *Department of Gastroenterological Surgery, Tokyo Women's Medical College, Tokyo, Japan*

N. HARADA • *Department of Gastroenterological Surgery, Tokyo Women's Medical College, Tokyo, Japan*

T. HATORI • *Department of Gastroenterological Surgery, Tokyo Women's Medical College, Tokyo, Japan*

RALPH H. HRUBAN • *Department of Pathology, The Johns Hopkins Hospital, Baltimore, MD*

T. IMAIZUMI • *Department of Gastroenterological Surgery, Tokyo Women's Medical College, Tokyo, Japan*

C. D. JOHNSON • *Southampton General Hospital, University of Southampton, UK*

SCOTT E. KERN • *The Johns Hopkins University School of Medicine, Baltimore, MD*

YOSHIFUMI KAWARADA • *First Department of Surgery • Mie University School of Medicine, Tsu City, Japan*

MURRAY KORC • *Division of Endocrinology and Metabolism, University of California, Irvine, CA*

JEFFREY E. LEE • *Department of Surgery, M. D. Anderson Cancer Center, University of Texas, Houston, TX*

NICHOLAS R. LEMOINE • *Oncology Unit, Imperial Cancer Research Fund, Hammersmith Hospital, Royal Postgraduate Medical School, London, UK*

DANIEL S. LONGNECKER • *Department of Pathology, Dartmouth-Hitchcock Medical Center, Dartmouth Medical School, Lebanon, NH*

CHRISTOPHER A. MOSKALUK • *The Johns Hopkins University School of Medicine, Baltimore, MD*

TATSUSHI NAGANUMA • *First Department of Surgery • Mie University School of Medicine, Tsu City, Japan*

TRILOK PAREKH • *Department of Pathology, The Stanley Kaplan Cancer Center, New York University Medical Center, New York, NY*

PETER W. T. PISTERS • *Department of Surgery, M. D. Anderson Cancer Center, University of Texas, Houston, TX*

DAVID W. RATTNER • *Department of Surgery, Massachusetts General Hospital, Harvard Medical School, Boston, MA*

TYVIN A. RICH • *Department of Therapeutic Radiology and Oncology, University Hospital, Charlottesville, VA*

CARLOS ROLLHAUSER • *Division of Gastroenterology and Nutrition, Department of Medicine, George Washington University Medical Center, Washington, DC*

MARGARET SCHWARZE • *Department of Surgery, Massachusetts General Hospital, Harvard Medical School, Boston, MA*

ROBBERT J. C. SLEBOS • *Department of Pathology, The Johns Hopkins Hospital, Baltimore, MD*

WILLIAM M. STEINBERG • *Division of Gastroenterology and Nutrition, Department of Medicine, George Washington University Medical Center, Washington, DC*

M. SUZUKI • *Department of Gastroenterological Surgery, Tokyo Women's Medical College, Tokyo, Japan*

MARGARET A. TEMPERO • *Department of Medicine, Eppley Cancer, University of Nebraska, Omaha, NE*

ROBB E. WILENTZ • *Department of Pathology, The Johns Hopkins Hospital, Baltimore, MD*

RICHARD C. K. WONG • *Gastroenterology Division, Brigham and Women's Hospital, Boston, MA*

I
Etiology and Pathogenesis

Molecular Genetics of Pancreatic Carcinoma

Christopher A. Moskaluk and Scott E. Kern

INTRODUCTION

The application of modern molecular biological techniques to the study of human tumors in the past two decades has demonstrated that cancer is a genetic disease. Structural alterations in genomic DNA (point mutation, gene rearrangement, and gene deletion), which result in alterations in protein coding sequences or their expression, have been found in every human neoplasm studied. The finding of these genetic alterations in invasive cancers and in their histologically identifiable neoplastic precursor lesions, but not in the nonneoplastic tissues from which they arose, is consistent with the theory that neoplastic progression is the result of the clonal evolution of cellular populations accompanying a selection for mutations *(1,2)*. Germ-line mutations in specific genes are also responsible for many cases in which there is a familial predisposition to cancer *(3)*, further underscoring the genetic basis of cancer.

The preponderance of evidence suggests that the genes that are frequently mutated in primary tumors have been selected for during the process of tumorigenesis, by result of the alterations conferring an increased growth potential to the tumor cells. In the case of an oncogene, the increased growth potential is caused by a dominant effect of the mutant gene product. In the case of a tumor-suppressor gene, it is caused by the loss of a negative regulatory effect. In the case of DNA repair genes, the loss of effective DNA repair leads to mutations in both oncogenes and in tumor-suppressor genes. Generally, more than one regulatory pathway has to be disabled in a cell in order to confer a full malignant phenotype, and this has been termed the "multihit" or "multistep" process of tumorigenesis *(4)*.

The deletion or mutation of the coding sequence of a gene is an irreversible event that fundamentally changes the function of that gene on the tumor cell. For the purposes of this review, the focus will be primarily on the recent advances in understanding the genetic alterations of ductal adenocarcinoma of the pancreas, which accounts for the majority of pancreatic neoplasms in humans. Pancreatic carcinoma has very recently gone from being one of the most poorly characterized to one of the most highly characterized tumors in terms of molecular genetic changes. These advances have implications for the diagnosis and treatment of pancreatic cancer, as well as aiding in our understanding of the neoplastic process in general.

ONCOGENES

Oncogenes are those genes whose biologic activity is increased by mutation. They are classically considered to be members of growth factor signaling pathways. Normal cellular genes (termed proto-oncogenes) become activated by point mutation, by gene amplification, which produces multiple copies of the gene, and by fusion to other genes and their regulatory elements. The most intensively studied oncogene has been the *K-ras* oncogene.

K-ras

Since the first report of the detection of *K-ras* mutations in 21 of 22 primary pancreatic adenocarcinomas (95%) *(5)*, numerous investigators have verified this finding in both primary carcinomas and in cell lines derived from pancreatic carcinomas, with frequencies ranging from 71 to 100% *(6)*. This is the highest reported prevalence of *K-ras* mutation in any tumor type *(7)*. *K-ras* is a member of the membrane-associated guanine nucleotide-binding protein family involved in signal transduction of growth-promoting effectors from the cell surface *(8)*. Mutations in codons 12, 13, or 61 of *K-ras* transform it into an oncogene, because these mutations impair the intrinsic GTPase activity of the gene product, causing it to remain constitutively active for signal transduction in its GTP-bound form. In pancreatic carcinoma, the vast majority of mutations occur in codon 12; only a handful of codon 13 mutations have been reported. *K-ras* mutations are fairly ubiquitous in pancreatic cancer, and they have not been shown to be correlated with tumor stage or patient survival. The finding of *K-ras* mutations in preinvasive pancreatic duct lesions (discussed in Tumor Progression in Pancreatic Carcinoma) suggests that this genetic alteration is probably not only essentially required in pancreatic adenocarcinoma, but also that it is an early event in neoplastic progression. The high prevalence of *K-ras* mutation in pancreatic neoplasia, including early stage disease, has made this a favored marker for the eventual development of diagnostic tests (*see* Chapter 6).

Other Known Oncogenes

There is no convincing genetic proof that another oncogene is involved in pancreatic tumorigenesis. A single case of MYC gene amplification in a primary pancreatic carcinoma has been reported *(9)*, but this has not been confirmed. Similarly, cytogenetic analysis has not implicated either the MYC or other oncogene loci as frequent sites of rearrangement *(10–12)*.

An area of the genome containing the putative oncogene *AKT2* (a protein–serine/threonine kinase) has been reported to be infrequently amplified, as seen in 2 of 18 pancreatic cell lines and 1 of 10 primary tumor specimens by Southern blot hybridization and fluorescence *in situ* hybridization *(13)*. Amplification of *AKT2* has been confirmed by others.

There have been many reports of increased expression of growth factors and their receptors in pancreatic cancer, utilizing immunohistochemistry and quantitative RNA analysis. However, studies that included cases of chronic pancreatitis also have reported increased expression of growth factor receptors in reactive nonneoplastic cells. Evidence of DNA amplification, gene rearrangement, or gene mutation of growth factor receptors has not been found.

Evidence for Yet-Uncharacterized Oncogenes

It is possible that activation of other proto-oncogenes besides *K-ras* are significantly involved in pancreatic carcinoma. There are four usual mechanisms of proto-oncogene activation: point mutation of the coding sequence, gene fusion with the coding sequence of another gene, amplification of copy number of the entire coding sequence, or up-regulation of gene transcription by translocation of the gene to the site of an active promoter/enhancer region. The first mechanism generally is detected by DNA sequence analysis of genomic coding sequences, and it requires knowledge of the specific gene to be analyzed, because nonspecific global screening assays for activated oncogenes are not very efficient. No new oncogenes have been identified in pancreatic carcinoma using these techniques.

The last three mechanisms of oncogene activation described above involve gross rearrangements of chromosomes, and can be detected by cytogenetic and *in situ* hybridization analysis. A large number of pancreatic cancers have been analyzed cytogenetically by Griffin et al. *(11,12)*, identifying chromatin fragments suggestive of double-minute chromosomes in 8 of 36 primary pancreatic carcinomas *(11)*. Double-minute chromosomes are a cytogenetic sign of DNA amplification. The presence of candidate oncogenes on double-minute chromosomes from pancreatic carcinoma has not yet been reported, but appears to be a fruitful field for further investigation. However, no consistent chromosomal translocation events have been identified that would be compatible with a common gene or promoter/enhancer fusion event. Thus, additional oncogenes may play a role in the development of pancreatic neoplasia, but these remain to be identified and characterized.

TUMOR-SUPPRESSOR GENES

Tumor-suppressor genes are those genes that play a normal role in negative regulation of cellular proliferation, but whose inactivation by mutation aids the emergence of neoplastic cell populations. These genes are inactivated by point mutations and by deletion, and both normal copies are usually found to be inactivated in tumors. The most commonly mutated genes in human cancer include the *p53* and *p16* genes.

p53

Inactivation of the *p53* gene is a common event in pancreatic carcinoma. *p53* mutations have been reported in 58–100% (average 78%) of pancreatic carcinoma cell lines *(14–18)*, in 75% of pancreatic xenografts *(19)*, and in up to 70% of primary pancreatic carcinomas *(14–16,20–24)*. The majority of mutations reported have been transitions (pyrimidine to pyrimidine or purine to purine) in the evolutionary conserved domains of the gene. Transversion mutations (pyrimidine to purine or purine to pyrimidine) are more commonly found in tumors highly associated with cigarette smoking, and this finding suggests that the documented increased risk of pancreatic carcinoma in smokers may be mediated by an effect other than direct DNA damage to the *p53* gene by tobacco carcinogens. In two studies, a relatively high prevalence (21 and 32%) *(15,21)* of small intragenic mutations in the *p53* gene in pancreatic cancers was noted, suggesting that unique mutational mechanisms may be at work in pancreatic carcinoma.

Some reports have shown a difference in the prevalence of *p53* mutations between cell lines and primary neoplasms, but this may reflect several artifacts. The first possibility is that there could be a selection bias for the establishment of cell lines in tumors with particular mutations, but there has been no evidence in pancreatic cancer for this phenomenon. The second possibility is that some methods used to detect gene mutations could lack adequate sensitivity for the analysis of primary tumors. Most pancreatic carcinomas induce an intense nonneoplastic stromal and inflammatory reaction, and, as a result, the neoplastic cells may often constitute the minority of the cells in the sample. In one study, even after careful cryostat dissection to enrich for neoplastic cells, only 7 of 33 cases of primary pancreatic tumors could be enriched to the level of 50% tumor cellularity *(25)*. Since a mutated allele represents only half of the possible sequences in a diploid cell, a tumor cellularity of 50% corresponds to a mutant/wild-type percentage of 33 or 25%, depending on whether or not the second allele is deleted in the tumor cells. This low level of mutant alleles may be below the threshold of many assay systems, particularly since tumor cellularity in primary tumors is usually far below 50% *(25)*.

p53 is a nuclear protein to which numerous activities have been attributed. Biochemically, the majority of evidence suggests that p53 acts as a DNA-binding transcriptional activator to stimulate the production of particular genes *(26–28)*. Biologically, p53 acts at a G1/S checkpoint, postponing DNA replication after certain cell stresses, such as DNA damage. If DNA damage has occurred, this delay presumably could give repair mechanisms the opportunity to work *(29)*. p53 also plays a biologic role in the induction of the apoptotic pathway of cell death *(30)*. The potential loss of these two important controls of the cellular life cycle (initiation of replication and induction of cell death) suggests that the inactivation of p53 by mutation may be a pivotal event in many tumors that allows the development of cancer of the pancreas.

*p16*INK4/MTS1/CDKN2

Caldas et al. *(31)* were the first to demonstrate that the *p16* gene is frequently inactivated in pancreatic cancer. Homozygous deletions involving the *p16* gene were found in 41% of a panel of xenografted pancreatic cancers and cell lines, and intragenic *p16* mutations were found in an additional 38% of cases. A subset of primary tumors were analyzed to control for artifacts of engraftment, and were found to have the same changes as the xenografts. Subsequent studies have verified these results, with rates of homozygous deletion of 46 and 50% *(32,33)* and rates of intragenic mutation of 30 and 34% *(33,34)*. These studies indicate that *p16* is inactivated in about 80% of pancreatic adenocarcinomas.

p16 is a part of a family of proteins that bind to cyclin–CDK complexes and inhibit the promotion of the cell cycle. p16 binds specifically to CDK4, and prevents that protein from phosphorylating the RB protein. The RB protein in the hypophosphorylated state inhibits the G1/S transition. Thus, inactivation of p16 by mutation disregulates an important cell cycle checkpoint *(35)*.

One remarkable aspect of the inactivation of *p16* is that half of the inactivations of *p16* involved a homozygous deletion, which at the time may have represented the highest rate of homozygous deletion described for a tumor-suppressor gene. Previous to this, homozygous deletions were known to involve some tumor-suppressor genes, but they were felt to be relatively rare events. One possible explanation for this phenomenon would be that a second tumor-suppressor gene is present in the vicinity of *p16*, and that homozygous deletions are selected for because they inactivate both genes. A gene closely related to *p16*, *p15 (MTS2)*, is located within 20 kilobases of *p16 (36,37)*, and it is involved by many of the homozygous deletions that inactivate *p16*. However, when *p15* was examined for evidence of mutation or transcriptional inactivation in carcinomas that did not involve the gene in a homozygous deletion, no abnormalities were detected *(32,38)*, making it unlikely that it is a second locus of tumor suppression. Thus, the explanation for the high rate of *p16* homozygous deletion remains to be elucidated. In related experiments, no abnormalities in coding sequence or transcriptional levels were detected in two other CDK inhibitors, *p18* and *p27*, in pancreatic adenocarcinomas *(32,38)*.

Recently, mutations in the *CDK4* gene that prevent the binding of wild-type *p16* gene product to *CDK4* have been reported in a melanoma cell line, and *CDK4* mutations have been suggested to be the cause of some cases of familial melanoma *(39,40)*. Although the possibility of CDK4 alteration was an attractive hypothesis to explore in cases of pancreatic carcinoma having wild-type *p16* genes, a study of nine pancreatic carcinomas with wild-type *p16* status found only wild-type *CDK4* sequences *(41)*. Similarly, the RB gene has been shown to be mutated in a small percentage of pancreatic carcinomas (*see* Other Tumor-Suppressor Genes), but the expected association among RB mutational status and *p16* wild-type pancreatic cancers has not been reported.

DPC4

As part of a global allelotype analysis of pancreatic carcinoma, an extremely high rate of chromosomal loss was detected on chromosomal arm 18q *(42)*. During this analysis, a number of homozygous deletions on 18q were identified. These deletions excluded *DCC*, the only known candidate tumor-suppressor gene on that chromosomal arm, as the locus of presumed tumor suppression *(43)*. Subsequent positional cloning and analysis of this locus led to the discovery of the putative tumor-suppressor gene *DPC4* (Deleted in Pancreatic Carcinoma, locus 4). *DPC4* was found to be inactivated by homozygous deletion in 30% of a panel of pancreatic cancer xenografts and cell lines. An additional 22% of tumors (not exhibiting homozygous deletions) were found to harbor potentially inactivating intragenic mutations, which were not present in control normal tissue. These findings are strong evidence that loss of *DPC4* activity is involved in at least 50% of pancreatic adenocarcinomas.

The *DPC4* gene product has homology to the MAD family of proteins, which are involved in signal transduction from the TGF-β superfamily of extracellular ligands *(44)*. A domain of the DPC4 protein has been shown to be active in transcriptional activation assays *(45)*, and *DPC4* may be one of the mediators in a TGF-β related signal. TGF-β has been shown in many model systems to downregulate growth of epithelial cells; inactivation of such a negative growth regulatory pathway represents an obvious candidate for tumor suppression *(46)*. A correlation between *DPC4* mutational status and the response of growth suppression to TGF-β has not been reported, however.

Alterations in the *DPC4* tumor-suppressor gene appear to occur most commonly in pancreatic and colorectal adenocarcinomas. Although *DPC4* was found to be inactivated in 15% of colitis-associated and sporadic colorectal carcinomas *(47,48)*, a survey study of 338 tumors from 12 anatomic sites found *DPC4* alterations to be uncommon (<10%) in other tumor types *(49)*. Other analyses have verified this finding *(50–52)*. Thus, inactivation of *DPC4* appears to be relatively specific for pancreatic cancer.

Other Tumor-Suppressor Genes

From the preceding discussion, it appears that of the known tumor-suppressor genes *p16, p53*, and *DPC4* are each inactivated in at least half of all pancreatic carcinomas. A number of other tumor-suppressor genes have been assayed in pancreatic carcinoma and have not been found to be mutated, or to be involved in frequent allelic loss in as significant a percentage of tumors.

Although an initial report of 10 cases indicated that the *APC* gene may be mutated in pancreatic carcinomas *(53)*, subsequent studies on 28 *(54)*, 33 *(25)*, and 39 *(55)* pancreatic cancers or cell lines found no demonstrable somatic mutations. This finding is of interest, since *APC* is one of the most frequently mutated genes in colorectal carcinomas, and it might have been expected that the pancreas, a gastrointestinal organ of endodermal origin, would also have a high rate of involvement of this gene in epithelial neoplastic transformation. This is a further indication of a mutational spectrum in pancreatic carcinoma that is distinct from those of other gastrointestinal neoplasms.

Mutations in the *RB* gene occur in pancreatic adenocarcinoma, but apparently at a low rate. Two studies found no evidence of RB protein loss in a total of 47 cases of primary adenocarcinoma studied by immunohistochemistry *(25,56)*. Similarly, a mutational screen of the *RB* gene in 14 pancreatic carcinoma cell lines failed to detect mutations in the coding sequence. In perhaps the most definitive study to date, Huang et al. *(57)* found evidence of loss of *RB* expression by immunohistochemistry in two of 32 archival paraffin-embedded specimens, and in 1 of 30 frozen tissue specimens of primary adenocarcinoma. Three of the 30 cancers with frozen tissue samples were found to have tumor-specific allele changes by single-strand conformation analysis, and DNA sequencing of two of these three cases revealed one truncating mutation and one missense mutation. The conclusion from this body of work is that *RB* inactivation plays a role in only a small minority of pancreatic ductal carcinomas.

The analysis of the role that the putative tumor-suppressor *DCC* gene plays in pancreatic carcinoma is complicated by several factors. The first is that *DCC* is 1.4 megabases in length, making it one of the largest genes known, and making direct analysis of the entire coding region difficult. Most studies have relied on indirect evidence for involvement of this gene in pancreatic tumorigenesis: the presence of genetic deletion in the *DCC* locus, or loss of detectable RNA production. *DCC* is located within one megabase of *DPC4* at 18q21.1 *(48)*, and, as described earlier, *DPC4* is known to be a target of inactivation in pancreatic cancer *(49,58)*. Since *DPC4* inactivation can be detected in only 50% of pancreatic carcinomas, and since *18q* is involved by heterozygous mutation in at least 89% of pancreatic carcinomas, it is conceivable that a second target of tumor suppression is present on *18q*. If *DCC* were this second target of mutation on this chromosomal arm, it might be expected that at least some of the frequent homozygous deletions that inactivate *DPC4* should have extended the relatively short distance to *DCC*, thereby inactivating both genes and conferring an increased growth advantage. Yet no such homozygous deletions were detected in a panel of tumor xenografts *(43)*. The final complication of our understanding of the role of *DCC* in pancreatic cancer is that there are conflicting reports in the literature regarding loss of *DCC* expression in pancreatic cancer, even when the same cell lines are tested by different groups *(18,56,59)*. The uncertainty over the role of *DCC* in the pathogenesis of pancreatic cancer will probably only be resolved with the development of better tests for intragenic mutations in this large gene.

JV18-1 (MADR2, SMAD2), a gene with homology to *DPC4*, has been localized to the same locus (18q21) as *DPC4 (60)*. This gene has been found to be somatically mutated in <10% of colorectal carcinomas, thus fulfilling minimal criteria for a candidate tumor-suppressor gene. No mutations of *JV18-1* have been reported in pancreatic cancer, and none were found in a protein truncation assay of 36 pancreatic tumors (unpublished data).

Evidence for Additional Tumor-Suppressor Genes

As a generalization, the majority of tumor-suppressor gene loci are inactivated by deletion of at least one allele. The presence of a deletion in one of two paired alleles is most commonly assayed by analyzing polymorphic genetic markers for loss of heterozygosity (LOH) in tumors, when compared to normal tissue from the same patient. In the most complete survey of polymorphic markers ("allelotype") in pancreatic carcinoma to date, the three chromosomal arms exhibiting the greatest frequency of LOH were 9p (89%), 17p (100%), and 18q (89%) *(42)*. These arms correspond to the location of the three tumor-suppressor genes known to be inactivated in the highest degree in pancreatic carcinoma: *p16* (9p), *p53* (17p), and *DPC4* (18q). This correlation validates the use of allelotypes in identifying probable loci of tumor-suppressor genes. With this premise in mind, eight other chromosomal arms exhibit LOH frequencies of >50%, and represent possible loci of tumor-suppressor genes: 1p, 6p, 6q, 8p, 12q, 13q, 21q, and 22q. Of these chromosomal arms, 1p, 6q, and 8p are corroborated in cytogenetic studies as loci of frequent DNA loss and rearrangement *(10–12)*, and perhaps are promising sites of as-yet uncharacterized tumor-suppressor genes for pancreatic carcinoma.

HOMOZYGOUS DELETIONS IN PANCREATIC CARCINOMA

Pancreatic carcinoma has one of the highest incidences of homozygous deletion reported for any tumor type. The *p16* gene is inactivated by homozygous deletion in 41% of carcinomas *(31)*, and the *DPC4* gene is inactivated by homozygous deletion in 30% of carcinomas *(58)*. Although the *BRCA2* gene is infrequently mutated in pancreatic carcinoma, it was the discovery and mapping of a small (<180 kb) homozygous deletion at this locus in a pancreatic carcinoma xenograft that led to the rapid localization of this tumor-suppressor gene *(61–63)*. Sixty-four percent of pancreatic cancers have a known homozygous deletion, and 19% are known to have at least two of them *(43)*. The significance of this high rate of homozygous deletion is unclear, but provides an opportunity for fruitful speculation.

Pancreatic cancers may not be more susceptible to homozygous deletion than are other carcinomas. The majority of homozygous deletions in pancreatic carcinomas have been detected through use of a tumor xenograft system, which is optimal for the finding of such deletions *(31,43,61)*. As noted under the discussion of the *p53* gene, the molecular analysis of primary tumor masses of pancreatic carcinoma is complicated by the presence of significant amounts of normal tissue. Since the assays for homozygous deletion involve the absence of a signal, the presence of nonneoplastic genomic DNA makes the interpretation of such tests difficult; thus, the majority of analyses carried out on primary tumors may not detect them, because of contaminating normal tissue. In fact, the genes that are reported to be homozygously deleted in pancreatic carcinoma at a significant rate, *p16* and *DPC4*, are also known to be homozygously deleted in other tumor types when assayed in cell lines and/or tumor xenografts *(36,49)*. The *p53* gene, which is not commonly homozygously deleted in other tumors, is likewise not commonly homozygously deleted in pancreatic carcinoma, even when assayed in tumor xenografts and cell lines *(15)*. Therefore, the relatively high rate of homozygous deletion detected in pancreatic carcinoma may be a reflection of the propensity of the type of genes commonly mutated in pancreatic carcinoma to undergo homozygous deletion in general, and in the use of tumor xenografts to study this neoplasm. This hypothesis may be confirmed as tumor xenograft banks become more common in the molecular analyses of other tumor types.

The discovery that homozygous deletions are not infrequent in pancreatic carcinoma may be of interest to more than just the molecular biologist. Homozygous deletions inactivate neighboring "innocent bystander" genes, as well as the targeted tumor-suppressor genes, resulting in clones lacking functional copies of these genes. Unless the deleted genes can be compensated by redundant protein function, homozygous deletions establish an irreversible absolute biochemical difference between neoplastic and nonneoplastic cells. The knowledge of the sum total of these differences may be useful in devising tumor-specific chemotherapeutic agents. An example of a potential therapeutic target is the methylthioadenosine phosphorylase *(MTAP)* gene, which is located near the *p16* gene *(36)*. The *MTAP* gene is included in up to one-half of the homozygous deletions that inactivate *p16*, and hence is deleted in approx 20% of all pancreatic carcinomas *(43)*. The *MTAP* gene product functions in the purine salvage pathway; its inactivation establishes an absolute biochemical difference between the metabolic pathways of neoplastic and nonneoplastic cells that may be utilized in designing agents that are toxic specifically to tumor cells, or its inactivation may be used to explain differences in chemosensitivity seen among individual tumors *(64)*. The characterization of other genes in the vicinities of *p16*, of *DPC4*, and of additional future hotspots of homozygous deletion, may suggest additional metabolic pathways that can be targeted for the development of specific chemotherapeutic agents *(43)*.

CELL CYCLE CONTROL IN PANCREATIC CARCINOMA

All of the genes most frequently mutated in pancreatic carcinoma are suspected of playing a role in the control of the cell cycle. The cell cycle is regulated by the family of cyclin-dependent protein kinase (CDK) complexes at several defined checkpoints. Cyclins are regulatory proteins that bind to CDKs and activate the kinase activity. These complexes are upregulated by specific phosphorylation events, and downregulated by the binding of CDK-inhibitory proteins, which include *p16*, *p15*, and the *p53*-activated gene, *p21*. Active cyclin CDK complexes catalyze specific protein phosphorylation events that eventually result in promotion of the cell cycle.

Although the entire activation pathway has not been elucidated, *K-ras* mutation provides a constitutive drive for cell replication. *K-ras* has been shown to activate the Raf-1/MAP kinase pathway, which eventually leads to changes in gene expression of transcription factors known to play a role in cell proliferation. Progression through a critical G1 checkpoint is controlled by the *p16*/CDK4/RB pathway. As a CDK inhibitor, *p16* acts as a brake on cell proliferation, by preventing the cyclin D/CDK4 complex from phosphorylating *RB*. Hypophosphorylated *RB* binds and sequesters such factors as E2F, and phosphorylation of *RB* causes the release of these factors. Inactivation of either *p16* or *RB* allows disregulated cell-cycle progression. The cell cycle is also negatively regulated by the CDK inhibitor *p21* at multiple checkpoints. *p21* expression is induced by the *p53* gene product; hence, *p53* gene inactivation decreases the presence of a global negative regulator of cell proliferation *(65)*. Finally, although the exact function of *DPC4* is unknown, its structural homology with other MAD proteins suggests that it lies in a TGF-β superfamily pathway. Multiple effects on cell cycle components following TGF-β treatment have been reported in experimental systems, including *RB* hypophosphorylation and induction of CDK-inhibitor gene expression, and it is possible that mutation of *DPC4* abrogates a negative regulatory effect on the cell cycle.

Although details of the specific effects of the genetic mutations identified in pancreas cancer remain to be worked out, it is clear that disregulation of the cell cycle is a central event in pancreatic neoplasia. These results also point to the fact that cell cycle control in pancreatic ductal cells tends to be inactivated in multiple regulatory pathways. This suggests that there is especially tight control over proliferation in normal pancreatic ducts, which must be overcome in malignant transformation.

DNA REPLICATION ERROR PHENOTYPE

In addition to oncogenes and tumor-suppressor genes, a third broad class of genes involved in neoplasia is composed of the mismatch repair genes. The role that the DNA mismatch repair (MMR) enzymes play in carcinogenesis has been elucidated by the discovery that mutations in such genes are responsible for the hereditary nonpolyposis colorectal carcinoma (HNPCC) syndrome, and for the replication error phenotype (RER) observed in tumors *(66)*. RER phenotype was first appreciated by the finding of new alleles among the highly polymorphic microsatellite repeats assayed by PCR. The most commonly used microsatellites are comprised of multiple repeats of the dinucleotide $(CA)_n$, which are prone to polymerase slippage during DNA replication. In the absence of an intact DNA repair mechanism, these slippage errors are the source of altered microsatellite alleles. The finding of such shifts of allele size has been used in many studies as a marker for the replication error phenotype, and have been correlated with mutations in MMR genes in sporadic carcinomas, as well as those occurring in the setting of HNPCC *(67–70)*.

There are conflicting reports on the prevalence of the RER phenotype in pancreatic carcinoma. One group from Japan reported a prevalence of replication error phenotype in six of nine (66.7%) tumors tested *(71)*, but another group from the United States reported that in analysis of thousands of informative microsatellite assays performed on five nonoverlapping patient subsets of different epidemiologic risk categories, only one tumor exhibited such as phenotype, for a prevalence of <1% *(31,42,43,72)*. Such dramatic differences in prevalence are difficult to reconcile. It reflects either differences in experimental technique and interpretation, or it may be the result of dramatically different rates of replication error phenotype in the two populations studied.

MOLECULAR GENETICS OF FAMILIAL PANCREATIC CARCINOMA

The genetic bases of several familial carcinoma syndromes have recently been discovered. Most familial cancer syndromes are first identified through families having a propensity to develop a specific form of neoplasm, or a limited set of neoplasms. In this regard, familial clustering of pancreatic carcinoma has been observed, with some pedigrees suggestive of an autosomal dominant inheritance factor *(73)*. For example, the authors established a National Familial Pancreatic Tumor Registry at The Johns Hopkins Hospital in 1994, and have already identified over 60 families in which there is an aggregation of pancreatic cancer *(74)*. Additionally, a case-controlled study showed that 7.8% of 179 pancreatic carcinoma patients had a positive family history of pancreatic carcinoma, compared to only 0.6% of controls *(75)*. It is therefore likely that an inherited genetic component underlies some fraction of pancreatic carcinoma.

Germ-line mutations in the *p16* tumor-suppressor gene have been linked to the development of pancreatic carcinomas in two families, with a highly penetrant autosomal dominant mode of transmission for pancreatic carcinoma. In these two families, the germ line *p16* mutation cosegregated with the cancer trait *(41,76)*. In a related finding, some kindred with familial atypical multiple-mole melanoma (FAMMM) syndrome, with germ line *p16* mutations, have been found to have a higher than expected prevalence of pancreatic carcinoma *(77–79)*. Although development of pancreatic carcinoma is increased in these kindred, it is not a highly penetrant trait. The reasons for why a germ-line *p16* mutation can predispose different families to different incidences of pancreatic cancer is unclear; however, it has been noted that the majority of high-incidence families have mutations in the extreme 3′ portion of the gene, suggesting that there is a domain-specific effect *(41)*. Germ-line mutations in *p16* may, however, account for <5% of such pancreatic carcinoma-prone pedigrees *(41)*. A closely related type of genetic lesion, a mutation in the *p16*-binding domain of CDK4, was not identified in 21 kindred with pancreatic carcinoma syndrome *(41)*.

Studies of germline mutations in patients with pancreatic cancer also suggest that our definitions of "sporadic" and "familial" pancreatic cancers are imprecise. Goggins et al. *(80)* recently examined a panel of 41 adenocarcinomas of the pancreas for *BRCA2* mutations. Four of the 41 cancers had loss of one allele and a mutation of the second, and three of these four *BRCA2* mutations were germ-line. Remarkably, none of the patients with germ-line mutations in *BRCA2* had family histories that would suggest a familial clustering of cancer. Thus, some germ-line mutations in tumor-suppressor genes can have incomplete penetrance for the trait, and can be responsible for many apparently sporadic forms of pancreatic cancer. An excess of pancreatic cancer can also be seen among families with hereditary breast cancer caused by *BRCA2* mutations *(81–83)*.

As a final note, an attractive candidate gene for familial pancreatic cancer, *DPC4*, was screened in 11 kindred with a familial aggregation of pancreatic carcinoma by complete gene sequencing *(84)*. No mutations were found, which makes it unlikely that *DPC4* mutation accounts for an appreciable fraction of this syndrome.

TUMOR PROGRESSION IN PANCREATIC CARCINOMA

The concept of a molecular genetic tumor progression was first established in human colorectal carcinoma. In this tumor model, increasing numbers of genetic alterations were identified in various premalignant precursor lesions of increasing histologic severity, with the largest number of alterations occurring in malignant neoplasms *(85)*. Pancreatic adenocarcinoma is derived from the epithelial cells lining the pancreatic ducts, and proliferative noninvasive epithelial lesions are commonly found as microscopic lesions in ducts adjacent to the infiltrating carcinomas. Although such a scenario invites a direct comparison to the adenoma–carcinoma sequence of colorectal carcinoma, there are certain difficulties in the field of pancreatic carcinoma that have prevented a clear understanding of premalignant precursor lesions to date.

To begin, proliferative pancreatic duct lesions have a variety of histologic appearances, with varying degrees of cytologic atypia. There is as yet no uniform nomenclature for these lesions, but, most commonly, the term "hyperplasia" (with nonpapillary and papillary subtypes) is used to describe duct lesions with no or mild cytologic atypia, and "atypical papillary hyperplasia" or "carcinoma *in situ*" to describe duct lesions with moderate-to-marked cytologic atypia *(86)*. Since these lesions can be found in pancreata resected for chronic pancreatitis with no concomitant carcinoma, as well as in pancreata with cancer, there has been a debate regarding which, if any, of these proliferative lesions are neoplastic rather than reactive in nature. To further complicate the issue, noninvasive lesions that form grossly visible masses within the ducts ("intraductal papillary neoplasms"), or form cystic spaces ("cystadenomas") occur, and are generally regarded as neoplasms, although histologically the epithelial cells in these lesions closely resemble those of the microscopic duct lesions. Unfortunately, there is insufficient clinical data to firmly establish the significance of these lesions in pancreatic tumorigenesis, a result in part of the difficulty in assessing pancreatic ducts *in situ* before pancreatectomy.

Molecular techniques can, however, be used to determine the nature of these duct lesions. A molecular model of tumor progression would predict that the premalignant precursor lesions of cancer should consist of clonal expansions of cells containing some of the mutations found in malignant neoplasms. This model predicts, therefore, that the pancreatic duct lesions that are precursor lesions to carcinoma should harbor some of the same mutations found in infiltrating pancreatic carcinoma. Several studies have been performed using *K-ras* analysis, and have borne out this concept. Irrespective of whether or not the organ contains cancer, most recent studies have shown that most papillary and atypical duct lesions, even some displaying minimal cytologic atypia, contain *K-ras* mutations *(87–91)*. *K-ras* mutations have also been found in over half of noninvasive intraductal papillary neoplasms and mucinous cystic neoplasms *(96–99)*. Indeed, in the 1996 study by Tada et al., pancreata from 138 autopsy specimens were examined from patients with no evidence of pancreatic disease, and epithelial duct lesions were identified in 86%. *K-ras* mutations were found in duct lesions in 12 of 38 specimens (32%) selected at random. Since *K-ras* mutation is almost ubiquitous in pancreatic cancer, there is an obvious and important role for this genetic lesion in pancreatic carcinogenesis. However, it also suggests that the risk of malignant progression of each such lesion must be low.

A complete understanding of tumor progression in pancreas cancer will entail additional studies of these duct lesions, with additional genetic markers. At present, no molecular genetic analyses other than those of the *K-ras* gene have been reported on microscopic duct lesions. One last clue to the role of various genes in tumor progression comes from the study by Hoshi et al. *(92)* in which no *p53* mutations were found in 16 cases of benign mucinous tumors of the pancreas; but 4 of 20 ductal pancreatic carcinomas were found to be mutated in *p53*, suggesting a role for *p53* in the clinical aggressiveness of pancreatic epithelial neoplasms.

IS DUCTAL ADENOCARCINOMA GENETICALLY DISTINCT FROM OTHER PANCREATIC TUMORS?

The short answer is yes, given the preliminary data. Ductal adenocarcinoma is derived from the epithelium lining pancreatic ducts and ductules; however, neoplasms derived from the pancreatic acini (acinar cell carcinoma) and the islets of Langerhans (islet cell neuroendocrine carcinomas) also occur. *K-ras* mutation occurs so frequently in pancreatic ductal adenocarcinoma that it can serve as a signature mutation for the neoplasm. In two studies that assayed the *K-ras* gene in acinar cell carcinoma, mutations were found in one of 16 and none of 11 neoplasms examined, respectively *(93,94)*. Similar results were found in analyses of pancreatic endocrine tumors, in which no *K-ras* mutations were found in 45 neoplasms examined *(20,95)*. In addition, only one *p53* mutation was found in 12 pancreatic endocrine neoplasms in the same study that found a 51% prevalence of *p53* mutation in pancreatic ductal adenocarcinoma. The differences in the mutation profiles of these neoplasms, compared to ductal adenocarcinoma, indicate that different molecular mechanisms underlie their pathways to malignancy.

An important question to be answered is whether these genetic differences are caused by differences in mutagenic events, or whether tissue-specific epigenetic mechanisms are permissive for different sets of gene mutations. In the first hypothesis, for instance, exposure of the duct epithelium to a different set or higher concentration of mutagenic compounds (carcinogens from cigarette smoke, activated pancreatic enzymes?, biliary secretions?) would explain its higher rate of neoplastic transformation when compared to other pancreatic cell types. Alternatively, the pancreatic epithelium may undergo a higher rate of proliferation, allowing DNA damage to be fixed as base mutations or genetic deletion at a higher rate. In the second hypothesis, mutation of genes occurs at the same rate in all of the pancreatic tissue, but the duct epithelium is permissive to alterations of cell proliferation and behavior caused by these mutations, but the other tissues are not. The elucidation of these questions will help explain why 90% of human pancreas cancers are of duct origin, yet only about 10% of all pancreatic cells are duct cells *(96)*.

CONCLUSIONS AND FUTURE DIRECTIONS

The characterization of molecular genetic changes in pancreatic carcinoma confirm the multihit model of carcinogenesis, in that four or more genes are altered in at least one-third of pancreatic adenocarcinomas *(19)*. Control of the cell cycle appears to be the preferred target of genetic disruption in pancreatic carcinoma. Evidence suggests, however, that additional genes may also be targets of mutation. Hence, future efforts will focus on the discovery of new cancer-related genes and of regulatory pathways that are disrupted when these genes are mutated.

With the more complete cataloging of the molecular changes in pancreatic carcinoma, and with future improvements in mutation-detection technology, many important questions may be addressed. First, is pancreatic carcinoma a genetically homogeneous or a genetically heterogeneous disease? That is, will the majority of cancers have the same mutation profile, or will there be two or more distinct sets of mutation groups? Can these profiles be used to develop a screening test for the earlier, potentially curable stages? If different mutation groups exist, are they actually functionally equivalent in terms of regulatory pathways that are disrupted? For instance, it will be of interest to see if the rare pancreatic cancers with RB mutations behave essentially the same as cancers with the more common p16 mutation. Can knowledge of these pathways lead to the rational and efficient design of effective chemotherapeutics, or help us to optimize radiotherapy? How common are the predisposing germline mutations in the general population, and what should be recommended for those who carry these risk genes? The pancreas may prove an important model system to answer these questions of general importance to cancer biology.

REFERENCES

1. Nowell P. Molecular events in tumor development, N Engl J Med 1988; *319:*575–577.
2. Kern SE. Clonality: more than just a tumor-progression model. J Natl Cancer Inst 1993; *85:*1020–1021.
3. Knudson AG. Antioncogenes and human cancer. Proc Natl Acad Sci USA 1993; *90:*10,914–10,921.
4. Knudson AG. Hereditary cancer: two hits revisited. J Cancer Res Clin Oncol 1996; *122:*135–140.
5. Almoguerra C, Shibata D, Forrester K, Martin J, Arnheim N, and Perucho M. Most human carcinomas of the exocrine pancreas contain mutant c-K-ras genes. Cell 1988; *53:*549–554.
6. Hruban RH, van Mansfeld ADM, Offerhaus GJA, van Weering DHJ, Allison DC, Goodman SN, et al. K-ras oncogene activation in adenocarcinomas of the human pancreas: a study of 82 carcinomas using a combination of mutant-enriched polymerase chain reaction analysis and allele-specific oligonucleotide hybridization. Am J Pathol 1993; *143:*545–554.
7. Bos JL. Ras oncogenes in human cancer: a review. Cancer Res 1989; *49:*4682–4689.
8. Maruta H and Burgess AW. Regulation of the Ras signalling network: bioessays. 1994; *16:*489–496.
9. Yamada H, Sakamoto H, Taira M, Nishimura S, Shimosato Y, Terada M, and Sugimura T. Amplifications of both c-Ki-ras with a point mutation and c-myc in a primary pancreatic cancer and its metastatic tumors in lymph nodes. Jpn J Cancer Res 1986; *77:*370–375.
10. Johansson B, Bardi G, Heim S, Mandahl N, Mertens F, Bak-Jensen E, Andren-Sandberg A, and Mitelman F. Nonrandom chromosomal rearrangements in pancreatic carcinomas. Cancer 1992; *69:*1–8.
11. Griffin CA, Hruban RH, Morsberger LA, Ellingham T, Long PP, Jaffee EM, et al. Consistent chromosome abnormalities in adenocarcinoma of the pancreas. Cancer Res 1995; *55:*2394–2399.
12. Griffin CA, Hruban RH, Long PP, Morsberger LA, Douna-Issa F, and Yeo CJ. Chromosome abnormalities in pancreatic adenocarcinoma. Genes, Chrom, Cancer 1994; *9:*93–100.
13. Cheng JQ, Ruggeri B, Klein WM, Sonoda G, Altomare DA, Watson DK, and Testa JR. Amplification of AKT2 in human pancreatic cancer cells and inhibition of AKT2 expression and tumorigenecity by antisense RNA. Proc Natl Acad Sci USA 1996; *93:*3636–3641.

14. Berrozpe G, Schaeffer J, Peinado MA, Reak FS, and Perucho M. Comparative analysis of mutations in the p53 and K-ras genes in pancreatic cancer. Int J Cancer 1994; *58:*185–191.

15. Redston MS, Caldas C, Seymour AB, Hruban RH, da Costa L, Yeo CJ, and Kern SE. p53 mutations in pancreatic carcinoma and evidence of common involvement of homocopolymer tracts in DNA microdeletions. Cancer Res 1994; *54:*3025–3033.

16. Suwa H, Yoshimura T, Yamaguchi N, Kanehira K, Manabe T, Imamura M, Hiai H, and Fukumoto M. K-ras and p53 alterations in genomic DNA and transcripts of human pancreatic adenocarcinoma cell lines. Jpn J Cancer Res 1994; *85:*1005–1014.

17. Ruggeri B, Zhang SY, Caamano J, DiRado M, Flynn SD, and Klein-Szanto AJP. Human pancreatic carcinomas and cell lines reveal frequent and multiple alterations in the p53 and Rb-1 tumor-suppressor genes. Oncogene 1992; *7:*1503–1511.

18. Simon B, Weinel R, Höhne M, Watz J, Schmidt J, Körtner G, and Arnold R. Frequent alterations of the tumor suppressor genes p53 and DCC in human pancreatic carcinoma. Gastroenterology 1994; *106:*1645–1651.

19. Rozenblum E, Schutte M, Goggins M, Hahn SA, Lu J, Panzer S, et al. Natural relationships among tumor-suppressive pathways: application of pancreatic cancer model. Cancer Res 1997; *57:*1731–1734.

20. Pellegata S, Sessa F, Renault B, Bonato M, Leone BE, Solcia E, and Ranzani GN. K-ras and p53 gene mutations in pancreatic cancer: ductal and nonductal tumors progress through different genetic lesions. Cancer Res 1994; *54:*1556–1560.

21. Weyrer K, Feichtinger H, Haun M, Weiss G, Ofner D, Weger AR, Umlauft F, and Grunewald K. p53, Ki-ras, and DNA ploidy in human pancreatic ductal adenocarcinomas. Lab Invest 1996; *74:*279–289.

22. Scarpa A, Capelli P, Mukai K, Zamboni G, Oda T, Iacono C, and Hirohashi S. Pancreatic adenocarcinomas frequently show p53 gene mutations. Am J Pathol 1993; *142:*1534–1543.

23. Nakamori S, Yashima K, Murakami Y, Ishikawa O, Ohigashi H, Imaoka S, et al. Association of p53 gene mutations with short survival in pancreatic adenocarcinoma. Jpn J Cancer Res 1995; *86:*174–181.

24. Casey G, Yamanaka Y, Friess H, Kobrin MS, Lopez ME, Buchler M, Beger HG, and Korc M. p53 mutations are common in pancreatic cancer and are absent in chronic pancreatitis. Cancer Lett 1993; *69:*151–160.

25. Seymour AB, Hruban RH, Redston M, Caldas C, Powell SM, Kinzler KW, Yee CJ, and Kern SE. Allelotype of pancreatic adenocarcinoma. Cancer Res 1994; *54:*2761–2764.

26. Kern SE, Pietenpol JA, Thiagalingam S, Seymour A, Kinzler KW, and Vogelstein B. Oncogenic forms of p53 inhibit p53-regulated gene expression. Science 1992; *256:*827–830.

27. Kern SE, Kinzler KW, Bruskin A, Jarosz D, Friedman P, Prives C, and Vogelstein B. Identification of p53 as a sequence-specific DNA-binding protein. Science 1991; *252:*1708–1711.

28. Kern SE, Kinzler KW, Baker SJ, Nigro JM, Rotter V, Levine AJ, et al. Mutant p53 proteins bind DNA abnormally in vitro. Oncogene 1991; *6:*131–136.

29. Kastan MB, Onyekwere O, Sidransky D, Vogelstein B, and Craig RW. Participation of p53 protein in the cellular response to DNA damage. Cancer Res 1991; *51:*6304–6311.

30. Yonish-Rouach E, Resnitzky D, Lotem J, Sachs L, Kimchi A, and Oren M. Wild-type p53 induces apoptosis of myeloid leukaemic cells that is inhibited by interleukin-6. Nature 1991; *352:*345–347.

31. Caldas C, Hahn SA, da Costa LT, Redston MS, Schutte M, Seymour AB, et al. Frequent somatic mutations and homozygous deletions of the p16 (MTS1) gene in pancreatic adenocarcinoma. Nature Genetics 1994; *8:*27–31.

32. Naumann M, Savitskaia N, Eilert C, Schramm A, Kalthoff H, and Schmiegel W. Frequent codeletion of p16/MTS1 and p15/MTS2 and genetic alterations in p16/MTS1 in pancreatic tumors. Gastroenterology 1996; *110:*1215–1224.

33. Liu Q, Yan YX, McClure M, Nakagawa H, Fujimura F, and Rustgi AK. MTS-1 (CDKN2) tumor suppressor gene deletions are a frequent event in esophagus squamous cancer and pancreatic adenocarcinoma cell lines. Oncogene 1995; *10:*619–622.
34. Bartsch D, Shevlin DW, Tung WS, Kisker O, Wells SAJ, and Goodfellow PJ. Frequent mutations of CDKN2 in primary pancreatic adenocarcinomas. Genes Chromosom Cancer 1995; *14:*189–195.
35. Yang R, Gombart AF, Serrano M, and Koeffler HP. Mutational effects on the p16INK4a tumor suppressor protein. Cancer Res 1995; *55:*2503–2506.
36. Kamb A, Gruis NA, Weaver-Feldhaus J, Liu Q, Harshman K, Tavtigian SV, et al. A cell cycle regulator potentially involved in genesis of many tumor types. Science 1994; *264:*436–440.
37. Jen J, Harper JW, Bigner SH, Bigner DD, Papadopoulos N, Markowitz S, et al. Deletion of *p16* and *p15* genes in brain tumors. Cancer Res 1994; *54:*6353–6358.
38. Rozenblum E, Schutte M, and Kern SE. *INK4* genes in pancreatic carcinoma. Oncol Rep 1996; *3:*743–745.
39. Wölfel T, Hauer M, Schneider J, Serrano M, Wölfel C, Klehmann-Hieb E, et al. A p16INK4a-insensitive CDK4 mutant targeted by cytolytic T lymphocytes in a human melanoma. Science 1995; *269:*1281–1284.
40. Zuo L, Weger J, Yang Q, Goldstein AM, Tucker MA, Walker GJ, et al. Germline mutations in the p16INK4a binding domain of CDK4 in familial melanoma. Nature Genet 1996; *12:*97–99.
41. Moskaluk CA, Hruban RH, Lietman AS, Smyrk T, Fusaro L, Fusaro R, et al. Novel germline p16INK4a mutation in familial pancreatic carcinoma. Hum Mutat (in press), 1998.
42. Hahn SA, Seymour AB, Hoque ATMS, Schutte M, da Costa LT, Redston MS, et al. Allelotype of pancreatic adenocarcinoma using a xenograft model. Cancer Res 1995; *55:*4670–4675.
43. Hahn SA, Hoque ATMS, Moskaluk CA, daCosta LT, Schutte M, Rozenblum E, et al. Homozygous deletion map at 18q21.1 in pancreatic cancer. Cancer Res 1996; *56:*490–494.
44. Sekelsky JJ, Newfeld SJ, Raftery LA, Chartoff EH, and Gelbart WM. Genetic characterization and cloning of Mothers against dpp, a gene required for decapentaplegic function in *Drosophila melanogaster.* Genetics 1995; *139:*1347–1358.
45. Liu F, Hata A, Baker JC, Doody J, Carcamo J, Harland RM, and Massague J. A human Mad protein acting as a BMP-regulated transcriptional activator. Nature 1996; *381:*620–623.
46. Alexandrow MG and Moses HL. Transforming growth factor beta and cell cycle regulation. Cancer Res 1995; *55:*1452–1457.
47. Hoque ATMS, Hahn SA, Schutte M, and Kern SE. *DPC4* gene mutation in colitis-associated neoplasia. Gut (in press), 1996.
48. Thiagalingam S, Lengauer C, Leach FS, Schutte M, Hahn SA, Overhauser J, et al. Evaluation of candidate tumour suppressor genes on chromosome 18 in colorectal cancers. Nat Genet 1996; *13:*343–346.
49. Schutte M, Hruban RH, Hedrick L, Molnar'Nadasdy G, Weinstein CL, Bova GS, et al. *DPC4* in various tumor types. Cancer Res 1996; *56:*2527–2530.
50. Nagatake M, Takagi Y, Osada N, Uchida K, Mitsudomi T, Saji S, et al. Somatic in vivo alterations of the DPC4 gene at 18q21 in human lung cancers. Cancer Res 1996; *56:*2718–2720.
51. Kim SK, Fan Y, Papadimitrakopoulou V, Clayman G, Hittleman WN, Hong WK, Lotan R, and Mao L. DPC4, a candidate tumor suppressor gene, is altered infrequently in head and neck squamous cell carcinoma. Cancer Res 1996; *56:*2519–2521.
52. Barrett MT, Schutte M, Kern SE, and Reid BJ. Allelic loss and mutational analysis of the DPC4 gene in esophageal adenocarcinoma. Cancer Res (in press), 1996.
53. Horii A, Nakatsuru S, Miyoshi Y, Ichii S, Nagase H, Ando H, et al. Frequent somatic mutations of the APC gene in human pancreatic cancer. Cancer Res 1992; *52:*6696–6698.

54. McKie AB, Filipe ML, and Lemoine NR. Abnormalities affecting the APC and MCC tumour suppressor gene loci on chromosome 5q occur frequently in gastric cancer but not in pancreatic cancer. Int J Cancer 1993; *55:*598–603.

55. Yashima K, Nakamori S, Murakami Y, Yamaguchi A, Hayashi K, Ishikawa O, Konishi Y, and Sekiya T. Mutations of the adenomatous polyposis coli gene in the mutation cluster region: comparison of human pancreatic and colorectal cancers. Int J Cancer 1994; *59:*43–47.

56. Barton CM, McKie AB, Hogg A, Bia B, Elia G, Phillips SM, Ding SF, and Lemoine NR. Abnormalities of the RB1 and DCC tumor suppressor genes: uncommon in human pancreatic adenocarcinoma. Mol Carcinog 1995; *13:*61–69.

57. Huang L, Lang D, Geradts J, Obara T, Klein-Szanto AJ, Lynch HT, and Ruggeri BA. Molecular and immunochemical analyses of RB1 and cyclin D1 in human ductal pancreatic carcinomas and cell lines. Mol Carcinog 1996; *15:*85–95.

58. Hahn SA, Schutte M, Hoque ATMS, Moskaluk CA, da Costa LT, Rozenblum E, et al. DPC4, a candidate tumor-suppressor gene at 18q21.1. Science 1996; *271:*350–353.

59. Höhne MW, Halatsch M-E, Kahl GE, and Weinel RJ. Frequent loss of expression of the potential tumor suppressor gene DCC in ductal pancreatic adenocarcinoma. Cancer Res 1992; *52:*2616–2619.

60. Riggins GJ, Thiagalingam S, Rozenblum E, Weinstein CL, Kern SE, Hamilton SR, et al. Mad-related genes in the human. Nat Genet 1996; *13:*347–349.

61. Schutte M, da Costa LT, Hahn SA, Moskaluk C, Hoque ATMS, Rozenblum E, et al. A homozygous deletion identified by representational difference analysis in pancreatic carcinoma overlaps the BRCA2 region. Proc Natl Acad Sci USA 1995; *92:*5950–5954.

62. Schutte M, Rozenblum E, Moskaluk CA, Guan X, Hoque ATMS, Hahn SA, et al. An integrated high-resolution physical map of the DPC/BRCA2 region at chromosome 13q12-13. Cancer Res 1995; *55:*4570–4574.

63. Wooster R, Bignell G, Lancaster J, Swift S, Seal S, Mangion J, et al. Identification of the breast cancer susceptibility gene BRCA2. Nature 1995; *378:*789–792.

64. Chen Z-H, Zhang H, and Savarese TM. Gene deletion chemoselectivity: codeletion of the genes for p16INK4, methylthioadenosine phosphorylase, and the α- and β-interferons in human pancreatic cell carcinoma lines and its implications for chemotherapy. Cancer Res 1996; *56:*1083–1090.

65. El-Deiry WS, Tokino T, Velculescu VE, Levy DB, Parsons R, Trent JM, et al. WAF1, a potential mediator of p53 tumor suppression. Cell 1993; *75:*817–825.

66. Modrich P. Mismatch repair, genetic stability, and cancer. Science 1994; *266:*1959–1960.

67. Liu B, Nicolaides NC, Markowitz S, Willson JK, Parsons RE, Jen J, et al. Mismatch repair gene defects in sporadic colorectal cancers with microsatellite instability. Nat Genet 1995; *9:*48–55.

68. Ionov Y, Peinado MA, Malkhosyan S, Shibata D, and Perucho M. Ubiquitous somatic mutations in simple repeated sequences reveal a new mechanism for colonic carcinogenesis. Nature 1993; *363:*558–561.

69. Aaltonen LA, Peltomäki P, Leach FS, Sistonen P, Pylkkänen L, Mecklin J-P, et al. Clues to the pathogenesis of familial colorectal cancer. Science 1993; *260:*812–816.

70. Thibodeau SN, Bren G, and Schaid D. Microsatellite instability in cancer of the proximal colon. Science 1993; *260:*816–819.

71. Han H-J, Yanagisawa A, Kato Y, Park J-G, Kato Y, and Nakamura Y. Genetic instability in pancreatic cancer and poorly differentiated type of gastric cancer. Cancer Res 1993; *53:*5087–5089.

72. Schutte M and Kern SE. The molecular genetics of pancreatic adenocarcinoma. In: Neoptolemos J. P. and Lemoine N. R. (eds), Pancreatic cancer: molecular and clinical advances, Blackwell, Oxford, 1996; pp. 115–132.

73. Lynch HT, Fusaro L, Smyrk TC, Watson P, Lanspa S, and Lynch JF. Medical genetic study of eight pancreatic cancer-prone families. Cancer Invest 1995; *13:*141–149.

74. World-Wide Web address hppt://www.med.jhu.edu/pancreas/registry.htm.
75. Ghadirian P, Boyle P, Simard A, Baillargeon J, Maisonneuve P, and Perret C. Reported family aggregation of pancreatic cancer within a population-based case-control study in the Francophone community in Montreal, Canada. Int J Pancreatol 1991; *10:*183–195.
76. Whelan AJ, Bartsch D, and Goodfellow PJ. Brief report: a familial syndrome of pancreatic cancer and melanoma with a mutation in the CDKN2 tumor-suppressor gene. N Engl J Med 1995; *333:*975–977.
77. Goldstein AM, Fraser MC, Struewing JP, Hussussian CJ, Ranade K, Zametkin DP, et al. Increased risk of pancreatic cancer in melanoma-prone kindreds with p16INK4 mutations. N Engl J Med 1995; *333:*970–974.
78. Gruis NA, Sandkuiji LA, van der Velden PA, Bergman W, and Frants RR. CDKN2 explains part of the clinical phenotype in Dutch familial atypical multiple-mole melanoma (FAMMM) syndrome families. Melanoma Res 1995; *9:*169–177.
79. Ciotti P, Strigini P, and Bianchi-Scarra G. Familial melanoma and pancreatic cancer. N Engl J Med 1996; *334:*469–470.
80. Goggins M, Schutte M, Lu J, Moskaluk CA, Weinstein CL, Petersen GM, et al. Germline *BRCA2* gene mutations in patients with apparently sporadic pancreatic carcinomas. Cancer Res 1996; *56:*5360–5364.
81. Berman DB, Costalas J, Schultz DC, Grana G, Daly M, and Godwin AK. A common mutation in BRCA2 that predisposes to a variety of cancers is found in both Jewish Askenazi and non-Jewish individuals. Cancer Res 1996; *56:*3409–3414.
82. Phelan CM, Lancaster JM, Tonin P, Gumbs C, Cochran C, Carter R, et al. Mutation analysis of the *BRCA2* gene in 49 site-specific breast cancer families. Nature Genet 1996; *13:*120–122.
83. Thorlacius S, Olafsdottir G, Tryggvadottir L, Neuhausen S, Jonasson JG, Tavtigian SV, et al. A single *BRCA2* mutation in male and female breast carcinoma families from Iceland with varied cancer phenotypes. Nature Genet 1996; *13:*117–119.
84. Moskaluk CA, Hruban RH, Schutte M, Lietman AS, Smyrk T, Fusaro L, et al. Genomic sequencing of DPC4 in the analysis of familial pancreatic carcinoma. Diag Mol Pathol 1997; *6:*85–90.
85. Vogelstein B, Fearon ER, Hamilton SR, Kern SE, Preisinger AC, Leppert M, et al. Genetic alterations during colorectal-tumor development. N Engl J Med 1988; *319:*525–532.
86. Kozuka S, Sassa R, Taki T, Masamoto K, Nagasawa S, Saga S, Hasegawa K, and Takeuchi M. Relation of pancreatic duct hyperplasia to carcinoma. Cancer 1979; *43:*1418–1428.
87. Yanagisawa A, Ohtake K, Ohashi K, Hori M, Kitagawa T, Sugano H, and Kato Y. Frequent c-Ki-ras oncogene activation in mucous cell hyperplasias of pancreas suffering from chronic inflammation. Cancer Res 1993; *53:*953–956.
88. Caldas C, Hahn SA, Hruban RH, Redston MS, Yeo CJ, and Kern SE. Detection of K-ras mutations in the stool of patients with pancreatic adenocarcinoma and pancreatic ductal hyperplasia. Cancer Res 1994; *54:*3568–3573.
89. DiGiuseppe JA, Hruban RH, Offerhaus GJA, Clement MJ, van den Berg FM, Cameron JL, and van Mansfeld ADM. Detection of K-ras mutations in mucinous pancreatic duct hyperplasia from a patient with a family history of pancreatic carcinoma. Am J Pathol 1994; *144:*889–895.
90. Tabata T, Fujimori T, Maeda S, Yamamoto M, and Saitoh Y. The role of Ras mutation in pancreatic cancer, precancerous lesions, and chronic pancreatitis. Int J Pancreatol 1993; *14:*237–244.
91. Tada M, Ohashi M, Shiratori Y, Okudairi T, Komatsu Y, Kawabe T, et al. Analysis of K-ras gene mutation in hyperplastic duct cells of the pancreas without pancreatic disease. Gastroenterology 1996; *110:*227–231.
92. Hoshi T, Imai M, and Ogawa K. Frequent K-ras mutations and absence of p53 mutations in mucin-producing tumors of the pancreas. J Surg Oncol 1994; *55:*84–91.

93. Hoorens A, Lemoine NR, McLellan E, Morohoshi T, Kamisawa T, Heitz PU, et al. Pancreatic acinar cell carcinoma. An analysis of cell lineage markers, p53 expression, and Ki-ras mutation. Am J Pathol 1993; *143:*685–698.

94. Terhune PG, Heffess CS, and Longnecker DS. Only wild-type c-Ki-ras codons 12, 13, and 61 in human pancreatic acinar cell carcinomas. Mol Carcinog 1994; *10:*110–114.

95. Yashiro T, Fulton N, Hara H, Yasuda K, Montag A, Yashiro N, et al. Comparison of mutations of ras oncogene in human pancreatic exocrine and endocrine tumors. Surgery 1993; *114:*758–763.

96. Lynch HT. Genetics and pancreatic cancer. Arch Surg 1994; *129:*266–268.

Role of Polypeptide Growth Factors and Their Receptors in Human Pancreatic Cancer

Murray Korc

INTRODUCTION

Carcinoma of the pancreas is the fifth leading cause of cancer death in the Western world *(1–2)*. The 1-yr overall survival rate in patients with pancreatic carcinoma is approx 12%; the 5-yr overall survival is approx 3–5% *(1–2)*. The diagnosis of pancreatic cancer is frequently established at an advanced stage, when the majority of patients are not candidates for surgery. Furthermore, nonsurgical treatment for pancreatic cancer is generally ineffective, because of the tumor's propensity to metastasize, and because of the resistance of pancreatic cancer cells to cytotoxic agents. Considerable effort has been directed, therefore, at understanding the molecular alterations that occur in this disorder, with the hope that this will lead to improved diagnostic and therapeutic modalities.

Overexpression of growth factors and their receptors has been implicated in the excessive growth of malignant cells *(3)*. Furthermore, some growth factors, such as members of the transforming growth factor beta family, may inhibit cell proliferation *(4)*. Loss of responsiveness to their growth-inhibitory signals may also contribute to enhanced cancer cell growth, as discussed in Chapter 5 *(4)*. This review will focus on the role in pancreatic cancer of polypeptide growth factors and their receptors, whose activation generally enhances cell proliferation.

GENERAL OVERVIEW OF POLYPEPTIDE GROWTH FACTORS

Polypeptide growth factors are produced by many different cells, often acting at or near their site of expression through autocrine and paracrine mechanisms (Fig. 1). Certain growth factors may also act prior to their release from the cell, either by exerting effects at intracellular sites via a so-called intracrine mechanism, or by acting prior to release from the cell surface via a so-called juxtacrine mechanism (Fig. 1). Growth factors are also abundant in the systemic circulation, from where they can exert effects on numerous target cells. Furthermore, the human pancreas consists of acinar cells, duct cells, and endocrine cells, which are grouped into islets and dispersed throughout the

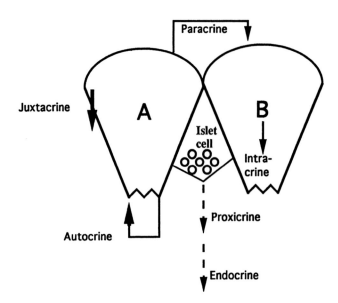

Fig. 1. Potential mechanisms for growth factor actions in pancreatic cancer. Overexpression of certain ligands, such as TGF-α (in cell A), can lead to EGF receptor activation via autocrine, paracrine, or juxtacrine mechanisms. Juxtacrine effects are exerted by the TGF-α precursor, which is a transmembrane protein that can bind and activate the EGF receptor. Overexpression of other ligands, such as bFGF (in cell B), can lead to activation of FGF receptors via autocrine, paracrine, or intracrine mechanisms. Intracrine effects may be exerted by the overexpressed bFGF inside the cancer cells. The pancreas also contains thousands of islet cells that release polypeptide hormones and growth factors into an intrapancreatic circulation that normally bathes the exocrine cells prior to draining into the pancreatic vein. Insulin, which is stored in the secretory granules (shown as small circles) of the β cell, can exert proxicrine effects on the exocrine cells and on pancreatic cancer cells prior to its arrival in the systemic circulation, where it acts as an endocrine hormone. IGF-II may act on pancreatic cancer cells via a similar proxicrine pathway.

exocrine tissue. These hormone-producing islets range widely in size, and receive as much as 20% of the intrapancreatic blood flow. Although the venous effluent from the larger islets bypasses the surrounding exocrine tissue, the effluent from the smaller islets, which are more numerous, is discharged into an intrapancreatic portal circulation that passes through the exocrine tissue *(5)*. Consequently, a large portion of the exocrine pancreas is exposed to high levels of islet-derived hormones and growth factors, which may act on the exocrine cells via a so-called proxicrine mechanism (Fig. 1).

EPIDERMAL GROWTH FACTOR AND RELATED PEPTIDES

The epidermal growth factor (EGF) receptor is activated by a family of peptides that includes EGF, transforming growth factor alpha (TGF-α), heparin-binding EGF-like growth factor (HB-EGF), amphiregulin, and betacellulin *(6)*. All five growth factors share amino-acid-sequence homology, posses six cysteine residues in the same relative positions as EGF, and are produced as precursor molecules *(6)*. These precursors insert into the cell membrane prior to undergoing proteolytic cleavage to yield the mature growth factor.

EGF and TGF-α are potent mitogens toward a variety of cell types that express the EGF receptor. Although they tend to exert similar biological actions in many cells, quantitative and qualitative differences have been reported. Thus, TGF-α exerts greater stimulatory effects than EGF with respect to calcium mobilization from fetal rat long bones, angiogenesis in the hamster cheek pouch model, skin-wound healing, induction of cell ruffling and migration, and anchorage-independent growth of certain human pancreatic cancer cell lines *(7)*. In addition, the inhibitory effects of EGF and TGF-α on norepinephrine-induced contraction in arterial strips is diminished following repeated exposure to EGF, but not to TGF-α *(8)*.

In contrast to EGF and TGF-α, HB-EGF, betacellulin, and amphiregulin are heparin-binding *(6)*. HB-EGF was originally purified from the conditioned medium of U937 macrophage-like cells *(9)*. It functions in its transmembrane precursor form as an internalization receptor for diphtheria toxin *(9)*. Mature HB-EGF has a highly hydrophilic domain with high affinity toward heparin and heparan sulfate at its N-terminal end. It has an EGF-like domain that is approx 40% homologous with human EGF and TGF-α at the C-terminal end, and it is a known mitogen for smooth muscle cells, fibroblasts, keratinocytes, and hepatocytes *(6)*.

Betacellulin is the most recently identified member of the EGF-like ligands. It was initially purified from the conditioned medium of a malignant beta cell line established from the pancreas of a transgenic mice expressing the SV40 large T-antigen under regulation of the insulin promoter *(10)*. Mature human betacellulin, cloned from MCF-7 human breast cancer cells, is 80% homologous with mouse betacellulin *(11)*. Betacellulin and EGF are equipotent with respect to their mitogenic effects in Balb c/3T3 fibroblasts, and with respect to binding to EGF receptor overexpressing A431 cells *(11)*.

Amphiregulin is the only growth factor in this group with a hydrophilic region at its amino terminal end and two putative nuclear targeting sequences *(12)*. It was originally isolated from conditioned medium of MCF-7 breast carcinoma cells that were treated with 12-*O*-tetradecanoylphorbol-13-acetate *(13)*. It binds to DNA and is present in the nuclei of certain cells *(13)*. It is an autocrine factor for normal human mammary epithelial cells, and it enhances the growth of normal fibroblasts, keratinocytes, and some ovarian and pituitary tumor cell lines *(6)*.

Members of the EGF family are mitogenic toward many cell types that express the EGF receptor. They are capable of autoinduction and cross-induction *(14)*. For example, TGF-α induces the expression of TGF-α, HB-EGF, and amphiregulin mRNA levels *(14)*. However, these EGF-like ligands do not localize in exactly the same cellular site in the pancreatic cancers. Thus, EGF immunoreactivity is most commonly present in the supranuclear region of the duct-like cancer cells; TGF-α tends to be present preferentially at the apical aspect of these cells; amphiregulin is either present in the nucleus or exhibits a diffuse cytoplasmic distribution; and HB-EGF may be found in a membranous, cytoplasmic, or apical distribution *(15–17)*. These observations imply specific roles for each of these growth factors in pancreatic cancers in vivo.

Several lines of evidence suggest that members of the EGF family have an important role in pancreatic malignant transformation. First, all five ligands and the EGF receptor are expressed at high levels in the cancer cells within the pancreatic tumor mass

(15–19). Second, HB-EGF, EGF, TGF-α, and amphiregulin enhance the proliferation of cultured human pancreatic cancer cell lines *(17,19–20).* Third, coexpression of the EGF receptor and either EGF or TGF-α is associated with decreased survival in patients with pancreatic cancer *(21).* Fourth, the EGF receptor often colocalizes with EGF and TGF-α in these cancers *(21),* suggesting that the ligands exert autocrine effects on the pancreatic cancer cells. Fifth, the cytoplasmic localization of amphiregulin in pancreatic cancer cells is associated with more aggressive disease *(17).* Sixth, anti-TGF-α antibodies or amphiregulin antisense oligonucleotides suppress the growth of pancreatic cancer cells *(22).* These observations suggest that pancreatic cancer cells derive a growth advantage as a result of excessive activation of the EGF receptor by EGF and EGF-like ligands, and raise the possibility that agents that suppress the expression of these ligands, and/or block the signaling pathways that they activate, may serve as novel therapies in pancreatic cancer.

EPIDERMAL GROWTH FACTOR
RECEPTOR AND RELATED RECEPTORS

The EGF receptor consists of an extracellular ligand-binding domain, a transmembrane domain, and an intracellular domain that possesses intrinsic tyrosine kinase activity *(23).* Following ligand binding, the EGF receptor undergoes dimerization, which is essential for activation of its mitogenic signaling pathways. The dimerized EGF receptors are then auto- and transphosphorylated on tyrosine residues, and the phosphorylated residues become the sites of association of effector proteins containing *src* homology 2 (SH2) motifs *(24–26).* Thus, growth factor-related binding protein 2 (GRB2) associates with the homolog of son-of-sevenless (SOS), which in turn associates with activated *ras*-GTP, which translocates raf-1 to the cell membrane. Raf-1 is a serine–threonine kinase that induces the phosphorylation of MAP kinase kinase, which in turn induces the phosphorylation of MAP kinase *(27).* Activated MAP kinase translocates to the nucleus and induces the phosphorylation of the protein products of *jun* and *fos* nuclear protooncogenes *(27).* Other regulatory proteins that are also activated following ligand binding include phospholipase C-gamma (PLC-γ) and phosphatidylinositol-3-kinase (PI 3-kinase).

In addition to undergoing dimerization, the EGF receptor heterodimerizes with several closely related receptors *(28,29),* known as EGF receptor type 2 (HER-2 or c-*erb*B-2), HER-3 (c-*erb*B-3) and HER-4 (c-*erb*B-4). HER-3 is ostensibly devoid of intrinsic tyrosine kinase activity and undergoes tyrosine phosphorylation following heterodimerization with either the activated EGF receptor or activated HER-2 *(28,29).* It then associates efficiently with PI 3-kinase, thereby enhancing the mitogenic potential of the EGF receptor.

Human pancreatic ductal adenocarcinomas exhibit high levels of the EGF receptor, HER-2, and HER-3 *(15,30–33).* Northern blot analysis and/or *in situ* hybridization studies indicate that the increase in EGF receptor, HER-2, and HER-3 immunoreactivity is a result of overexpression of the respective mRNA moieties *(15,30–32).* Although the concomitant presence of the EGF receptor with either EGF or TGF-α is associated with a shorter postoperative survival period in patients with pancreatic cancer, EGF receptor or HER-2 expression is not associated with a worse prognosis *(21,31).* In contrast, expression of HER-3 is associated with decreased patient survival *(32).* Taken together, these observations suggest that the EGF receptor and HER-3 may have an especially important role in contributing to pancreatic cancer cell growth.

Overexpression of the EGF receptor, its ligands, and related receptors has also been observed in chronic pancreatitis, as discussed in Chapter 3 of this book. However, in chronic pancreatitis, this overexpression is not associated with an altered gene background, as is observed in pancreatic cancer. Thus, pancreatic cancer in humans is associated with a comparatively high rate (75–95%) of K-*ras* oncogene mutations *(34–36)*. K-*ras* plays a pivotal role in signal transduction pathways that are activated following binding of a variety of ligands to their specific cell-surface receptors. It possesses intrinsic GTPase activity, which is attenuated when K-*ras* is mutated, resulting in enhanced mitogenic signaling through K-*ras*-dependent pathways of the type that are activated by the EGF receptor *(37)*.

In addition to K-*ras* mutations, these cancers harbor mutations in the *p53* and *DPC4* tumor suppressor genes *(38–40)*, and exhibit alterations in cell-cycle-associated kinases, such as *p16 (41)*. Pancreatic cancers also express high levels of mdm-2, whose protein product inhibits wild-type *p53* functions *(42,43)*. Thus, mdm-2 may have the potential to induce cellular proliferation in pancreatic cancer in the absence of *p53* mutations. *p53* is not mutated in chronic pancreatitis, and mdm2 expression is not increased in this disorder *(39,42)*. Taken together, these observations suggest that the absence of these alterations may preclude chronic pancreatitis from frequently transforming into pancreatic cancer. Conversely, their presence in the pancreatic carcinomas may allow the overexpression of certain growth factors and their receptors to confer on the cancer cells a unique growth advantage.

The most direct evidence for the importance of the EGF receptor in pancreatic cancer derives from studies in which EGF receptor-dependent signaling is blocked by expression of a truncated EGF receptor cDNA in PANC-I cells, which heterodimerizes with the endogenous EGF receptor *(44)*. Although this cell line harbors both a K-*ras* mutation and a *p53* mutation, blockade of EGF receptor signaling with the truncated receptor markedly attenuates the growth of this cell line and enhances its sensitivity to *cis*-platinum *(44)*.

FIBROBLAST GROWTH FACTORS AND THEIR RECEPTORS

Another example of a family of growth factors that are often mitogenic and that activate transmembrane tyrosine kinase receptors is represented by the fibroblast growth factor (FGF) family. To date, this family consists of nine homologous polypeptide growth factors that have an affinity for heparin and glycosaminoglycans, and that participate in the regulation of biological processes in numerous cell types *(45)*. In addition to being mitogenic, FGFs are motogenic, promote angiogenesis, and modulate cell differentiation and tissue repair. The best characterized members of this family are acidic FGF (aFGF or FGF1) and basic FGF (bFGF or FGF2). Other members are numbered as FGF-3 through FGF-9. FGF-3 is also known as int-2, FGF-7 is also known as keratinocyte growth factor or KGF, FGF-8 is also known as androgen-induced growth factor, and FGF-9 is also known as glia-activating factor *(45)*.

There are four distinct high-affinity transmembrane tyrosine kinase FGF receptors that function as signaling molecules to mediate the effects of FGFs, as well as low-affinity receptors that are devoid of signaling capabilities, but which act to enhance ligand presentation to the high-affinity receptors *(46)*. These high-affinity receptors have been designated as FGFR-1, -2, -3, and -4. Their extracellular domains generally have three immunoglobulin-like (Ig-like) regions; their intracellular tyrosine kinase domains are separated into two contiguous regions.

As a result of alternative splicing, a number of variant FGF receptors have been described for FGFR-1, -2, and -3, including some that have lost the first Ig-like region in the extracellular domain, resulting in the generation of a 2 Ig-like form. The presence of an intron–exon boundary in the third Ig-like loop (domain III) allows for the generation of three alternative Ig-like domains in this carboxy-terminal region (domains IIIa, IIIb, IIIc) of FGFR. The IIIa splice form yields a secreted FGF-binding protein, the IIIb splice form is expressed in epithelial cell types, and expression of the IIIc splice form is restricted to mesenchymal cell types *(46)*. These splice variants may have important functions that dictate the responsiveness of certain cell types to FGFs. In addition, the receptor for KGF (KGFR) is a splice variant of FGFR-2, exhibiting a unique IIIc domain and a high affinity for both KGF and aFGF *(46)*.

Human pancreatic cancer cell lines express variable levels of FGF-1–5, and -7, and coexpress one or another of the known high-affinity FGF receptors *(47)*. Furthermore, aFGF and bFGF are overexpressed in human pancreatic cancers, as determined by immunohistochemistry, *in situ* hybridization, Northern blot analysis, and immunoblotting studies *(48)*. Although the presence of bFGF in the cancer cells is associated with shorter postoperative patient survival, aFGF expression does not correlate with patient survival *(48)*. The reasons for these differences between aFGF and bFGF are not known. It is established, however, that both aFGF and bFGF lack a signal peptide, and are therefore concentrated within their cells of origin. In contrast to aFGF, there are multiple isoforms of bFGF that range in size from 18 to 24 kDa *(49)*. Often, these are produced in the same cell from a single mRNA species as a result of different initiation sites. Furthermore, the shorter 18 kDa bFGF moiety is generated as a result of initiation of translation at the AUG codon, and is predominantly localized in the cytosol, but is also found at the cell surface, and extracellularly, following secretion via a distinct cellular mechanism that is not fully understood. The higher mol forms of bFGF are generated as a result of initiation at CUG codons, and often preferentially localize in the nucleus. Nuclear localization is caused, in part, by the presence of arginine residues at their amino terminal ends. Production of multiple bFGF isoforms with at least two different cellular localization sites raises the possibility that each of these isoforms may exert specific functions. For example, the intracellularly secreted forms of bFGF may exert intracrine effects that may lead to enhanced mitogenic signaling *(49)*. These observations are especially relevant to pancreatic cancer, inasmuch as human pancreatic cancers frequently exhibit the high-mol forms of bFGF *(48)*.

Human pancreatic cancers express high levels of the 2 Ig-like form of FGFR-1, as determined by RNase protection assays and polymerase chain reaction analysis. By immunohistochemistry and by *in situ* hybridization, FGFR-1 is abundant in the duct-like cancer cells *(50)*. In contrast, the 3 Ig-like form predominates in the normal pancreas, where it is especially abundant in the acinar cells *(50)*. These observations again suggest that there is a potential for excessive autocrine and paracrine activation of FGF-dependent pathways in human pancreatic cancer, and raise the possibility that the 2 Ig-like form of FGFR-1 may have an especially important role in mediating this aberrant stimulation. In support of this hypothesis, expression of a truncated FGFR-1 cDNA in PANC-1 cells markedly inhibits the growth of these cells *(51)*.

INSULIN AND INSULIN-LIKE
GROWTH FACTORS AND THEIR RECEPTORS

Insulin-like growth factor I (IGF-I) is a mitogenic polypeptide that regulates cell cycle progression *(52)*. It is produced by many different cell types, and it has been implicated in a variety of malignancies *(52)*. In contrast to IGF-I, insulin is synthesized and secreted exclusively by the beta cells in the endocrine islets; its release into the circulation is tightly controlled by circulating glucose levels *(53)*. Insulin's main function is to control glucose homeostasis, and it participates in the regulation of a variety of metabolic pathways in many different cells; it has only been infrequently implicated in human malignancies. A third member of this family is insulin-like growth factor-II (IGF-II), a polypeptide that exhibits structural homology to proinsulin and IGF-I *(52)*. IGF-II also exerts growth promoting and metabolic effects *(52)*. Like IGF-I, IGF-II may function as an autocrine and paracrine growth factor in a variety of mesenchymal and epithelial tumors *(54,55)*.

As in the case of other polypeptide hormones and growth factors, the first step in the initiation of insulin, IGF-I, or IGF-II actions is dependent on their binding to their own specific cell-surface receptors. Both the insulin and IGF-I receptors are heterotetrameric proteins that possess intrinsic tyrosine kinase activity *(52)*. Both receptors activate insulin receptor substrate-1 (IRS-1), an important multisite docking protein implicated in mitogenic signaling, and which mediates the metabolic effects of the IGF-I and insulin *(56)*. In contrast, the IGF-II receptor is a single-chain transmembrane protein, identical to the mannose 6-phosphate receptor *(57)*. It appears to be devoid of signaling capabilities. However, IGF-II can exert mitogenic effects, because it binds and activates the IGF-I receptor *(52)*.

There are additional potential interactions between these ligands and their receptors. Thus, insulin, IGF-I, and IGF-II bind to the insulin receptor. However, the affinity of the insulin receptor toward IGF-I or IGF-II is considerably less than toward insulin *(52)*. Conversely, the affinity of the IGF-I receptor toward insulin or IGF-II is considerably less than toward IGF-I *(52)*. In many instances, the high levels of insulin in cultured-cell systems are sufficient to activate the IGF-I receptor, and insulin exerts mitogenic effects in these cells by activating the IGF-I receptor. The IGF-II receptor binds IGF-I and IGF-II, but does not bind insulin *(52)*. A syndrome of extrapancreatic tumor hypoglycemia has been correlated with the production of large quantities of pro-IGF-II, also known as big IGF-II, which causes hypoglycemia by increasing glucose uptake into muscle, and by suppressing hepatic glucose release *(52,58)*.

Recent studies have suggested that IGF-I has a role in pancreatic cancer. Thus, both IGF-1 and its receptor are overexpressed in human pancreatic cancers, raising the possibility that IGF-I may act via autocrine and paracrine mechanisms to enhance pancreatic cancer cell growth *(59)*. Indeed, four lines of evidence indicate that the IGF-I receptor mediates mitogenic signaling in pancreatic cancer cells, and that this effect is important in vivo. First, the proliferative effects of IGF-I in pancreatic cancer cell lines is inhibited by α-IR3, a specific anti-IGF-I receptor antibody *(59)*. Second, the growth of cultured human pancreatic cancer cells is inhibited by IGF-I receptor antisense oligonu-

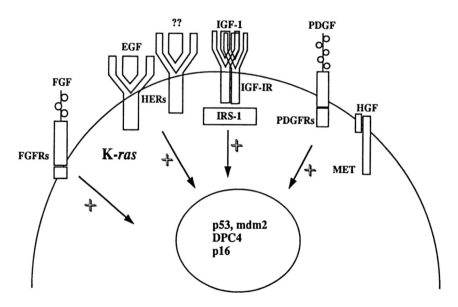

Fig. 2. Interactions among growth factors, oncogenes, and tumor-suppressor genes in pancreatic cancer. Overexpression of the EGF receptor (HERs) family as well as the EGF family of ligands and related known (such as cripto) and unknown (??) ligands, the 2 Ig-like form of FGFR-1, and possibly other FGF receptors (FGFRs) and multiple FGFs, IGF-I receptor (IGF-IR), its ligand IGF-1, and its downstream signaling molecule IRS-1, the hepatocyte growth factor receptor MET and its ligand, both types of the PDGF receptor, and the B-chain of PDGF combine to lead to aberrant activation of tyrosine kinase-dependent pathways and enhanced cell proliferation. Growth stimulation through IGF-IR, and, subsequently, IRS-1, is also enhanced by islet cell-derived insulin and IGF-II. Activation of mitogenic pathways is magnified as a consequence of mutations in the K-ras oncogene and cell-cycle-associated kinases, such as p16. Concurrently, there is loss of negative growth constraints because of p53 tumor-suppressor gene mutations or excessive expression of the mdm-2 gene, and mutations in the DPC4 gene. The net result is enhanced cell proliferation and loss of negative constraints on cell growth.

cleotides *(59)*. Third, *in situ* hybridization studies have shown that, in the normal pancreas, IGF-I is only expressed in the stromal elements *(59)*. In contrast, in the pancreatic cancers, IGF-1 mRNA is abundant in both the cancer cells and the surrounding stroma *(59)*. Fourth, IGF-I receptor activation leads to phosphorylation of IRS-1, an important regulatory protein that mediates the growth-promoting effects of insulin and IGF-1 *(56)*. IRS-1 is also overexpressed in pancreatic cancer *(60)*, indicating that there is an enhanced potential for excessive activation of IGF-I receptor-dependent signaling pathways in this disorder.

IGF-II and insulin also appear to have a role in pancreatic cancer. Although neither polypeptide is expressed at high levels in this malignancy, both insulin and IGF-II are present in the endocrine islets *(61)*. Following their release into the intrapancreatic circulation, they may act via proxicrine mechanisms to activate the overexpressed IGF-I receptor in the pancreatic tumors. In addition, IGF-II may act by binding the IGF-II receptor, which is also overexpressed in pancreatic cancers *(62)*. This receptor participates in the uptake and transport of lysosomal enzymes, internalization, activation and/or degradation of other mannose-6-phosphate-containing proteins, and internalization and degradation of IGF-II *(57)*. It has also been implicated in enhancing cell motility, and in the activation of the TGF-β1 precursor *(63,64)*. Therefore, it is possible that overexpression of the IGF-II receptor in pancreatic cancers may enhance cancer cell motility and activate the overexpressed TGF-β1, thereby contributing to tumor growth and invasion *(65)*.

ADDITIONAL GROWTH FACTORS AND THEIR RECEPTORS IN HUMAN PANCREATIC CANCER

Human pancreatic cancers frequently overexpress the B-chain of platelet-derived growth factor (PDGF), both types of PDGF receptors, hepatocyte growth factor and its receptor c-MET, and the EGF-like ligand, cripto, whose receptor is yet to be identified *(66–69)*. Together with the gene alterations described above, the overexpression of multiple ligands and their tyrosine kinase receptors, and their abundance in pancreatic islets, imply an important role for these molecules in pancreatic cancer cell growth (Fig. 2). It is therefore likely that therapeutic modalities aimed at abrogating the excessive activation of their mitogenic signaling pathways will ultimately have a clinical role in this deadly disorder.

ACKNOWLEDGMENT

Supported by NIH grants CA-40162 and DK-44948.

REFERENCES

1. Gudjonsson B. Cancer of the pancreas. 50 years of surgery. Cancer 1987; *60:*2284–2303.
2. Warshaw AL and Ferandez-Del Castillo C. Pancreatic carcinoma. N Engl J Med 1992; *326:*455–465.
3. Aaronson SA. Growth factors and cancer. Science 1991; *254:*1146–1153.
4. Kingsley DM. (1994) The TGF-β superfamily: new members, new receptors, and new genetic tests of function in different organisms. Genes Dev 1994; *8:*133–146.
5. Henderson JR and Daniel PM. A comparative study of the portal vessels connecting the endocrine and exocrine pancreas, with a discussion of some functional implications. Quart J Exp Physiol Cog Med Sci 1979; *64:*267–275.
6. Massague J and Pandiella A. Membrane-anchored growth factors. Ann Rev Biochem 1993; *62:*515–541.
7. Korc M, Chandrasekar B, and Shah GN. Differential binding and biological activities of epidermal growth factor and transforming growth factor a in a human pancreatic cancer cell line. Cancer Res 1991; *51:*6243–6249.
8. Gan BS, Hollenberg MD, MacCannell KL, Lederis K, Winkler ME, and Derynck R. Distinct vascular actions of epidermal growth factor-urogastrone and transforming growth factor-α. J Phar Exp Ther 1987; *242:*331–337.
9. Fen Z, Dhadly MS, Yoshizumi M, Hilkert RJ, Quertermous T, Eddy RL, Hows TB, and Lee M-E. Structural organization and chromosomal assignment of the gene encoding the human heparin-binding epidermal growth factor-like growth factor/diphteria toxin receptor. Biochemistry 1993; *32:*7932–7938.
10. Shing Y, Christofori D, Hanahan D, Ono Y, Sasada R, Igarashi K, and Folkman J. Betacellulin: a mitogen from pancreatic b cell tumors. Science 1993; *259:*1604–1607.
11. Watanabe T, Shintani A, Nakata M, Shing Y, Folkman J, Igarashi K, and Sasada R. Recombinant human betacellulin. Molecular structure, biological activities, and receptor interaction. J Biol Chem 1994; *269:*9966–9973.

12. Plowman GD, Green JM, McDonald VL, Neubauer MG, Disteche CM, Todaro GJ, and Shoyab M. The amphiregulin gene encodes a novel epidermal growth factor-related protein with tumor-inhibitory activity. Mol Cell Biol 1990; *10:*1969–1981.

13. Johnson GR, Saeki T, Gordon AW, Shoyab M, Salomon DS, and Stromberg K. Autocrine action of amphiregulin in a colon carcinoma cell line and immunocytochemical localization of amphiregulin in human colon. J Cell Biol 1992; *10:*1969–1981.

14. Barnard JA, Graves-Deal R, Pittelkow MR, DuBois R, Cook P, Ramsey GW, et al. Auto- and cross-induction within the mammalian epidermal growth factor-related peptide family. J Biol Chem 1994; *269:*22817–22822.

15. Korc M, Chandrasekar B, Yamanaka Y, Friess H, Buchler M, and Beger HG. Overexpression of the epidermal growth factor receptor in human pancreatic cancer is associated with concomitant increases in the levels of epidermal growth factor and transforming growth factor alpha. J Clin Invest 1992; *90:*1352–1360.

16. Ebert M, Yokoyama M, Kobrin MS, Friess H, Lopez ME, Buchler MW, Johnson GR, and Korc M. Induction and expression of amphiregulin in human pancreatic cancer. Cancer Res 1994; *54:*3959–3962.

17. Yokoyama M, Ebert M, Funatomi H, Friess H, Büchler MW, Johnson GR, and Korc M. Amphiregulin is a potent mitogen in human pancreatic cancer cells: correlation with patient survival. Int J Oncol 1995; *6:*625–631.

18. Yokoyama M, Funatomi H, Kobrin MS, Ebert M, Friess H, Buchler MW, and Korc M. Betacellulin, a member of the epidermal growth factor family, is overexpressed in human pancreatic cancer. Int J Oncol 1995; *7:*825–829.

19. Kobrin MS, Funatomi H, Friess H, Büchler MW, and Stathis P. Induction and expression of heparin-binding EGF-like growth factor in human pancreatic cancer. Biochem Biophys Res Commun 1994; *202:*1705–1709.

20. Smith JJ, Derynck R, and Korc M. Production of transforming growth factor α in human pancreatic cancer cells: evidence for a superagonist autocrine cycle. Proc Natl Acad Sci USA 1987; *84:*7567–7570.

21. Yamanaka Y, Friess H, Kobrin MS, Buchler M, Beger HG, and Korc M. Coexpression of epidermal growth factor receptor and ligands in human pancreatic cancer is associated with enhanced tumor aggressiveness. Anticancer Res 1993; *13:*565–570.

22. Funatomi H, Itakura J, Ishiwata T, Pastan I, Thompson SA, Johnson GR, and Korc M. (1997) Amphiregulin antisense oligonucleotide inhibits the growth of T3M4 human pancreatic cancer cells and sensitizes the cells to EGF receptor targeted therapy. Int J Cancer 1997; *72:*512–517.

23. Prigent SA and Lemoine NR. The type 1 (EGFR-related) family of growth factor receptors and their ligands Prog Growth Factor Res 1992; *4:*1–24.

24. Schlessinger J and Ullrich A. Growth factor signaling by receptor tyrosine kinases. Neuron 1992; *9:*383–391.

25. Pawson T and Schlessinger J. SH2 and SH3 domains. Curr Biol 1993; *3:*434–442.

26. Cadena DL and Gill GN. Receptor tyrosine kinases. FASEB J 1992; *6:*2332–2337.

27. Ahn AG. The MAP kinase cascade Discovery of a new signal transduction pathway. Mol Cell Biochem 1993; *127:*201–209.

28. Soltoff SP, Carraway III KL, Prigent SA, Gullick WG, and Cantley LC. ErbB3 is involved in activation of phosphatidylinositol 3-kinase by epidermal growth factor. Mol Cell Biol 1994; *14:*3550–3558.

29. Carraway KL and Cantley LC. A Neu acquaintance for ErbB3 and ErbB4: a role for receptor heterodimerization in growth signaling. Cell 1994; *78:*5–8.

30. Lemoine NR, Hughes CM, Barton CM, Poulsom R, Jeffery RE, Kloppel G, Hall PA, and Gullick WJ. The epidermal growth factor receptor in human pancreatic cancer. J Pathol 1992; *166:*7–12.

31. Yamanaka Y, Friess H, Kobrin MS, Buchler M, Kunz J, Beger HG, and Korc M. Overexpression of HER-2/neu oncogene in human pancreatic carcinoma. Hum Pathol 1993; *24:*1127–1134.

32. Friess H, Yamanaka Y, Kobrin MS, Do D, Buchler MW, and Korc M. Enhanced erbB-3 expression in human pancreatic cancer correlates with tumor progression. Clin Cancer Res 1995; *1:*1413–1420.

33. Lemoine NR, Lobresco M, Leung H, Barton C, Hughes CM, Prigent SA, Gullick WJ, and Kloppel G. The erbB-3 gene in human pancreatic cancer. J Pathol 1992; *168:*269–273.

34. Almoguera C, Shibata D, Forrester K, Martin J, Arnheim N, and Perucho M. Most human carcinomas of the exocrine pancreas contain mutant c-K-ras genes. Cell 1988; *53:*549–554.

35. Grunewald K, Lyons J, Frohlich A, Feichtinger H, Weger RA, Schwab G, Janssen JWG, and Bartram CR. High frequency of Ki-ras codon 12 mutations in pancreatic adenocarcinomas. Int J Cancer 1989; *43:*1037–1041.

36. Pellegata NS, Sessa F, Rneut B, Bonato B, Leone BE, Solcia E, and Ranzani GN. K-ras and p53 gene mutation in pancreatic cancer: ductal and nonductal tumors progress through different genetic lesions. Cancer Res 1994; *54:*1556–1560.

37. Bos JL. Ras oncogenes in human cancer: a review. Cancer Res 1989; *49:*4682–4689.

38. Barton CM, Staddon SL, Hughes CM, Hall PA, O'Sullivan C, Kloppel G, et al. Abnormalities of the p53 tumour suppressor gene in human pancreatic cancer. Br J Cancer 1991; *64:*1076–1082.

39. Casey G, Yamanaka Y, Friess H, Kobrin MS, Lopez ME, Buchler M, Beger HG, and Korc M. p53 Mutations are common in pancreatic cancer and are absent in chronic pancreatitis. Cancer Lett 1993; *69:*151–160.

40. Hahn SA, Schutte M, Shansul Hoque ATM, Moskaluk CA, da Costa LT, Fischer A, et al. DPC4, a candidate tumor suppressor gene at human chromosome 18q21.1. Science 1996; *268:*350–353.

41. Goldstein AM, Fraser MC, Struewing JP, Hussussian CJ, Ranade K, Zametkin DP, et al. Increased risk of pancreatic cancer in melanoma-prone kindreds with pl6INK4 mutations. New Engl J Med 1995; *333:*970–974.

42. M Ebert, M Yokoyama, MS Kobrin, H Friess, MW Büchler, and M Korc. Increased MDM2 expression and immunoreactivity in human pancreatic ductal adenocarcinoma. Int J Oncol 1994; *5:*1279–1284.

43. Haines DS, Landers JE, Engle LJ, and George DL. Physical and functional interaction between wild-type p53 and mdm2 proteins. Mol Cell Biol 1994; *14:*1171–1178.

44. Wagner M, Cao T, Lopez ME, Hope C, Van Nostrand K, Korbin MS, et al. Expression of a truncated EGF receptor is associated with inhibition of pancreatic cancer cell growth and enhanced sensitivity to cisplatinum. Int J Cancer 1996; *68:*782–787.

45. Mason IJ. The ins and outs of fibroblast growth factors Cell 1994; *78:*547–552.

46. Jaye M, Schlessinger J, and Dionne C. Fibroblast growth factor receptor tyrosine kinases: molecular analysis and signal transduction. Biochim Biophys Acta 1992; *1135:*185–199.

47. Leung HY, Gullick WJ, and Lemoine NR. Expression and functional activity of fibroblast growth factors and their receptors in human pancreatic cancer. Int J Cancer 1994; *59:*667–675.

48. Yamanaka Y, Friess H, Buchler M, Beger HG, Uchida E, Onda M, Kobrin MS, and Korc M. Overexpression of acidic and basic fibroblast growth factors in human pancreatic cancer correlates with advanced tumor stage. Cancer Res 1993; *53:*5289–5296.

49. Estival A, Monzat V, Miquel K, Gaubert F, Hollande E, Korc M, Vaysse N, and Clemente F. Differential regulation of fibroblast growth factor (FGF) receptor-1 mRNA and protein by two molecular forms of basic FGF. J Biol Chem 1996; *271:*5663–5670.

50. Kobrin MS, Yamanaka Y, Friess H, Lopez ME, and Korc M. Aberrant expression of the type I fibroblast growth factor receptor in human pancreatic adenocarcinomas. Cancer Res 1993; *53:*4741–4744.

51. Wagner M, Kan M, Lopez ME, and Korc M. Suppression of fibroblast growth factor receptor signaling inhibits pancreatic cancer cell growth in vivo and in vitro. Gastroenterology, in press.

52. Le Roith D. Insulin-like growth factors. N Engl J Med 1997; *336:*633–640.

53. Korc M. Normal function of the endocrine pancreas. In: Go VLW, DiMagno EP, Gardner JD, Lebenthal E, Reber HA, and Scheele GA (eds), The pancreas: biology, pathobiology and disease, Raven, New York, 1993; pp. 751–758.

54. Daughaday WH. Editorial: The possible autocrine/paracrine and endocrine roles of insulin-like growth factors of human tumors. Endocrinology 1990; *127:*14.

55. Macaulay VM. Insulin-like growth factors and cancer. Br J Cancer 1992; *65:*311–320.

56. Cheatham B and Kahn CR. Insulin action and the insulin signaling network. Endocr Rev 1995; *16:*117–142.

57. Nissley P, Kiess W, and Sklar MM. The insulin-like growth factor II/mannose 6-phosphate receptor. In: LeRoith G (ed.), Insulin-like growth factors: molecular and cellular aspects. CRC, Boca Raton, FL, 1991; pp. 111–150.

58. Zapf J. Role of insulin-like growth factor II and IGF binding proteins in extrapancreatic tumor hypoglycemia. Horm Res 1994; *42:*20–26.

59. Bergmann U, Funatomi H, Yokoyama M, Beger HG, and Korc M. Insulin-like growth factor I overexpression in human pancreatic cancer: evidence for autocrine and paracrine roles. Cancer Res 1995; *55:*2007–2011.

60. Bergmann U, Funatomi H, Kornmann M, Beger HG, and Korc M. Increased expression of insulin receptor substrate-1 in human pancreatic cancer. Biochem Biophys Res Commun 1996; *220:*886–890.

61. Bergmann U, Funatomi H, Kornmann M, Ishiwata T, Beger HG, and Korc M. Insulin-like growth factor II activates mitogenic signaling in pancreatic cancer cells via IRS-1: *in vivo* evidence for an islet-cancer cell axis. Int J Oncol 1996; *9:*487–492.

62. Ishiwata T, Bergmann U, Kornmann M, Lopez M, Beger HG, and Korc M. Altered expression of insulin-like growth factor II receptor in human pancreatic cancer. Pancreas 1997; 15:367–373.

63. Minniti CP, Kohn EC, Grubb JH, Sly WS, Oh Y, Muller HL, Rosenfeld RG, and Helman LJ. The insulin-like growth factor II (IGF-II)/mannose 6-phosphate receptor mediates IGF-II-induced motility in human rhabdomyosarcoma cells. J Biol Chem 1992; *267:*9000–9004.

64. Saperstein LA, Jirtle RL, Farouk M, Thompson HJ, Chung KS, and Meyers WC. Transforming growth factor-beta 1 and mannose 6-phosphate/insulin-like growth factor II receptor expression during intrahepatic bile duct hyperplasia and biliary fibrosis in the rat. Hepatology 1994; *19:*412–417.

65. Friess H, Yamanaka Y, Buchler M, Ebert M, Beger HG, Gold LI, and Korc M. Enhanced expression of transforming growth factor-beta isoforms in human pancreatic cancer correlates with decreased survival. Gastroenterology 1993; *105:*1846–1856.

66. Ebert M, Yokoyama M, Friess H, Kobrin MS, Buchler MW, and Korc M. Induction of platelet-derived growth factor A and B chains and over-expression of their receptors in human pancreatic cancer. Int J Cancer 1995; *62:*529–535.

67. Ebert M, Yokoyama M, Friess H, Buchler MW, and Korc M. Coexpression of the c-*met* proto-oncogene and hepatocyte growth factor in human pancreatic cancer. Cancer Res 1994; *54:*5775–5778.

68. Di Renzo MF, Poulsom R, Olivero M, Comoglio PM, and Lemoine NR. Expression of the Met/hepatocyte growth factor receptor in human pancreatic cancer. Cancer Res 1995; *55:*1129–1138.

69. Friess H, Yamanaka Y, Büchler M, Beger HG, Kobrin MS, Tahara E, and Korc M. Cripto, a member of the epidermal growth factor family, is over-expressed in human pancreatic cancer and chronic pancreatitis. Int J Cancer 1994; *56:*668–674.

3

Growth Factors and Growth Factor Receptors in Chronic Pancreatitis, and the Relation to Pancreatic Cancer

Helmut Friess, Pascal Berberat, and Markus W. Büchler

INTRODUCTION

Chronic pancreatitis is an inflammatory disease of the pancreas that leads to persistent and progressive morphological and functional alterations of the whole organ and in its terminal state severe exocrine and endocrine insufficiencies are present. *(1–3)*. Morphologically, chronic inflammation of the pancreas is also associated with pancreatic head enlargement, calcifications of the parenchyma, cysts, necrosis, and pancreatic stones *(4–6)*. The continuous tissue destruction and subsequent remodeling causes finally the two major clinical symptoms: upper abdominal pain and maldigestion.

Although many studies have attempted to clarify the pathobiological mechanisms of pain generation in chronic pancreatitis, all proposed hypotheses are still controversial. Theories of pain pathogenesis have included focal acute inflammation of the pancreas, increased intraductal pressure, extrapancreatic causes like common bile duct or duodenal stenosis, and postprandial pancreatic hyperstimulation caused by decreased secretion capacity and the insufficient functioning of the so-called negative-feedback mechanism *(7,8)*. However, none of these concepts can conclusively explain the pain syndrome in these patients. Recent studies using modern molecular biology techniques, such as *in situ* hybridization, have led to the postulation that direct alterations of nerves and changes in neurotransmitters might cause pain in patients with chronic pancreatitis *(9–11)*. There is great expectation that the availability of new molecular methods will help to complete our understanding of pain generation in chronic pancreatitis in coming years.

The second leading symptom in patients with chronic pancreatitis is maldigestion, which is generally caused by the loss of exocrine parenchyma. However, the mechanisms which lead to the destruction of the exocrine pancreas and the replacement of pancreatic acinar and ductal cells by fibrosis are not known. In the past, several independent pathophysiological concepts of chronic pancreatitis were introduced by different research groups, but there is still disagreement over which of them is the most valid explanation for the morphological changes that occur in chronic pancreatitis *(12–15)*. The most-favored concept postulates that alcohol overconsumption causes a reduction in the secretion of lithostatin, a protein that stabilizes the pancreatic juice and inhibits the formation of protein plugs; it is believed that protein plugs are then formed, which lead to obstruction of the pancreatic ductal system and, subsequently, to a chronic inflammation in the pancreas *(12)*. Other proposed causes include recurrent attacks of acute pancreatitis, with subsequent necrosis, periductular fibrosis, ductal obstruction, and continuous fibrosis *(13)*, the direct toxic effect of alcohol and its metabolites on pancreatic acinar and ductal cells *(14)*, and direct damage of the pancreatic parenchyma by increased levels of free radicals caused by reduced hepatic detoxification *(15)*. However, none of these concepts can conclusively explain the morphological, functional, and clinical picture of chronic pancreatitis *(16)*. Therefore, additional mechanisms must be involved in the pathogenesis of chronic pancreatitis. We favor a new hypothesis of inflammatory destruction that causes pain and exocrine/endocrine failure. Recently, we have reported that there exists a correlation between inflammatory cell infiltrates, pain, and changes in and around pancreatic nerves *(17)*. Exocrine and endocrine pancreatic destruction and fibrotic replacement seems to be additionally influenced by activated lymphocytes and by activation of nonpancreatic proteolytic systems *(18,19)*.

The fast-developing field of molecular biology, with its new techniques and knowledge about fundamental biological mechanisms, has enabled clinicians to gain deeper insight into the pathophysiology of human diseases in the past decade. However, the molecular mechanisms that contribute to the histomorphological changes in chronic pancreatitis are still not known. Bockman and coworkers *(20)* reported in 1992 that transgenic mice, which overexpress transforming growth factor alpha (TGF-α) in the pancreas, develop morphological pancreatic changes that are comparable to those found in chronic pancreatitis in humans: The pancreata of these mice were macroscopically firm and enlarged. Microscopically, there was a high degree of fibrosis and dedifferentiation of pancreatic acinar cells into tubular structures. These findings provided the first hint that growth factors and growth factor receptors may play a role in the morphological changes that occur in chronic pancreatitis.

Using modern molecular biology techniques, such as Northern blot analysis, *in situ* hybridization, immunoblotting, and Southern blot analysis, and histological approaches, such as immunohistochemistry, the authors have tried to determine over the past 4 yr whether expression and distribution of growth factors and growth factor receptors occurs in chronic pancreatitis. In addition, the authors have tried to evaluate whether changes in the expression of these factors might influence the development of chronic pancreatitis.

The following review will summarize some of the authors' and other researchers' findings on the role of growth factors and growth factor receptors in chronic pancreatitis in humans.

THE EPIDERMAL GROWTH FACTOR (EGF) RECEPTOR, C-*ERBB*-2 AND C-*ERBB*-3 IN CHRONIC PANCREATITIS

The EGF receptor, also known as human EGF receptor I (HER-1), is a transmembrane 180 kDa protein that exhibits tyrosine kinase activity by its intracellular domain *(21–23)*. The EGF receptor belongs to a growth factor family that also includes c-*erb*B-2 (HER-2) *(24,25)*, c-*erb*B-3 (HER-3) *(26)*, and c-*erb*B-4 (HER-4) *(27)*. They share significant amino-acid-sequence homology, possessing six cystine residues in the same relative position. All these growth factor receptors are activated by specific ligands. Through binding of ligands to the extracellular domain of the receptor, which provide a complicated tertiary structure consisting of 25 disulfide bonds, the intracellular tyrosine kinase is activated, leading to the phosphorylation of various intracellular substrates, such as phospholipase C-gamma, and to tyrosine autophosphorylation *(21,23)*. Several ligands have been found during the past two decades that bind and activate the EGF receptor. These include EGF, TGF-α, amphiregulin, betacellulin, and heparin-binding EGF *(28–32)*. All five polypeptides are generated by proteolytic cleavage of the extracellular domains of precursor molecules, which possess a hydrophobic transmembrane domain and an intracellular domain as their receptors. The activation of the EGF receptor by EGF and TGF-α has been studied extensively. Binding of EGF to the receptor first induces dimerization of the receptor, which seems to be its functional state, and then leads both to phosphorylation of intracellular substrates by the tyrosine kinase domain and to the internalization of the ligand–receptor complex (receptor-mediated endocytosis) *(33)*. During this process, the receptors are quickly removed from the surface of the cell and the cell can consequently not be stimulated by further exogenous growth factors (refractory period, also called receptor downregulation). EGF is recycled and released from the cytoplasm in the extracellular space for further activation of the EGF receptor. The activation of the EGF receptor by TGF-α is approx 100× stronger than activation of EGF. However, following internalization of the EGF-receptor–TGF-α complex, TGF-α is degraded in the cytoplasm *(34)*.

The exact function of EGF in vivo is not yet completely clear. It seems to have a physiological effect as an autocrine and paracrine growth factor in tissue renewal and wound repair, and to play a role in milk production and as a growth-promoting agent for the newborn, as well as to have some function in the male reproductive system *(35,36)*.

Using Northern blot analysis, we found low levels of EGF receptor, EGF, and TGF-α mRNA expression *(37–39)*. *In situ* hybridization with specific cRNA probes revealed that EGF receptor, EGF, and TGF-α mRNA transcription takes place in acinar and ductal cells in the normal pancreas. TGF-α mRNA grains were present at comparatively high values in the normal pancreas. All three mRNA moieties were preferentially localized at the apical portion of ductal cells. In acinar cells, the mRNA grains of all three species were present in the basal portion *(37–39)*.

In tissue samples obtained from patients with chronic pancreatitis, expression of EGF receptor, EGF, and TGF-α mRNA was increased, but amylase mRNA values were considerably decreased when compared with the normal controls *(39)*. Densitometry of the Northern blot membranes revealed that 70% of the chronic pancreatitis samples exhibited a 5.7-fold increase in EGF-receptor values, and 74% of the chronic pancreatitis samples showed a six-fold increase of TGF-α mRNA, compared with the normal controls *(39)*. *In situ* hybridization demonstrated a readily evident increase in EGF receptor, EGF, and TGF-α mRNA both in remaining acinar cells and ductal cells in the chronic pancreatitis samples. Quantitative video image analysis of the *in situ* hybridization data from normal and chronic pancreatitis tissue samples showed that there were 23-fold and four-fold increases of EGF receptor and TGF-α mRNA values, respectively, in the chronic pancreatitis tissues, compared to the normal pancreas *(39)*. mRNA grains were localized in exocrine pancreatic cells, but not in the stroma or in fibroblasts.

c-*erb*B-2 analysis in the normal pancreas and in chronic pancreatitis tissue samples was performed using Southern blot analysis, Northern blot analysis, *in situ* hybridization, and immunohistochemistry. Northern blot analysis of RNA samples extracted from normal pancreases, and from patients with chronic pancreatitis, revealed low levels of c-*erb*B-2 mRNA expression in the normal pancreas *(40,41)*. In contrast, some of the chronic pancreatitis samples exhibited markedly increased c-*erb*B-2 mRNA expression; others had c-*erb*B-2 mRNA levels comparable with those of normal controls. Analysis of the clinical data of the chronic pancreatitis patients revealed that patients with pancreatic head enlargement had increased c-*erb*B-2 mRNA levels; patients without pancreatic head enlargement did not exhibit enhanced c-*erb*B-2 mRNA expression in the resected pancreas. Densitometric analysis of the Northern blots indicated that, by comparison with the normal pancreas, there was a 4.5-fold increase (range: 1.7–8.7) in c-*erb*B-2 mRNA levels in chronic pancreatitis tissues of patients with pancreatic head enlargement. No aberrant mRNA transcripts were found in any of the normal or chronic pancreatitis samples *(40)*. Linear regression analysis of the fold increases in c-*erb*B-2 mRNA levels with the vertical pancreatic head diameter of the pancreas showed a significant positive correlation ($y = -2.9 + 1.3 \times X$, $r = 0.82$; $p < 0.001$). When expression analysis of the EGF receptor was performed in the same chronic pancreatitis samples, only 54% of the chronic pancreatitis samples with pancreatic head enlargement exhibited enhanced expression *(40)*. In addition, 42% of the chronic pancreatitis patients with no enlargement of the vertical pancreatic head diameter showed marked overexpression of the EGF receptor.

In situ hybridization in the normal pancreas demonstrated specific c-*erb*B-2 mRNA grains in acinar and ductal cells *(40)*. In chronic pancreatitis tissue samples without pancreatic head enlargement, the number of specific *in situ* hybridization grains was comparable to that of the normal controls *(40)*. In contrast, patients with pancreatic head enlargement exhibited consistently higher levels of c-*erb*B-2 mRNA *in situ* hybridization grains in the remaining pancreatic acinar and ductal cells. Comparative video image analysis of the *in situ* hybridization signals in the normal pancreas, and in chronic pancreatitis tissues with and without pancreatic head enlargement, indicated that, in tissue samples of patients with pancreatic head enlargement, c-*erb*B-2 mRNA grains were 4.8-fold higher ($p < 0.001$) than in the other two groups.

To investigate whether overexpression of c-*erb*B-2 is caused by gene amplification, as has been reported in many mammary cancers, Southern blot analysis was performed in the same normal and chronic pancreatitis samples that were used in Northern blot analysis and in the *in situ* hybridization experiments. Following digestion of genomic DNA with the restriction enzymes *Eco*RI and *Bg*III, no aberrant DNA bands or gene amplifications were observed *(40)*.

By immunohistochemistry using a highly specific monoclonal antibody against the c-*erb*B-2 protein (p185), the authors found weak-to-moderate immunoreactivity in a focal pattern in some acinar and ductal cells in the normal pancreas (Fig. 1A) *(40)*. Chronic pancreatitis samples of patients without pancreatic head enlargement (Fig. 1B) exhibited a staining pattern that was comparable to that in the normal controls *(40)*. In contrast, a diffuse increase in c-*erb*B-2 immunoreactivity was present in acinar and ductal cells in tissues obtained from chronic pancreatitis patients with pancreatic head enlargement. Immunoreactivity was mostly located in the cytoplasm of the cells (Fig. 1C). In addition, most regions with pseudoductular structures exhibited intense c-*erb*B-2 immunostaining. In areas with fibrosis, only some of the fibroblasts were positive for c-*erb*B-2. However, in the fibrosis there was no difference in staining intensity and frequency between chronic pancreatitis patients with and without enlargement of the pancreatic head.

c-*erb*B-3, the third member of the EGF receptor family, was studied in chronic pancreatitis, in comparison with pancreatic cancer and normal controls *(42)*. In all samples of normal pancreas, low levels of c-*erb*B-3 mRNA expression were present. In chronic pancreatitis, 24% of the samples exhibited enhanced c-*erb*B-3 mRNA expression. By immunohistochemistry, c-*erb*B-3 immunoreactivity was found only in ductal cells *(42)* in the normal pancreas (Fig. 2A). Centroacinar cells and most ductal cells in the intralobular and interlobular ducts showed faint-to-moderate c-*erb*B-3 immunostaining (Fig. 2A). In chronic pancreatitis samples, faint-to-moderate c-*erb*B-3 immunoreactivity was present in the remaining acinar and ductal cells (Fig. 2B). In addition, regions with pseudoductal metaplasia exhibited moderate-to-intense c-*erb*B-3 immunostaining; in fibrotic tissues, no immunostaining for c-*erb*B-3 was detectable.

CRIPTO IN CHRONIC PANCREATITIS

The cripto gene encodes a 188-amino-acid polypeptide growth factor that was originally cloned from cell lines of an undifferentiated human teratocarcinoma *(43,44)*. In its central region, it shows strong structural homology to EGF and TGF-α *(44)*. Therefore, cripto belongs to the EGF family of growth factors. In contrast to EGF and TGF-α, cripto does not bind to the EGF-receptor. Functional studies with teratocarcinoma cell lines have demonstrated that shutting off the cripto gene leads to cell differentiation *(44)*. These findings suggest that cripto is associated with an undifferentiated cell state.

The expression and distribution of cripto was analyzed in chronic pancreatitis, parallel to pancreatic cancer. By Northern blot analysis, a four-fold increase ($p < 0.02$) of the cripto mRNA levels was found in the chronic pancreatitis samples *(45)*, compared with normal controls. The increase in mRNA expression was not caused by gene amplification or gene rearrangement, as confirmed by Southern blot analysis *(45)*. Neither *Eco*RI nor *Hin*dIII digestion of genomic DNA revealed any aberrant DNA fragments in the normal pancreas and in chronic pancreatitis samples. Cripto immunostaining in the normal pancreas was present in ductal cells, and only faintly in

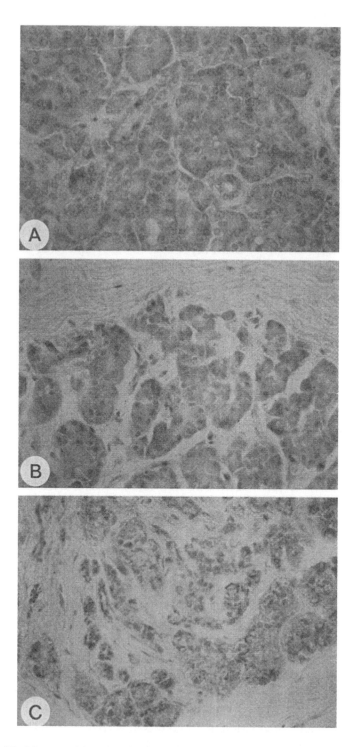

Fig. 1. c-*erb*B-2 immunohistochemical staining in the normal pancreas (**A**), and in chronic pancreatitis without (**B**), and with pancreatic head enlargement (**C**). In the normal pancreas, c-*erb*B-2 immunoreactivity was present in the cytoplasm of some acinar cells and ductal cells (A). In chronic pancreatitis patients without enlargement of the pancreatic head, c-*erb*B-2 immunostaining in the remaining acinar and ductal cells was comparable with that in the normal controls (B). In contrast, tissue samples obtained from chronic pancreatitis patients with pancreatic head enlargement exhibited increased c-*erb*B-2 immunoreactivity in the pancreas (C).

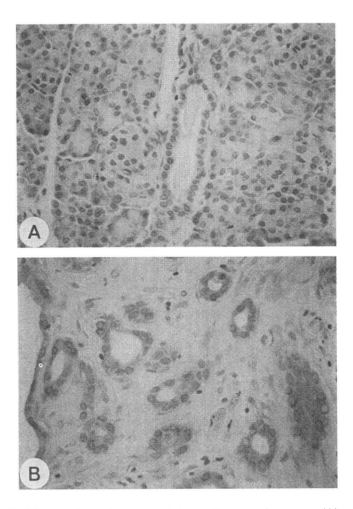

Fig. 2. c-*erb*B-3 immunohistochemical staining in the normal pancreas (**A**), and in chronic pancreatitis (**B**). In the normal pancreas, c-*erb*B-3 immunoreactivity was present in ductal cells and in central acinar cells. In chronic pancreatitis, the remaining acinar and ductal cells exhibited moderate-to-strong c-*erb*B-3 immunoreactivity.

a few acinar cells (Fig. 3A). Immunohistochemical analysis in chronic pancreatitis tissues revealed that the intensity of cripto immunostaining was closely related to the histomorphological damage of the exocrine pancreatic parenchyma. In chronic pancreatitis tissues, areas with minor histomorphological damage exhibited cripto immunostaining comparable to that of normal controls. In contrast, in atrophic acinar cells (Fig. 3B) and ductal cells, and in regions with ductal metaplasia (Fig. 3C), intense cripto immunoreactivity was present *(45)*.

ACIDIC FIBROBLAST GROWTH FACTOR (aFGF) AND BASIC FIBROBLAST GROWTH FACTOR (bFGF) IN CHRONIC PANCREATITIS

aFGF and bFGF belong to a second family of homologous polypeptide growth factors that influence various biological functions, such as cell differentiation, cell mi-

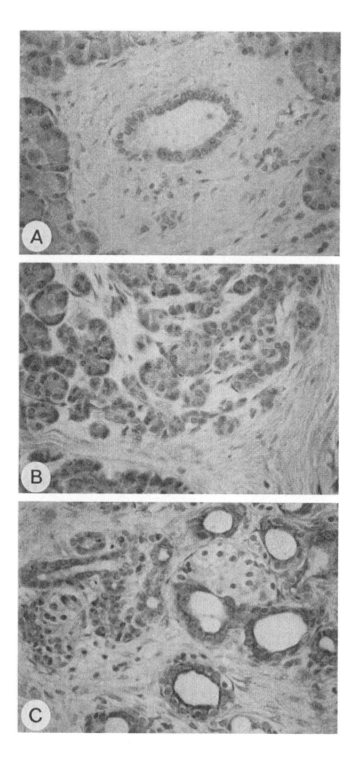

Fig. 3. Immunohistochemical staining of cripto in the normal pancrease (**A**), and in chronic pancreatitis (**B, C**). In the normal pancreas, cripto immunoreactivity was present in the cytoplasm of most ductal cells, and was very faint in a few acinar cells (A). In contrast, in chronic pancreatitis samples, acinar cells (B) and areas with ductal metaplasia (C) exhibited moderate-to-strong cripto immunoreactivity.

gration, and angiogenesis *(46–52)*. In addition, bFGF also seems to play an important role in tissue repair, by increasing the production of collagen and plasminogen activator *(53,54)*. Both growth factors exert chemotactic effects on fibroblasts and increase collagen production by these cells *(46,51,55)*. Fibroblast growth factors have a high affinity for heparin and glycosaminoglycans, which is important for their biological functions *(52)*. In addition to aFGF and bFGF, the fibroblast growth factor gene family currently includes FGF-3 (int-2), FGF-4 (Kaposi FGF), FGF-5, FGF-6, FGF-7 (keratinocyte growth factor), FGF-8 (androgen-induced growth factor), and FGF-9 *(48–52)*. The family members have between 30 and 70% of their amino-acid sequence in common. The prototypes aFGF and bFGF are found in abundance in the extracellular matrix, which seems to serve as a reservoir for FGFs. One theory suggests that, in this way, a "pool" of FGFs can quickly be mobilized in response to requirements such as cell migration, wound healing, and angiogenesis.

Like other growth factors, fibroblast growth factors transmit their messages to the target cells by binding to specific transmembrane receptors. At least five fibroblast growth factor receptors (FGFR) have been discovered: FGFR-1 (flg-1), FGFR-2 (bek), FGFR-3 (cek-2), FGFR-4 (flg-2), and FGFR-5. FGF receptors consist of two or three immunoglobulin-like regions in the extracellular domain, a short transmembraneous region, and an intracellular domain. The intracellular segment possesses tyrosine kinase activity that is separated into two contiguous regions. Binding of FGFs to their receptors requires the presence of heparin sulfate, which is usually found on the cell surface or in the extracellular matrix. First, the ligands bind with high affinity to heparin-like molecules; next, they bind to the cognate FGF receptors by forming a trimolecular complex that transmits the signal into the cell. The heparin-like molecules might present the FGFs to their receptors, or they may serve as strong stabilization factor in the ligand–receptor complex. Other studies have shown that the heparin-like molecules also increase the half-life of FGFs by preserving them for early proteolytic degradation *(47,48,51,52)*. Through different mRNA splicing, the distinct isoforms of FGFRs are generated. As mentioned above, FGF receptors belong to the tyrosine kinase receptor family, as do many other growth factor receptors. Like the ligands, the receptors also show a significant sequence homology. Additionally, they demonstrate an overlap concerning their binding specificity for the various FGFs *(51,52,56)*.

In humans, aFGF has been found in nerve tissue, heart, kidneys, prostate, and liver. In contrast, bFGF seems to be more ubiquitous in human tissues *(46,48,50,57,58)*. The presence of aFGF and bFGF and four of their high-affinity FGF receptors has already been reported in the normal human pancreas *(59)*. In addition, experimental studies in isolated rat pancreatic acini have demonstrated that aFGF and bFGF can stimulate amylase release. These observations raise the possibility that these growth factors might play a physiological role in the regulation of the exocrine pancreas.

In the normal human pancreas, Northern blot analysis has shown low levels of aFGF and bFGF mRNA expression *(60,61)*, and *in situ* hybridization analysis has revealed low levels of these grains in some pancreatic acinar and ductal cells *(61)*. Only faint aFGF and bFGF immunoreactivity was found in the cytoplasm of acinar and ductal cells in the normal pancreas; however, aFGF was present preferentially in ductal cells, and bFGF was more frequently found in acinar cells *(60,61)*.

In contrast, when the chronic pancreatitis samples were compared with normal controls, Northern blot analysis showed a significant increase of aFGF mRNA ($p < 0.01$) in 72% of the CP samples, and of bFGF mRNA in 91%. Densitometric analysis of the Northern blot signals indicated a 10-fold increase for aFGF and a 14-fold increase for bFGF. Linear regression analysis of the mRNA increases above control in aFGF, and bFGF mRNA levels of the individual chronic pancreatitis samples indicated that there was a significant positive correlation between the expression levels of these growth factors ($r = 0.88$; $p < 0.001$) *(61)*. The mRNA expression data obtained by Northern blot analysis could be confirmed by *in situ* hybridization. aFGF and bFGF mRNA expression were markedly increased in many acinar and ductal cells, especially when these cells exhibited atrophic changes. In regions of chronic pancreatitis samples exhibiting less damage of the parenchyma, the intensity and the frequency of aFGF and bFGF mRNA grains were slightly above those of normal controls. Furthermore, in the surrounding stroma and in the fibrotic regions, grains of both mRNA moieties were slightly elevated *(61)*.

Immunohistochemical staining, using specific monoclonal antibodies for aFGF and bFGF, demonstrated that aFGF (Fig. 4B,C) and bFGF (Fig. 5B,C) were markedly elevated in the chronic pancreatitis tissues. In the normal pancreas, some acinar cells and ductal cells of small ductules or larger interlobular ducts showed immunoreactivity for aFGF (Fig. 4A) and bFGF (Fig. 5A) at the apical aspect. In the chronic pancreatitis tissue samples, aFGF (Fig. 4B) and bFGF (Fig. 5B) immunoreactivity was intense for both factors in degenerating acinar and ductal cells, and in areas exhibiting pseudoductular metaplasia (Figs. 4C and 5C). In contrast, areas of chronic pancreatitis tissues with minor damage showed immunostaining in acinar and ductal cells that was only slightly increased when compared with normal controls. There was no immunoreactivity of aFGF and bFGF in the stroma or in the fibrosis in the chronic pancreatitis samples *(61)*.

TRANSFORMING GROWTH FACTOR
BETAS (TGF-βS) IN CHRONIC PANCREATITIS

Transforming growth factor betas (TGF-βs) and their homologues form a third important family of growth factors. They are stable, multifunctional polypeptide growth factors that belong to the TGF-β gene superfamily of regulatory polypeptides, which act as signaling molecules by binding to specific receptors located on the surface of the cell membrane *(62,63)*. TGF-βs are excreted as an inactive molecule, which has to be activated before it can bind to its specific cell membrane receptors. In mammalian cells, three isoforms of transforming growth factor beta exist: TGF-β1, TGF-β2, and TGF-β3. TGF-βs are multifunctional cytokines that play an important role in the regulation of cell growth, cell differentiation, angiogenesis, immunoreactions, and formation of the extracellular matrix *(64–67)*. TGF-βs have been demonstrated to be potent inhibitors of growth in many cell types, including epithelial, endothelial, neuronal, hemopoetic, and lymphoid cells *(63,67)*. In addition, TGF-βs can regulate biological processes by controlling gene transcription. In this way, TGF-βs stimulate the expression of extracellular matrix-forming proteins, and of several proteases that degrade extracellular matrix proteins, thereby controlling wound healing, cellular adhesion, and extracellular matrix deposition *(68,69)*.

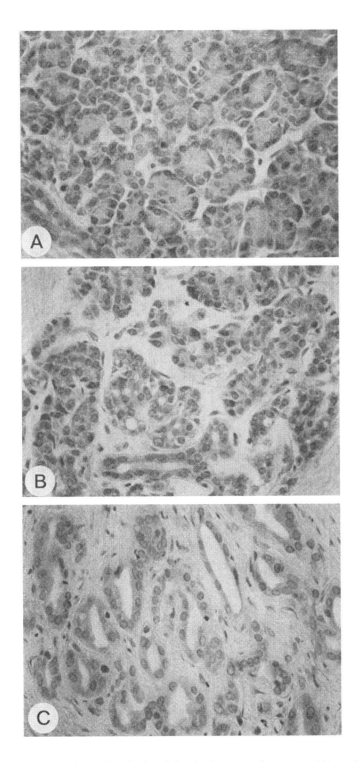

Fig. 4. aFGF immunohistochemical staining in the normal pancreas (**A**), and in chronic pancreatitis (**B, C**). In the normal pancreas (A), faint aFGF immunoreactivity was present in the cytoplasm of some acinar and ductal cells. In chronic pancreatitis, most atrophic acinar cells (B) and metaplastic ductal cells (C) exhibited moderate-to-strong aFGF immunoreactivity.

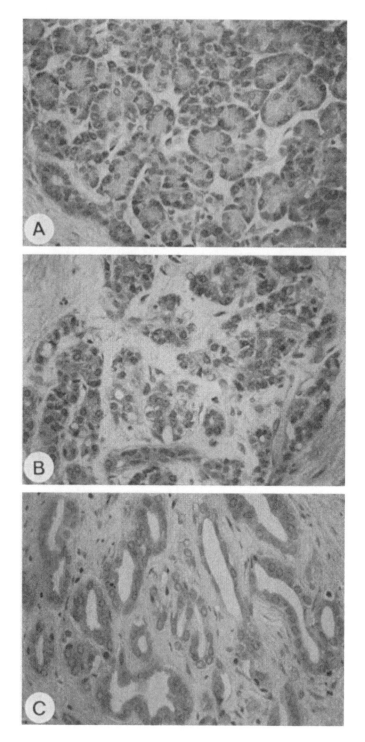

Fig. 5. bFGF immunohistochemical analysis in the normal pancreas (**A**), and in chronic pancreatitis (**B, C**). In the normal pancreas, faint bFGF immunostaining was present in the cytoplasm of some acinar and ductal cells (A). In chronic pancreatitis samples, moderate-to-intense bFGF immunoreactivity was present in most atrophic acinar cells (B), and in areas with ductal metaplasia (C).

TGF-β signaling occurs via specific cellsurface receptors. Three major TGF-β receptors (TβR) have been characterized in recent years; they have been named TGF-β receptor types I, II, and III *(70–73)*. Receptor types I and II are involved in signal transduction; the type III receptor is involved in storage of TGF-βs and their presentation to the signaling receptors *(71,73)*. Although only one subtype of TGF-β receptor type II has been identified, several subtypes of the TGF-β receptor type I have been characterized. TGF-β receptor type I ALK5 (TβR-I$_{Alk5}$), which is the most important type I TGF-β receptor subtype, mostly participates in maintaining the signaling pathway. Another TGF-β receptor type I subtype is TβR-I$_{SKR1}$, which plays a less important role in signal transduction than TβR-I$_{Alk5}$ *(62)*. Biochemical studies indicate that the TGF-β receptor type II activates signal transmission through an intracellular serine-threonine-kinase. However, signaling is dependent on the presence of TGF-β receptor type I. On the other hand, TGF-β receptor type II is necessary for binding of TGF-βs to the TGF-β receptor type I. The TGF-β signal is transduced through a heterodimeric receptor complex consisting of TGF-β receptor types I and II *(71,73)*. TGF-β receptor type III is a proteoglycan also known as betaglycan, and seems not to be directly involved in signal transmission. It participates in storage of TGF-βs and in the presentation of TGF-β isoforms to their signaling receptors *(72)*. A soluble form of TGF-β receptor type III was isolated in the serum and in the extracellular matrix of cultured fibroblasts. This soluble receptor can bind TGF-βs. TβR-III-bound TGF-β cannot simultaneously bind to the signaling TGF-β receptors. Therefore, TGF-β receptor type III can regulate the access of TGF-βs to the signaling receptors, thereby playing a central role in controlling interactions between TGF-βs and their signaling receptors *(74)*. In addition, TβR-III has a highly conserved serine- and threonine-rich cytoplasm domain, which might interact with TβR-I$_{ALK5}$ and TβR-II during signaling *(62,75)*.

In the normal human pancreas, low levels of TGF-β1, TGF-β2, and TGF-β3 mRNA were present. *In situ* hybridization showed TGF-β1, TGF-β2, and TGF-β3 mRNA grains in islet cells, acinar cells, and ductules, but rarely in larger ducts in the normal pancreas. In addition, TβR-I$_{ALK5}$, TβR-II, and TβR-III mRNA grains were present. *In situ* hybridization indicated that all three TGF-β receptors are transcribed in a few acinar and ductal cells within the normal pancreas. The strongest mRNA signals could be obtained by Northern blot analysis for TβR-III.

Immunostaining for TGF-β1, TGF-β2, TGF-β3, TβR-I$_{ALK5}$, and TβR-II demonstrated a distribution pattern similar to that shown by *in situ* hybridization. Independent analysis of chronic pancreatitis samples by other groups has also demonstrated strong immunostaining in the majority of ductal cells for TGF-β1, in the normal controls only single ductular and centroacinar cells exhibited TGF-β1 immunoreactivity. TGF-β1 immunoreactivity was especially present at the junctions between ductules and acini in the normal pancreas. In chronic pancreatitis samples, mononuclear cells and some fibroblasts exhibited TGF-β1 immunoreactivity in areas with inflammation and fibrosis *(76,77)*. Remnant islet cells showed diffuse TGF-β1 immunoreactivity in chronic pancreatitis tissues, in a pattern similar to that seen in the normal pancreatic samples.

The importance of TGF-β signaling in the formation of fibrosis is underlined by experiments in transgenic mice overexpressing TGF-β1 in the pancreas *(78)*. These animals develop accumulation of extracellular matrix in the pancreas that is histologically identical to chronic pancreatitis in humans. Therefore, upregulation of TGF-βs in the human pancreas seems to influence fibrogenesis, and might contribute indirectly to the ongoing destruction of the exocrine and endocrine parenchyma in humans.

CONCLUSIONS

This chapter has reported enhanced expression of a variety of growth factors and growth factor receptors in chronic pancreatitis *(39–41,45,61,70,76–78)*. These factors are produced in the remaining pancreatic acinar and ductal cells, as demonstrated by *in situ* hybridization and immunohistochemical staining. Immunohistochemistry showed that areas with a higher degree of pancreatic damage and areas with ductal metaplasia exhibited the strongest staining for these factors. These observations indicate that growth factors and growth factor receptors might influence the morphological changes that occur in chronic pancreatitis. Overexpression of many growth factors and growth factor receptors has also been reported previously in the literature on pancreatic cancer *(28,32,37,38,41,42,45,56,60,70)*, which leads to two crucial questions: Is chronic pancreatitis a risk disease for pancreatic cancer; and does pancreatic cancer develop from chronic pancreatitis lesions in the pancreas? Presently these important questions cannot be answered. However, there is clinical evidence that patients with chronic pancreatitis have a significantly higher risk of developing pancreatic cancer, which supports the hypothesis that pancreatic cancer might develop from chronic pancreatitis lesions in some patients *(80)*. In general, the fold increase of RNA expression of growth factors and growth factor receptors in chronic pancreatitis samples is lower than in pancreatic cancer samples, compared with normal controls. Therefore, quantitative differences in the expression levels of these factors seem to exist between cancer and chronic inflammation in the pancreas. However, it is not known if these differences in expression are of biologically great enough significance for the behavior of pancreatic cells to change their phenotype and to undergo malignant transformation.

The exact function of growth factors and growth factor receptors in chronic pancreatitis remains controversial. The concomitant overexpression of EGF-receptor and its ligand TGF-α suggests that TGF-α may excessively activate the EGF-receptor through autocrine/paracrine mechanisms *(39)*. In this way TGF-α may enhance ductal proliferation, modulate acinar cell functions, increase collagen production, and exert chemotactic effects on fibroblasts. This hypothesis is strongly supported by recent studies in transgenic mice overexpressing TGF-α in the pancreas *(20)*. These animals develop morphological pancreatic damage that is comparable to human chronic pancreatitis, except that no signs of inflammation are present. In addition to overexpressing members of the EGF-receptor family and the EGF family, many chronic pancreatitis samples exhibit increased aFGF and bFGF mRNA expression and protein levels *(61)*. aFGF and bFGF can also stimulate fibroblast proliferation and collagen synthesis, which might contribute to scarring in the pancreas *(46–51,79)*. Similar effects can be proposed for TGF-βs, which are enhanced in many chronic pancreatitis samples *(76,77)*. TGF-βs are strong inducers of fibrosis by stimulating collagen synthesis, and by inhibiting collagenases *(63,65–68,81)*. In other diseases associated with fibrosis, such as lung fibrosis, liver cirrhosis, and glomerulonephritis, the central role of TGF-βs in extracellular matrix production is well established. An area of great interest for future investigation is the expression pattern of growth factors and growth factor receptors in different stages of chronic pancreatitis. Our studies describe changes in these factors in advanced stages of chronic pancreatitis, when there have already been a number of severe complications that require surgical resection. However, studying chronic pancreatitis lesions in an early stage of chronic pancreatitis is normally not possible, because these patients do not require surgery. Thus, it is presently not possible to determine whether upregulation of growth factors and growth factor receptors has already begun to occur early on in the development of chronic pancreatitis.

Although many studies have focused in the past on the development of chronic pancreatitis, the pathophysiological mechanisms in chronic pancreatitis are mostly unknown *(12–19)*. Although it is believed that overconsumption of alcohol induces chronic pancreatitis, the initial cellular changes in acinar and ductal cells contributing to the disease have not been identified. It will be difficult to establish the sequential pathophysiological steps that occur in chronic pancreatitis, because, in addition to alcohol, there also seems to be a genetic predisposition that strongly influences the onset of the disease. Therefore, we have to focus on general pathways that are activated during the course of chronic pancreatitis. Upregulation of growth factors and growth factor receptors, which stimulate fibrogenesis, occurs in pancreatic acinar and ductal cells itself *(39,40,42,45,61,70,76–78)*. Future pathophysiological concepts of chronic pancreatitis may also have to consider alteration of growth factors and growth factor receptors as one important aspect in the pathophysiological process of chronic pancreatitis that might influence the morphological and clinical course of the disease.

REFERENCES

1. Sarles H, Bernard JP, Johnson C, and Chir M. Pathogenesis and epidemiology of chronic pancreatitis. Annu Rev Med 1989; *40:*453–468.
2. DiMagno EP, Layer P, and Clain JE. Chronic pancreatitis. In: Go VLW, DiMagno EP, Gardner JD, Lebenthal E, Reber HA, and Scheele GA, The exocrine pancreas: biology, pathobiology, and diseases. Raven, New York, 1993; pp. 665–706.
3. DiMagno EP. A short, elective history of exocrine pancreatic insufficiency and chronic pancreatitis. Gastroenterology 1993; *104:*1255–1262.
4. Friess H, Müller M, Ebert M, and Büchler MW. Chronic pancreatitis with inflammatory enlargement of the pancreatic head. Zentralblatt für Chirurgie 1995; *120:*292–297.
5. Bockman DE. Surgical anatomy of the pancreas and adjacent structures. In: Beger HG, Büchler M, and Malfertheiner P (eds), Standards in pancreatic surgery. Springer, Heidelberg–New York, 1993; pp. 1–9.
6. Oertel JE, Heffess CS, and Oertel YC. Pancreas. In: Sternberg SS (ed), Diagnostic surgical pathology, Raven, New York, 1989; pp. 1057–1093.
7. Di Magno EP, Layer P, and Clain JE. Chronic pancreatitis. In: Go VLW, Di Mango EP, Gardner JD, Lebenthal E, Reber HA, and Scheele GA (eds), The pancreas. Raven, New York, pp. 707–740.
8. Di Magno EP. Conservative management of chronic pancreatitis. In: Beger HG, Büchler M, Malfertheiner P (eds), Standards in pancreatic surgery. Springer, Heidelberg–New York, 1993; pp. 325–331.
9. Bockman DE, Büchler M, Malfertheiner P, and Beger HG. Analysis of nerves in chronic pancreatitis. Gastroenterology 1988; *94:*1459–1469.
10. Büchler M, Weihe E, Friess H, Malfertheiner P, Bockman E, Müller S, Nohr D, and Beger HG. Changes in peptidergic innervation in chronic pancreatitis. Pancreas 1992; *7:*183–192.
11. Weihe E, Nohr D, Müller S, Büchler M, Friess H, and Zentel HJ. The tachykinin neuroimmune connection in inflammatory pain. Ann NY Acad Sci 1991; *632:*283–295.

12. Sarles H, Dagorn JC, Giorgi D, and Bernard JP. Remaining pancreatic stone protein as "lithostatine". Gastroenterology 1990; *99:*900–905.
13. Klöppel G and Maillet B. Pseudocysts in chronic pancreatitis: a morphological analysis of 57 resection specimens and 9 autopsy pancreata. Pancreas 1991; *6:*266–274.
14. Noronha, M, Bordalo O, Dreiling DA. Alcohol and the pancreas. II. Pancreatic morphology of advanced alcoholic pancreatitis. Am J Gastroenterol 1981; *76:*120–124.
15. Braganza JM. Pancreatic disease: a casualty of hepatic "detoxification"? Lancet ii 1983; *8357:*1000–1003.
16. DiMagno EP. A short, eclectic history of exocrine pancreatic insufficiency and chronic pancreatitis. Gastroenterology 1993; *104:*1255–1262.
17. Di Sebastiano P, Fink Th, Weihe E, Friess H, Innocenti P, Beger HG, and Büchler MW. Immune cell infiltration and growth-associated protein-43 expression correlate with pain in chronic pancreatitis. Gastroenterology 1997; *112:*1648–1655.
18. Hunger R, Müller Ch, Zgraggen K, Friess H, and Büchler MW. Cytotoxic cells are activated in cellular infiltrates of alcoholic chronic pancreatitis. Gastroenterology 1997; *112:*1656–1663.
19. Friess H, Cantero H, Graber H, Tang WH, Guo XZ, Kashiwagi M, et al. Enhanced urokinase plasminogen activation in chronic pancreatitis suggests a role in its pathogenesis. Gastroenterology 1997; *113:*904–913.
20. Bockman DE and Merlino G. Cytological changes in the pancreas of transgenic mice overexpressing transforming growth factor. Gastroenterology 1992; *103:*1883–1892.
21. Ullrich A and Schlessinger J. Signal transduction by receptors with tyrosine kinase activity. Cell 1990; *61:*203–212.
22. Schlessinger J and Ullrich A. Growth factor signaling by receptor tyrosine kinases. Neuron 1992; *9:*383–391.
23. Yarden Y and Ullrich A. Molecular analysis of signal transduction by growth factors. Biochemistry 1988; *27:*3113–3119.
24. Coussens L, Yank-Feng TL, Liao YC, Chen E, Gray A, McGrath J, et al. Tyrosine kinase receptor with extensive homology to EGF receptor shares chromosomal location with neu oncogene. Science 1985; *230:*1132–1139.
25. Di Fiore PP, Pierce JH, Kraus MH, Segatto O, King CR, and Aaronson SA. erbB-2 is a potent oncogene when overexpressed in NIH/3T3 cells. Science 1987; *237:*178–182.
26. Kraus MH, Issing W, Miki T, Popescu NC, and Aaronson SA. Isolation and characterization of ERBB3, a third member of the ERBB/epidermal growth factor receptor family: evidence for overexpression in a subset of human mammary tumors. Proc Nat Acad Sci USA 1989; *86:*9193–9197.
27. Plowman GD, Green JM, McDonald VL, Neubauer MG, Disteche CM, Todaro GJ, and Shoyab M. The amphiregulin gene encodes a novel epidermal growth factor-related protein with tumor-inhibitory activity. Mol Cell Biol 1981; *10:*1969–1981.
28. Barton CM, Hall PA, Hughes CM, Gullick WJ, and Lemoine NR. Transforming growth factor alpha and epidermal growth factor in human pancreatic cancer. J Pathol 1991; *163:*111–116.
29. Ciccodicola A, Dono R, Obici S, Simeone A, Zollo M, and Persico MG. Molecular characterization of a gene of the 'EGF family' expressed in undifferentiated human NTERA2 teratocarcinoma cells. EMBO J 1989; *8:*1987–1991.
30. Higashiyama S, Abraham JA, Miller J, Fiddes JC, and Klagsbrun M. A heparin-binding growth factor secreted by macrophage-like cells that is related to EGF. Science 1991; *251:*936–939.
31. Plowman GD, Culouscou JM, Whitney GS, Green JM, Carlton GW, Foy L, Neubauer MG, and Shoyab M. Ligand specific activation of HER4/p180erbB4, a fourth member of the epidermal growth factor receptor family. Proc Nat Acad Sci USA 1993; *90:*1746–1750.

32. Prigent SA and Lemoine NR. The type 1 (EGFR-related) family of growth factor receptors and their ligands. Prog Growth Factor Res 1992; *4:*1–24.

33. Dautry-Varsat A and Lodish HF. How receptors bring proteins and particles into cells. Sci Am 1984; *250:*52–58.

34. Carpenter G and Cohen S. ^{125}I-labeled human epidermal growth factor: binding, internalization, and degradation in human fibroblasts. J Cell Biol 1976; *71:*159–163.

35. Carpenter G. Epidermal growth factor is a major factor-promoting agent in human milk. Science 1980; *210:*198–199.

36. Tsutsumi O, Kurachi H, and Oka T. A physiological role of epidermal growth factor in male reproductive function. Science 1986; *233:*975–977.

37. Korc M, Chandrasekar B, Yamanaka Y, Friess H, Büchler M, and Beger HG. Overexpression of the epidermal growth factor receptor in human pancreatic cancer is associated with concomitant increases in the levels of epidermal growth factor and transforming growth factor alpha. J Clin Invest 1992; *90:*1352–1360.

38. Yamanaka Y, Friess H, Kobrin MS, Büchler M, Beger HG, and Korc M. Coexpression of epidermal growth factor receptor and ligands in human pancreatic cancer is associated with enhanced tumor aggressiveness. Anticancer Res 1993; *13:*565–570.

39. Korc M, Friess H, Yamanaka Y, Kobrin M, Büchler MW, and Beger HG. Chronic pancreatitis is associated with increased concentrations of epidermal growth factor receptor, transforming growth factor alpha and phospholipase C gamma. Gut 1994; *35:*1468–1473.

40. Friess H, Yamanaka Y, Büchler MW, Hammer K, Kobrin M, and Beger HG. A subgroup of patients with chronic pancreatitis overexpress the c-erbB-2 protooncogene. Ann Surg 1994; *220:*183–192.

41. Yamanaka Y, Friess H, Kobrin MS, Büchler M, Kunz J, Beger HG, and Korc M. Overexpression of HER2/neu oncogene in human pancreatic cancer. Hum Pathol 1993; *24:*1127–1134.

42. Friess H, Yamanaka Y, Kobrin SM, Do DA, Büchler MW, and Korc M. Enhanced erbB-3 expression in human pancreatic cancer correlates with tumor progression. Clin Cancer Res 1995; *1:*1413–1420.

43. Ciardiello F, Dono R, Kim N, Persico MG, and Salomon DS. Expression of cripto, a novel gene of the epidermal growth factor gene family, leads to in vitro transformation of a normal mouse mammary epithelial cell line. Cancer Res 1991; *51:*1051–1054.

44. Baldassarre G, Bianco C, Tórtora G, Ruggiero A, Moasser M, Dmitrovsky E, Bianco AR, and Ciardiello F. Transfection with a cripto anti-sense plasmid suppresses endogenous CRIPTO expression and inhibits transformation in a human embryonal carcinoma cell line. Int J Cancer 1996; *66:*538–543.

45. Friess H, Yamanaka Y, Büchler M, Kobrin MS, Tahara E, and Korc M. Cripto, a member of the epidermal growth factor family, is overexpressed in human pancreatic cancer and chronic pancreatitis. Int J Cancer 1994; *56:*668–674.

46. Burgess WH and Maciag T. The heparin-binding (fibroblast) growth factor family of proteins. Ann Rev Biochem 1989; *58:*575–606.

47. Damon DH, Lobb RR, D'Amore PA, and Wagner JA. Heparin potentiates the action of acidic fibroblast growth factor by prolonging its biological half-life. J Cell Physiol 1989; *138:*221–226.

48. Folkman J and Klagsbrun M. Angiogenic factors. Science 1987; *235:*442–447.

49. Gospoderowicz D, Neufeld G, and Schweigerer L. Molecular and biological characterization of fibroblast growth factor, an angiogenic factor which also controls the proliferation and differentiation of mesoderm and neuroectoderm derived cells. Cell Differ 1986; *19:*1–17.

50. Gospoderowicz D, Ferrara N, Schweigerer L, and Neufeld G. Structural characterization and biological functions of fibroblast growth factor. Endocr Rev 1987; *8:*95–114.

51. Klagsbrun M. The fibroblast growth factor family: structural and biological properties. Prog Growth Factor Res 1989; *1:*207–235.
52. Givol D and Yardon A. Complexity of FGF receptors: genetic basis for structural diversity and functional specificity. FASEB J 1992; *6:*3362–3369.
53. Moscatelli D, Presta M, and Rifkin DB. Purification of a factor from human placenta that stimulates capillary endothelial cell protease production, DNA synthesis and migration. Proc Nat Acad Sci 1986; *83:*2091–2095.
54. Saksela O, Moscatelli D, and Rifkin DB. The opposing effects of basic fibroblast growth factor and transforming growth factor-β on the regulation of plasminogen activator activity in capillary endothelial cells. J Cell Biol 1987; *105:*957–963.
55. Courty J, Loret C, Chevallier B, Moenner M, and Barritault D. Biochemical comparative studies between eye and brain derived growth factors. Biochemie 1987; *69:*511–516.
56. Kobrin MS, Yamanaka Y, Friess H, Lopez ME, and Korc M. Aberrant expression of the type I fibroblast growth factor receptor in human pancreatic adenocarcinomas. Cancer Res 1993; *53:*4741–4744.
57. Mori H, Maki M, Oishi K, Jaye M, Igarashi K, Yoshida O, and Hatanaku M. Increased expression of genes for basic fibroblast growth factor and transforming growth factor type 2 in human benign prostatic hyperplasia. Prostate 1990; *16:*71–80.
58. Schulze-Osthoff K, Risau W, Vollmer E, and Sorg C. *In situ* detection of basic fibroblast growth factor by highly specific antibodies. Am J Pathol 1990; *137:*85–92.
59. Friess H, Kobrin MS, and Korc M. Acidic and basic fibroblast growth factors and their receptors are expressed in the human pancreas. Pancreas 1992; *7:*737.
60. Yamanaka Y, Friess H, Büchler M, Beger HG, Uchida E, Onda M, Kobrin MS, and Korc M. Overexpression of acidic and basic fibroblast growth factors in human pancreatic cancer correlates with advanced tumor stage. Cancer Res 1993; *53:*5289–5296.
61. Friess H, Yamanaka Y, Büchler M, Beger HG, Do DA, Kobrin MS, and Korc M. Increased expression of acidic and basic fibroblast growth factors in chronic pancreatitis. Am J Pathol 1994; *144:*117–128.
62. Yingling JM, Wang XF, and Bassing CH. Signaling by the transforming growth factor-beta receptors. Biochim Biophys Acta 1995; *1242:*115–136.
63. Massague J. The transforming growth factor-beta family. Rev Cell Biol 1990; *6:*597–641.
64. Hebda PA. Stimulatory effects of transforming growth factor-beta and epidermal growth factor on epidermal cell outgrowth from porcine skin explant cultures. J Invest Dermatol 1988; *91:*440–445.
65. Massague J, Cheifetz S, Laiho M, Ralph DA, Weiss FMB, and Zentella A. Transforming growth factor-beta. Cancer Surveys 1992; *12:*81–103.
66. Roberts AB, Sporn MG, Assoian RK, Smith JM, and Roche NS. Transforming growth factor type-b: rapid induction of fibrosis and angiogenesis *in vivo* and stimulation of collagen formation *in vitro*. Proc Nat Acad Sci USA 1986; *83:*4167–4171.
67. Sporn MB and Roberts AB. Transforming growth factor-beta: recent progress and new challenges. J Cell Biol 1992; *119:*1017–1021.
68. Roberts AB and Sporn MB. Physiological actions and clinical applications of transforming growth factor-beta. Growth Factors 1993; *8:*1–9.
69. Roberts AB and Sporn MB. The transforming growth factor-beta. In: Sporn MB and Roberts AB (eds), Peptide growth factors and their receptors, vol. 95 of Handbook of experimental pharmacology. Springer-Verlag, New York, 1990; pp. 419–472.
70. Friess H, Yamanaka Y, Büchler M, Beger HG, Kobrin MS, Baldwin RL, and Korc M. Enhanced expression of the type II transforming growth factor-beta receptor in human pancreatic cancer cells without alteration of type III receptor expression. Cancer Res 1993; *53:*2704–2707.

71. Lin HY, Wang X-F, Ng-Eaton E, Weinberg RA, and Lodish HF. Expression cloning of the TGF-β type II receptor, a functional transmembrane serine/threonine kinase. Cell 1992; *68:*775–785.

72. Lopez-Casillas F, Cheifetz S, Doody J, Andres JL, Lane WS, and Massague J. Structure and expression of the membrane proteoglycan betaglycan, a component of the TGF-β receptor system. Cell 1991; *67:*785–795.

73. Wrana JL, Attisano L, Carcamo J, Zentella A, Doody J, Laiho M, Wang X-F, and Massague J. TGF-β signals through a heteromeric protein kinase receptor complex. Cell 1992; *71:*1003–1014.

74. Lopez-Casillas F, Wrana JL, and Massague J. Betaglycan presents ligand to the TGF beta signaling receptor. Cell 1993; *73:*1435–1444.

75. Yamashita H, Ichijo H, Grimsby S, Moren A, ten Dijke P, and Miyazono K. Endoglin forms a heteromeric complex with the signaling receptors for transforming growth factor-beta. J Biol Chem 1994; *269:*1995–2001.

76. Slater SD, Williamson RCN, and Foster CS. Expression of transforming growth factor-beta 1 in chronic pancreatitis. Digestion 1995; *56:*237–241.

77. Van Laethem JL, Deviere J, Resibios A, Rickaert F, Vertongen P, Ohtani H, et al. Localization of transforming growth factor beta 1 and its latent binding protein in human chronic pancreatitis. Gastroenterology 1995; *108:*1873–1881.

78. Van Laethem JL, Robberecht P, Resibios A, and Deviere J. Transforming growth factor beta promotes development of fibrosis after repeated courses of acute pancreatitis in mice. Gastroenterology 1996; *110:*576–582.

79. Estival A, Louvel D, Couderc B, Prats H, Hollande E, Vaysse N, and Clemente F. Morphological and biological modifications induced in a rat pancreatic acinar cancer cell line (AR4 2J) by unscheduled expression of basic fibroblast growth factors. Cancer Res 1993; *53:*1182–1187.

80. Lowenfels AB, Maisonneuve P, Cavallini G, Ammann RW, Lankisch PG, Andersen JR, et al. Pancreatitis and the risk of pancreatic cancer. International Pancreatitis Study Group. N Engl J Med 1993; *328:*1433–1437.

81. Border WA and Noble NA. Transforming growth factor beta in tissue fibrosis. N Engl J Med 1994; *331:*1286–1292.

4

Clues from Experimental Models

Daniel S. Longnecker

INTRODUCTION

Selecting or creating an animal model of carcinoma of the pancreas is a complex process. One must ask what is being modeled. The reflex response is "ductal adenocarcinoma," because this is the most common histologic type of pancreatic cancer. However, a recently revised classification of neoplasms of the exocrine pancreas in humans lists 17 major types and 11 subtypes *(1)*. These are grouped into three categories according to clinical behavior (benign, borderline, and malignant). The complexity is reduced somewhat by the fact that several histologic phenotypes have benign or borderline and malignant counterparts that apparently represent sequential steps in the development of a fully malignant phenotype. For example, one group includes mucinous cystadenoma, mucinous cystic tumor with moderate dysplasia, and mucinous cystadenocarcinoma. In such cases, one might anticipate that a single animal model would cover the spectrum of several types of human tumors.

Adding to the complexity is the fact that a given histologic type of carcinoma in the human may be heterogeneous in regard to molecular changes in oncogenes and tumor suppressor genes. For example, most but not all ductal adenocarcinomas harbor mutation of the c-K-*ras* gene *(2)*. About half of ductal carcinomas have lost normal function of the *p53* gene.

Against this challenging background, one animal model stands out because of the variety of relevant histologic types of neoplasms that it provides. This model was developed in Syrian golden hamsters by treating with *N*-nitrosobis(2-oxopropyl)amine (BOP) or with several structurally related compounds *(3)*. The most common neoplasms induced by BOP are ductal adenocarcinomas of the pancreas, although cystic mucinous neoplasms and intraductal papillary neoplasms also occur *(4,5)*. This single animal model mimics at least seven of the major histologic types listed in the new WHO classification, as well as several of the subtypes of ductal adenocarcinoma, e.g., mucinous noncystic carcinoma and adenosquamous carcinoma.

Several different chemicals have induced acinar cell adenocarcinomas in rats. The best-characterized of these models involves treating Lewis rats with azaserine *(6)*. The

Table 1
Selected Chemically Induced Animal Models of Carcinoma of the Pancreas[a]

| Carcinogen | Tumor | | | |
	Acronym	Species	Phenotype[b]	Refs.
N-nitrosobis(2-oxopropyl) amine	BOP	Hamster	Ductal	3
N-nitroso(2-hydroxypropyl)(2-oxopropyl)amine	HPOP	Hamster	Ductal	3
		Rat	Acinar	48
N-nitrosobis(2-hydroxypropyl) amine	BHP	Hamster	Ductal	3
		Rat	Acinar	73
N-methyl-N-nitrosourea	MNU	Guinea pig	Ductal	74
		Hamster	Ductal	75
N^δ-(N-methyl-N-nitrosocarbamoyl)-L-ornithine	MNCO	Hamster	Ductal, acinar	49
		Rat	Acinar	50
4-(methylnitrosamino)-1-(3-pyridyl)-1-butanone	NNK	Hamster	Ductal, acinar	14
		Rat	Acinar, ductal	76,77
7,12-dimethylbenz(a)anthracene	DMBA	Rat	Ductal	46
N-ethyl-N-nitrosoguanidine	ENNG	Dog	Ductal	13

[a] The major emphasis is on models in which the pancreas is the primary or a prominent site of carcinoma development. A few other chemicals have induced similar lesions in the pancreas, but with a low incidence and/or a high background of carcinomas in other organs.

[b] The phenotype listed first is most common when both ductal and acinar phenotypes are listed.

majority of the induced pancreatic neoplasms are of acinar cell type, although several subtypes are described *(7)*.

The majority of experimental studies of chemical carcinogenesis in the pancreas have utilized the hamster and rat models mentioned above, but several other models have been reported (Table 1). Their major characteristics have been reviewed *(8,9)* and they are not repeated here in detail, although specific reference will be made to some of these models in later sections. In addition to the chemically induced models, several transgenic mouse models have been developed for both exocrine and endocrine pancreatic neoplasms *(9,10)*. Several of the transgenic models of exocrine carcinoma are listed in Table 2.

CARCINOGEN DISTRIBUTION AND METABOLISM

The problem of developing animal models for carcinogenesis and carcinoma in the pancreas was actively approached, using chemical carcinogens, nearly 25 yr ago, before transgenic mouse technology was developed. Experimental approaches were based on different rationales. The basic question was how to target exogenous carcinogens to the pancreas, and a secondary question was whether the pancreas contained enzymes needed for activation of indirect acting carcinogens. Since more carcinomas arise in the head of the pancreas than in the body and tail, some investigators proposed that reflux of duodenal contents into the pancreatic duct might provide the most relevant route of exposure to ingested carcinogens. Similarly, reflux of bile might expose pancreatic ductal cells to carcinogens or their metabolites that are excreted in the bile.

Several investigators addressed the issue of targeting the pancreas by directly implanting or instilling the carcinogen into the pancreas or its duct system *(11–13)*. Since

Table 2
Transgenic Mouse Models of Exocrine Pancreatic Carcinoma

Transgene	Tumor phenotype	Refs.
Ela-1-SV40TAg	Acinar, Islet	*39,40*
Ela-1-*myc*	Acinar ± ductal metaplasia	*33,41*
Ela-1-SV40T × Ela-1–TGFα crosses	Acinar	*45*
Ela-1-*myc* × Ela-1–TGFα crosses	High grade acinar	*45*

two of the agents used in this approach required metabolic activation, these studies provided indirect evidence that the pancreas contains the enzymes required for metabolism of the carcinogens. Direct instillation of *N*-ethyl-*N*-nitrosoguanidine into the main pancreatic duct provided a method for inducing dysplasia and carcinoma in ductal epithelium in the head of the pancreas *(13)*. However, none of the models involving direct application of the carcinogen to the pancreas seems to have general relevance to the carcinogenesis in humans, because of the artificial route of exposure.

The author employed the approach of targeting the pancreas by utilizing known mutagens (putative carcinogens), which included an intact α-amino-acid residue in the molecular structure. The pancreatic acinar cells are known to transport and to avidly concentrate amino acids. This rationale led to development of the azaserine model in rats, and is also the basis of the less efficient and less useful model using N^{δ}-(*N*-methyl-*N*-nitrosocarbamoyl)-L-ornithine as a carcinogen. These carcinogens were given by intraperitoneal injection in carcinogenesis studies, and apparently reached the pancreas largely by absorption and distribution through the blood.

The models induced by BOP or its metabolic derivatives resulted from the systematic evaluation of the carcinogenicity of a series of dialkyl nitrosamines. Although low-dose regimens of BOP are highly selective for the induction of carcinomas in the pancreas, the basis for this targeting is unknown. BOP and related carcinogens are commonly given by subcutaneous injection, and appear to reach the pancreas via the blood. These carcinogens require metabolism to their active form, providing further support for the ability of the pancreas to activate carcinogens.

The tobacco-derived nitrosamine, 4-(methylnitrosamino)-1-(3-pyridyl)-1-butanone (NNK), has been given to hamsters. When it is given to pregnant dams by subcutaneous injection or intratracheal instillation, carcinomas of the pancreas have developed in a significant fraction of the offspring *(14)*. This model provides further evidence for vascular distribution as well as for transplacental transfer of the carcinogen.

One of the major conclusions from studies in animal models is that several different classes of chemicals reach the pancreas by the vascular route following absorption. Both acinar and ductal cells are affected in various models. None of the models has provided evidence that distribution of the carcinogen involves reflux of duodenal content or bile; however, some studies have suggested the possibility that active metabolites formed in the liver may be transferred to the pancreas via the circulation *(15)*.

If we extrapolate these results to considerations of the etiology of pancreatic cancer in humans, we must conclude that the pancreas might be affected by carcinogens following absorption from the skin, gastrointestinal tract, or respiratory tract. The latter two routes might pertain for exposure to carcinogens in tobacco, and may be relevant to the increased risk of pancreatic cancer in cigarette smokers. The experimental studies with NNK support this notion.

MECHANISMS OF CARCINOGENESIS

As indicated in the preceding section, animal models have provided evidence that procarcinogens can be activated in the pancreas. A variety of short-term in vivo and in vitro studies provide further support for the capability of both acinar *(16)* and ductal cells *(17)* to metabolize carcinogens. As is the case in other tissues, activated carcinogens are mutagenic DNA-damaging agents that in some cases have been shown to form specific DNA adducts *(18,19)*. As is noted below, mutations appear to be induced in specific oncogenes, such as c-K-*ras*. Several of the same carcinogen-metabolizing enzymes that are active in the liver are involved, and are inducible in the pancreas *(16)*.

Most of the experimental carcinogens that affect the pancreas are nitrosamines. This raises the suspicion that nitrosamines that are formed endogenously in the stomach *(20)* might be absorbed and affect the pancreas. Although this hypothesis is not supported by direct experimental evidence in the pancreas, it has not been adequately evaluated.

A recent review provides a summary of carcinogen metabolism in the pancreas *(21)*. From these studies, we can conclude that the pancreas can be affected by either direct- or indirect-acting carcinogens, but that agents in the latter category are more likely to reach and target cells in the pancreas. Although some agents may be activated in other sites (probably the liver), and then affect the pancreas, there is no dependence on this pathway or proof that it is of major importance in humans. The inducibility of enzymes in the pancreas by exogenous chemicals provides a mechanism for modulation of the initial steps of carcinogenesis by diet or dietary supplements. Ethanol induces carcinogen-activating enzymes in the liver, and may do so in the pancreas. This possibility is supported by the studies of NNK carcinogenesis by Schüller et al. *(14)* in which the incidence of pancreatic neoplasms in the offspring was enhanced by pretreatment of the dams with ethanol.

PRECURSOR LESIONS

Comparison of focal proliferative lesions in the pancreata of carcinogen-treated animals with lesions that are found in the human pancreas provides an approach for evaluating the significance of the latter lesions. These may include either sporadic lesions in pancreata from patients without pancreatic disease, or lesions from patients with chronic pancreatitis or pancreatic carcinoma. Such comparisons can provide a means to examine specific hypotheses regarding the origin and significance of the lesions.

Recent studies in this lab provide an example. As part of an evaluation of the rate of mutation of the c-K-*ras* gene in a series of focal lesions from human pancreas, workers here have focused on three categories of focal epithelial lesions, which may be described as nonpapillary ductal hyperplasia (also called flat hyperplasia, mucous cell hypertrophy, or mucus cell hyperplasia), papillary ductal hyperplasia, and adenomatoid ductal hyperplasia (also called adenomatous hyperplasia). In searching for examples of such lesions, which can be microdissected for isolation of DNA, workers confronted the fact that these three lesions are commonly closely associated. Nonpapillary and papillary hyperplasia frequently occur adjacent to one another in the same duct or in separate ducts within the same pancreas, and either may be closely associated with adenomatoid hyperplasia. The latter lesion is virtually always found either in close proximity to ductal hyperplasia, or in a pancreas in which ductal hyperplasia can be found nearby. These observations suggest that these three patterns of ductal change are closely related in origin. This tentative conclusion is reinforced by published reports that the rate of c-K-*ras* mutation is similar in nonpapillary and papillary ductal hyperplasia *(22)*, and by new data from studies here that showed a similar rate of c-K-*ras* mutation in adenomatoid and nonpapillary ductal hyperplasia (unpublished). Although the coincidence of such lesions in the human has sometimes been acknowledged *(1,23)*, the hypothesis that they represent a biologic continuum has not been emphasized or supported.

A group of pancreata from 23 HPOP-treated hamsters, which were provided by Dimitri Kokkinakis, were also under review for the presence of intraductal hyperplasia and the development of lesions that might qualify for a diagnosis of intraductal papillary-mucinous tumor (adenoma or borderline) as described in the revised WHO classification *(1; see* Table 3). This provided the opportunity to look for the association of nonpapillary ductal hyperplasia, papillary ductal hyperplasia, and adenomatoid ductal hyperplasia in the animal model. Of the 23 pancreata, 14 exhibited ductal hyperplasia, and 12 of these had associated adenomatoid type changes in small ducts or lobular tissue near the hyperplastic ducts (Fig. 1–3). None of the 9 pancreata without ductal hyperplasia contained adenomatoid lesions. The Fisher exact test indicates a level of significance of <0.005 for the association of ductal and adenomatoid hyperplasia. This offers support from the animal model for the hypothesized relationship of adenomatoid and ductal hyperplasia in the human.

The pancreata from the HPOP-treated hamsters also contained dilated pancreatic ducts containing mucus in the lumen and lined by papillary-mucinous epithelium, which seemed analogous to the intraductal papillary-mucinous adenoma and more advanced intraductal papillary-mucinous tumors of humans. The pancreases also contained cystic tumors comparable to mucinous cystic tumors, and mucinous cystadenocarcinoma as described in humans. One mucinous cystadenocarcinoma (Fig. 4A) had invasive areas that appeared ductal (Fig. 4B) as it invaded at the edge of the main tumor, and mucinous as it extended into the acinar tissue (Fig. 4C). This spectrum of changes has been described in the human *(1)*. Thus, in addition to the more common pattern of ductal adenocarcinoma that is commonly associated with the hamster model, we feel that nitrosamine-treated hamster can also model intraductal papillary-mucinous tumors and mucinous cystic tumors.

ABNORMALITIES OF SPECIFIC GENES

In contrast to the number evaluated in human pancreatic carcinomas, relatively few proto-oncogenes and tumor suppressor genes have been evaluated in experimentally induced pancreatic carcinomas from animals. Nonetheless, some striking parallels between animal and human tumors have been documented. For example, a large fraction (75–90%) of human pancreatic carcinomas have been shown to harbor c-K-*ras* mutations in codon 12, and a few cancers have a mutation in codon 13 *(2)*. The carcinomas in the nitrosamine-induced hamster model consistently show codon 12 mutations *(5,24–27)*, and a single spontaneously arising hamster carcinoma was found to have a

Table 3
**Revised WHO Histological Classification of Epithelial Tumors
of the Exocrine Pancreas**

1.1	*Benign*
1.1.1	Serous cystadenoma
1.1.2	Mucinous cystadenoma
1.1.3	Intraductal papillary-mucinous adenoma
1.1.4	Mature teratoma
1.2	*Borderline (Uncertain Malignant Potential)*
1.2.1	Mucinous cystic tumor with moderate dysplasia
1.2.2	Intraductal papillary-mucinous tumor with moderate dysplasia
1.2.3	Solid-pseudopapillary tumor
1.3	*Malignant*
1.3.1	Severe ductal dysplasia—carcinoma *in situ*
1.3.2	Ductal adenocarcinoma
1.3.2.1	Mucinous noncystic carcinoma
1.3.2.2	Signet ring cell carcinoma
1.3.2.3	Adenosquamous carcinoma
1.3.2.4	Undifferentiated (anaplastic) carcinoma
1.3.2.5	Mixed ductal–endocrine carcinoma
1.3.3	Osteoclast-like giant cell tumor
1.3.4	Serous cystadenocarcinoma
1.3.5	Mucinous cystadenocarcinoma
1.3.5.1	Noninvasive
1.3.5.2	Invasive
1.3.6	Intraductal papillary-mucinous carcinoma
1.3.6.1	Noninvasive
1.3.6.2	Invasive (papillary-mucinous carcinoma)
1.3.7	Acinar cell carcinoma
1.3.7.1	Acinar cell cystadenocarcinoma
1.3.7.2	Mixed acinar–endocrine carcinoma
1.3.8	Pancreatoblastoma
1.3.9	Solid-pseudopapillary carcinoma
1.3.10	Miscellaneous carcinomas

Adapted with permission from ref. *1*.

codon 13 mutation *(25)*. There is evidence that c-K-*ras* mutation arises at an early stage of carcinogenesis in hamsters (histologically, ductal hyperplasia), and is present in a higher fraction of severely dysplastic and frankly malignant lesions *(28)*. Attempts to base a transgenic mouse model on overexpression of c-K-*ras* in the pancreas resulted in the development of anaplastic carcinomas in utero that were so rapidly growing that the mice died in utero or shortly after birth, and no line could be established *(29)*. Thus, c-K-*ras* mutation is closely associated with pancreatic carcinoma both in humans and in some animal models.

In contrast, only 1 of 33 human pancreatic acinar cell carcinomas examined is reported to have a c-K-*ras* mutation *(30)*. This observation matches reports that azaser-

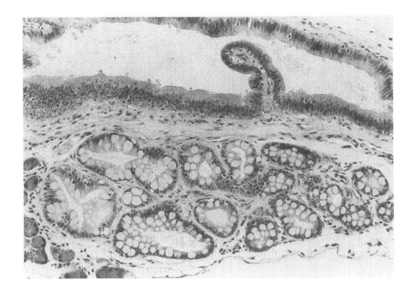

Fig. 1. Hyperplasia (mainly nonpapillary) in ductal epithelium (top) and adenomatoid hyperplasia in glands in an adjacent lobule (bottom) in a pancreas from a HPOP-treated hamster. Hematoxylin and eosin.

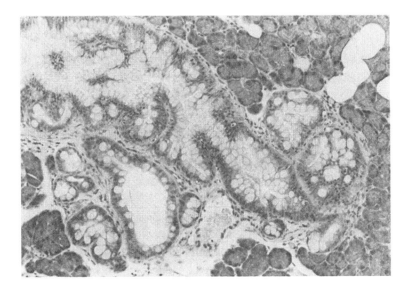

Fig. 2. Papillary hyperplasia (upper left, center) in a duct extending into adjacent glands or small ducts (lower left, right) from the pancreas of a HPOP-treated hamster. Hematoxylin and eosin.

ine-induced carcinomas in rats *(31,32)* and transgenic mouse acinar cell carcinomas *(33,34)* lack the c-K-*ras* mutation.

Hamster-model carcinomas have lacked evidence of p53 mutation in primary carcinomas *(27,35,36)*, although mutations were identified in cell lines or transplantable carcinomas. This stands in contrast to the report of the presence of such mutations in about

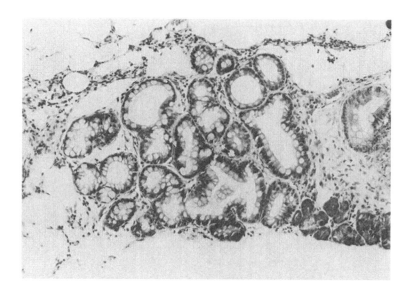

Fig. 3. Focus of adenomatoid ductal hyperplasia lying adjacent to a duct with papillary hyperplasia (out of the field to the right) from the pancreas of a HPOP-treated hamster. Hematoxylin and eosin.

50% of human pancreatic carcinomas, based on a composite figure derived from multiple studies *(37)*. One explanation could be that the hamster carcinomas harvested in vivo have been at an early stage of progression compared to most human carcinomas; an alternate explanation is that other tumor-suppressor genes are involved in the hamster. The latter view finds some support *(27)*.

The transgenic mouse models of pancreatic carcinoma, based on the elastase-1 promoter and the SV40 large T-antigen gene, can be regarded as a surrogate model for *p53* mutation. The elastase-1 promoter directs expression to islet and acinar cells at a young age, and exclusively to acinar cells in older animals *(38)*. Several lines based on this gene construct yield a high incidence of acinar cell carcinomas *(39,40)*, even though studies of human acinar cell carcinomas have failed to yield proof of mutation in the *p53* gene.

The elastase-1-*myc* transgenic mouse model yields acinar cell carcinomas with a high incidence of ductal metaplasia *(41)*. This model documents the power of *myc* overexpression to drive carcinogenesis in the pancreas, but it is unknown how frequently *myc* is overexpressed in human carcinomas. The carcinomas arising in the Ela-1-*myc* model have lacked c-K-*ras* mutation *(33)* which is of note because of the high incidence of ductal metaplasia.

Expression of TGF-α and overexpression of the EGF-receptor are documented in human pancreatic carcinomas and in BOP-induced hamster carcinomas *(42)*, but were absent in the azaserine-induced carcinomas in the rat *(43)*. The observation in human neoplasms provided part of the motivation for creation of a transgenic mouse model based on an elastase-1–TGF-α construct *(44)*. The resulting phenotype showed fibrosis with ductular complexes, but not carcinomas in the pancreas. The histologic appearance mimicked changes of chronic pancreatitis. However, when double transgenic mice were cre-

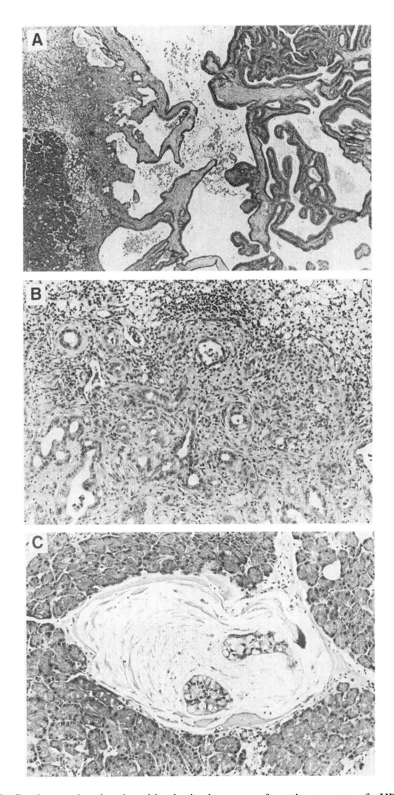

Fig. 4. Carcinoma showing three histologic phenotypes from the pancreas of a HPOP-treated hamster. **(A)** The main mass was a mucinous cystadenocarcinoma. **(B)** Invasion of fat at the margin of the cystadenocarcinoma shows the pattern of scirrhous ductal adenocarcinoma. **(C)** Invasion of adjacent acinar tissue shows noncystic mucinous pattern. Hematoxylin and eosin.

ated by crossing Ela-1–TGF-α mice with Ela-1-*myc* mice, there was a high yield of acinar cell carcinomas *(45)*.

Thus, the animal models offer direct or indirect support for the importance of mutant c-K-*ras*, *myc* overexpression, TGF-α overexpression, and EGF-receptor overexpression in the genesis or progression of pancreatic ductal carcinomas. Heterogeneity at the molecular level correlates with the tumor phenotypes in the case of c-K-*ras* mutation, which are characteristically present in ductal carcinomas in both humans and hamster models, and absent in acinar cell carcinomas in both humans and rat and mouse models.

NEOPLASTIC PHENOTYPES

Because multiple phenotypes of pancreatic neoplasms are found in humans and the spectrum of tumors encountered in individual animal models is narrower, modeling the complete spectrum of human neoplasms requires more than one animal model.

The human tumors can be grouped according to presumed cellular origin, as indicated in Table 3 *(1)*. The tumors of duct cell phenotype are largely modeled by the BOP-induced tumors in hamsters. This includes mucinous cystic tumors ranging from benign to malignant, intraductal papillary-mucinous tumors ranging from benign to malignant, ductal carcinoma *in situ*, ductal adenocarcinomas and most of its variants, such as adenosquamous carcinoma, and mucinous noncystic carcinoma. Some tumors are quite anaplastic, and many of them include minor populations of endocrine cells.

Both solid and cystic acinar cell adenocarcinomas are modeled by azaserine-induced neoplasms in rats and transgenic mouse models that employ the elastase-1 promoter. Both rat and mouse models have yielded tumor cell populations with ductal phenotype arising in acinar cell carcinomas. This observation, together with the observation of Bockman et al. *(46)* that the origin of DMBA-induced ductlike tumors is from acinar cells that have undergone ductal metaplasia raises the question as to whether some human carcinomas of ductal phenotype might have arisen from metaplastic acinar cells. Since animal and most human acinar cell carcinomas lack mutation of the c-K-*ras* gene, we have hypothesized that some of the human carcinomas of ductal phenotype that lack this mutation might be of acinar cell origin *(37)*. The rat and mouse models document that this occurs in animals.

Animal models have not yet provided examples of several rare types of pancreatic neoplasms, such as pancreatoblastoma, solid-pseudopapillary tumors, serous cystadenoma, and osteoblastic type giant cell tumors. The first two of these are likely to be of stem-cell origin, and might require the treatment of pregnant dams by chemicals to achieve a model. Alternately, a well-calculated transgenic construct might yield such a model. The elastase-1 promoter is expressed in both acinar and islet cells *(38)*. Very primitive neuroendocrine cells proliferate at the periphery of islets in young mice of the Bri-18 transgenic strain *(39)*. In older mice of this strain, one finds both insulinomas and a few somatostatinomas, as well as acinar cell tumors. Sandgren has noted the early proliferation of islet-associated cells in the Ela-1-*myc* transgenic model, although the ultimate tumor type arising from such early lesions appears to be exocrine *(41)*. This is the model that yields mixed acinar and ductal neoplasms, so it is quite possible that this model approaches the production of carcinomas of stem-cell origin, although the mouse tumors lack characteristic elements of human pancreatoblastoma.

Pour *(47)* has emphasized the role of islet-associated cells in the genesis of some of the carcinomas that arise in the BOP-hamster model. The origin of carcinomas from primitive, pluripotent cells provides an attractive explanation for the presence of both endocrine and exocrine cells in many human pancreatic adenocarcinomas that are predominantly of ductal phenotype.

SPECIES DIFFERENCES

One of the unanticipated findings in studies of pancreatic carcinoma in animals is the striking difference among species in response to chemical carcinogens. The cellular type of the tumor consistently differs in hamsters and rats in response to some of the same carcinogens (Table 1). Two examples serve to support this point. HPOP induces a spectrum of ductal tumors in hamsters that are similar to those induced by BOP. Although BOP has not been an effective carcinogen in rats, administration of HPOP to 2-wk-old rats induced acinar cell nodules, adenomas, and carcinomas that are generally similar to those induced by azaserine *(48)*. A second, similar example is provided by N^δ-(*N*-methyl-*N*-nitrosocarbamoyl)-L-ornithine, which induced ductal neoplasms in hamster *(49)* and acinar cell carcinomas in rats *(50)*. In general, it seems clear that acinar cells respond in rats, and that ductal cells are targeted in hamsters, although rare acinar cell carcinomas are found in carcinogen-treated hamsters. When ductlike tumors have occurred in rats *(11)*, the investigators concluded that they arose from metaplastic acinar cells *(46)*. Knowledge of response in other species is less complete, but it appears that mice respond similarly to rats.

The net result of these species differences is that there are separate models for carcinomas of ductal origin (hamster) and carcinomas of acinar cell origin (rat and mouse). Although they are rare, spontaneous carcinomas in hamster are ductal and in rats are acinar, so the models appear to be true to nature in each species. This implies that genetically based biologic factors strongly influence the response to carcinogenic stimuli. In general, the human pancreas appears to respond more like the hamster than like the rat, but, within the heterogeneity of humankind, we should anticipate considerable genetically influenced difference in the response to carcinogens. This may provide an explanation for the multiple histologic types of pancreatic cancer that are found in humans, and for racial differences in the phenotype of neoplasms that have been hypothesized *(51)*.

MODULATION BY DIET

A variety of diets have been shown to inhibit or promote the development of carcinomas in carcinogen-treated animals. Several examples will be cited, and other examples will be found in primary reports and prior reviews *(9,52)*.

The incidence of carcinomas in rats and mice fed standard laboratory chow diets is lower than that found in animals fed defined diets composed of purified ingredients, such as the AIN-76A formulation of the American Institute of Nutrition. While the mechanism of this "chow effect" is not defined, one common interpretation is that one or more micronutrients found in the natural product-based diet inhibits carcinogenesis, since the macronutrient content (fat, protein, and carbohydrate) and vitamin content in the purified diet are made similar to those found in chow. This effect is observed in rat *(53)* and mouse models *(52)*, but was not found in the hamster *(54)*.

A second well-documented dietary effect is promotion of pancreatic carcinogenesis by increased dietary fat content. These studies are often done using the AIN-76A diet that contains 5% corn oil, and modifications of this diet in which the level of corn oil or another fat is raised to 20 or 25%. They have been conducted in hamster, rat, and mouse models in several different laboratories. Despite the numerous studies of the "high fat effect," the mechanism remains unknown. One element may be total caloric intake, which is likely to be higher when high-fat diets are consumed, since simple caloric restriction has been demonstrated to reduce the incidence of pancreatic carcinomas in rat *(53)*. Another mechanism that has been postulated is alteration of prostaglandin synthesis *(55)*.

Promotion of carcinogenesis in the pancreas is documented in rats fed diets containing trypsin inhibitors. The trypsin inhibitors that have been used include natural ingredients, such as raw soya flour, isolates of soybean trypsin inhibitor, and a synthetic inhibitor *(56)*. The mechanism involves feedback control of pancreatic secretion through release of cholecystokinin (CCK) from the duodenum. In addition to stimulating pancreatic secretion, CCK is a growth hormone for the pancreas and can induce hyperplasia. CCK secretion is stimulated by peptide-releasing factors from the pancreas or intestine *(57)*. Dietary trypsin inhibitor (TI) protects the releasing peptide from degradation in the duodenal lumen, allowing its sustained action and prolonged CCK release. Carcinogen-induced nodules, and similar spontaneously arising foci of cells in the pancreas, overexpress CCK receptors *(58)*, and therefore presumably are stimulated to grow *(59)* and to progress to carcinomas. This effect may pertain primarily in rats, since analogous studies in the hamster model have yielded conflicting results *(9)*.

These and other well-documented dietary effects on pancreatic carcinogenesis in animals suggest that dietary content will influence pancreatic carcinogenesis in the human. Geographic and national differences in the incidence of pancreatic carcinoma may at least in part reflect dietary influences, and it seems likely that individual risk is influenced by diet. General dietary recommendations derived from these studies so far seem largely to match general recommendations based on experimental observations in other organ sites and epidemiologic studies in humans, i.e., to reduce dietary fat content, and to increase intake of natural products (fruits, vegetables, grains). In view of the demonstrated anticarcinogenic effects of certain trypsin inhibitors in experimental carcinogenesis models *(60)*, and the possible species specificity of the TI effect in rats, it is contraindicated to recommend avoidance of dietary TI in humans.

DIETARY ADDITIVES

A variety of dietary additives have been evaluated for activity in reducing the incidence of carcinomas in the animal models. Most additives have been evaluated in the BOP-hamster model, or the azaserine-rat model. A few additives have had a significant effect, e.g., certain synthetic retinoids *(61)*. Since most of these are published older studies, they are not reviewed here in detail (*see* reviews in ref. 8). They seem to document that there is some potential for specific dietary additives to inhibit the formation of cancers. A recent study in the BOP-treated hamster model of an agent, oltipraz, which induces phase II drug-metabolizing enzymes in the liver, provided evidence of inhibition of the development of carcinomas in the pancreas *(62)*. Results of a recent study on the effect of antioxidant micronutrients in the hamster model failed to show significant inhibition of carcinogenesis *(63)*. This suggests that natural inhibitors contained in diets that are high in vegetables and grains provide the level of protection that is available by making defined additions to purified diets. Thus, studies in the animal models do not yet provide a strong basis for recommendations beyond the general dietary guidelines noted above, but provide some hope that new dietary additives might be chemopreventive in the pancreas.

HORMONES

A variety of hormones have been shown to affect the rate of formation of carcinomas in animal models, or to alter the rate of growth of carcinoma-derived cell lines in culture *(9,64)*. Inconsistencies of effect are noted in different species, and the changes have not been explored equally in all models. There is sufficient information to support the contention that the development or growth of some tumors is influenced by hormones *(65,66)*, and to suggest that the response of individual tumors is likely to be heterogeneous. A variety of somatostatin analogs and receptor blockers for several trophic hormones have inhibited the growth of transplanted or primary or BOP-induced pancreatic carcinomas in animal models *(67)*. Promising results from the hamster model *(68)* have been evaluated in human cell lines *(69)*. Hormones that have been implicated by such studies include CCK, bombesin, gastrin, somatostatin, estrogen, and testosterone.

The promoting effect of feeding trypsin inhibitors to carcinogen-treated rats, discussed above, was presumed and subsequently documented to reflect the effect of CCK, a growth factor for acinar cells, in stimulating growth of the preneoplastic acinar cell lesions *(70)*. We noted that the carcinogen-induced foci responded more vigorously than normal pancreas in such studies *(71)*. This led to the hypothesis, now supported by several studies, that the acinar cell foci and nodules overexpress a CCK receptor *(58)*. Extension of this line of study has shown that the CCK-A receptor is overexpressed early during carcinogenesis in the azaserine rat model *(66)*, and that the CCK-B receptor can be overexpressed at a later stage in the carcinomas *(72)*. These studies pertain to tumors of acinar cell origin and they probably have limited relevance for the major fraction of human carcinomas that are of ductal phenotype. This view is supported by the inconsistency of findings in experimental studies of the effect of CCK and cerulein in the BOP-hamster model *(9)*.

To date, the outcomes of clinical trials based on hormonal manipulation have been disappointing. The failure to document clearly defined endocrine influences that can serve as the basis for hormonal therapy probably reflects the heterogeneity of human carcinomas. This problem may yield to approaches involving the recognition of specific molecular markers, e.g., receptor levels, that will predict the biologic response of individual neoplasms to clinical hormonal manipulations.

CONCLUDING COMMENTS

Three major needs stand out in the conquest of carcinoma of the pancreas at the public health and clinical level: approaches for prevention; the ability to diagnosis the cancers early when they are curable by surgery; and the need for effective adjuvant or systemic treatment for inoperable cases.

Animal models suggest that multiple factors are involved in the etiology of pancreatic cancer. Although the animal models demonstrate that a variety of chemical carcinogens can affect the pancreas, none of the specific agents identified can be implicated as one to which there is widespread exposure, with the exception of NNK. The models establish that the pancreas can be affected by carcinogens that reach it via the blood.

Dietary, chemopreventive, and hormonal factors have influenced carcinogenesis in the animal models. Some of these agents appear to have promoted the growth of spontaneously initiated foci, i.e., they have induced a low incidence of tumors in animals that were not exposed to a genotoxic carcinogen. The models provide an approach for further evaluation of both promoters and chemopreventive agents.

The hamster model, in particular, seems to be suitable for evaluation of several approaches to early diagnosis using biomarkers because of its morphologic and molecular similarities to human ductal adenocarcinomas. On the other hand, the small size of the animal precludes its use for realistic evaluation of imaging techniques that might be applied in the human. A dog model might better meet this need.

The hamster model is being used for evaluation of potential hormonal therapies. Because of the lack of a strong sex difference in the development of carcinomas in hamsters, there may be some question regarding the suitability of this model for evaluation of hormonal manipulations aimed at sex steroids or their receptors. On the other hand, the lack of a significant effect of CCK in this model suggests that it is closer to the human than rats models regarding the effect of CCK.

Several animal models in different species seem to be required to model the full spectrum of pancreatic malignancy in humans. This conclusion pertains to duplication of histologic types, as well as molecular changes and mechanisms of carcinogenesis. Evaluation of preventive and therapeutic agents seems also to require comparison of effects in several models.

ACKNOWLEDGMENT

All figures were prepared from histologic slides provided by Dimitri Kokkinakis.

REFERENCES

1. Klöppel G, Solcia E, Longnecker DS, Capella C, and Sobin, LH. Histologic typing of tumours of the exocrine pancreas. Springer-Verlag, New York, 1996.
2. Caldas C and Kern SE. K-*ras* mutation and pancreatic adenocarcinoma: state-of-the-art. Int J Pancreatol 1995; *18:*1–6.
3. Pour PM. Modification of tumor development in the pancreas. Prog Exp Tumor Res 1991; *33:*108–131.
4. Kokkinakis DM and Albores-Saavedra J. Orotic acid enhancement of preneoplastic and neoplastic lesions induced in the pancreas and liver of hamsters by N-nitroso(2-hydroxypropyl) (2-oxopropyl)amine. Cancer Res 1994; *54:*5324–5332.
5. Sugio K, Gazdar AF, Albores-Saavedra J, and Kokkinakis DM. High yields of K-ras mutations in intraductal papillary mucinous tumors and invasive adenocarcinomas induced by *N*-nitroso(2-hydroxypropyl)(2-oxopropyl)amine in the pancreas of female Syrian hamsters. Carcinogenesis 1996; *17:*303–309.
6. Longnecker DS. The azaserine-induced model of pancreatic carcinogenesis in rats. In: D. G. Scarpelli, J. K. Reddy and D. S. Longnecker (eds), Experimental pancreatic carcinogenesis, CRC, Boca Raton, FL, 1987; pp. 117–130.

7. Longnecker DS, Roebuck BD, Yager JD, Jr, Lilja HS, and Siegmund B. Pancreatic carcinoma in azaserine-treated rats: induction, classification and dietary modulation of incidence. Cancer 1981; *47:*1562–1572.

8. Longnecker DS. Experimental models of exocrine pancreatic tumors. In: Go VLW, Brooks FP, Di Magno EP, Gardner JD, Lebenthal E, and Scheele GA (eds), The exocrine pancreas: biology, pathobiology and diseases, Raven, New York, 1986; pp. 443–458.

9. Longnecker DS. Experimental models of exocrine pancreatic tumors. In: Go VLW, DiMagno EP, Gardner JD, Lebenthal E, Reber HA, and Scheele GA (eds), The exocrine pancreas: biology, pathobiology, and diseases, Raven, New York, 1993; pp. 551–564.

10. Longnecker DS. Experimental models of endocrine tumors of the pancreas. In: Mignon M, and Jensen RT (eds), Frontiers of gastrointestinal research, Karger, Basel, 1995; pp. 70–83.

11. Dissin J, Mills LR, Mains DL, Black O, and Webster PD. Experimental induction of pancreatic adenocarcinoma in rats. J Natl Cancer Inst 1975; *55:*857–864.

12. Corbett TH, Roberts BJ, Leopold WR, Peckham JC, Wilkoff LJ, Griswold DP, and Schabel FM, Jr, Induction and chemotherapeutic response of two transplantable ductal adenocarcinomas of the pancreas in C57BL/6 mice. Cancer Res 1984; *44:*714–726.

13. Kamano T, Tamura J, Uchida T, Kanno T, Sakakibara N, Tsutsumi M, Maruyama H, and Konishi Y. Studies by pancreatography of ductal changes induced by administration of pancreatic carcinogen in two dogs. Jpn J Clin Oncol 1991; *21:*282–286.

14. Schüller HM, Jorquera R, Reichert A, and Castonguay A. Transplacental induction of pancreas tumors in hamsters by ethanol and the tobacco-specific nitrosamine 4-(methylnitrosamino)-1-(3-pyridyl)-1-butanone. Cancer Res 1993; *53:*2498–2501.

15. Schaeffer BK, Wiebkin P, Longnecker DS, Coon CI, and Curphey TJ. DNA damage produced by *N*-nitrosomethyl(2-oxopropyl)amine (MOP) in hamsters and rat pancreas: a role for the liver. Carcinogenesis 1984; *5:*565–570.

16. Wiebkin P, Schaeffer BK, Longnecker DS, and Curphey TJ. Oxidative and conjugative metabolism of xenobiotics by isolated rat and hamster acinar cells. 1984; *12:*427–431.

17. Kokkinakis DM, Reddy MK, Norgle JR, and Baskaran K. Metabolism and activation of pancreas specific nitrosamines by pancreatic ductal cells in culture. Carcinogenesis 1993; *14:*1705–1709.

18. Kokkinakis DM and Subbarao V. The significance of DNA damage, its repair and cell proliferation during carcinogen treatment in the initiation of pancreatic cancer in the hamster model. Cancer Res 1993; *53:*2790–2795.

19. Zurlo J, Curphey TJ, and Longnecker DS. Identification of 7-carboxy-methylguanine in DNA from pancreatic acinar cells exposed to azaserine. Cancer Res 1982; *42:*1286–1288.

20. Konishi Y. Carcinogenic activity of endogenously synthesized N-nitrosobis(2-hydropropyl)amine in rats. IARC Sci Publ 1991; *105:*318–321.

21. Lawson T. and Kolar CH. Xenobiotic metabolism and toxic responses in pancreatic duct epithelial cells. In: Sirica AE and Longnecker DS (eds), Biliary and pancreatic ductal epithelia. Pathobiology and pathophysiology, Marcel Dekker, New York, 1997; pp. 443–455.

22. Yanagisawa A, Ohtake K, Ohashi K, Hori M, Kitagawa T, Sugano H, and Kato Y. Frequent c-Ki-ras oncogene activation in mucous cell hyperplasias of pancreas suffering from chronic inflammation. Cancer Res 1993; *53:*953–956.

23. Pour PM, Konishi Y, Klöppel G, and Longnecker DS (eds), Atlas of exocrine pancreatic tumors. Springer-Verlag, Tokyo, 1994.

24. Fujii H, Egami H, Pour P, and Pelling J. Pancreatic ductal adenocarcinomas induced in Syrian hamsters by *N*-nitrosobis(2-oxopropyl)amine contain a c-Ki-ras oncogene with a point-mutated codon 12. Mol Carc 1990; *3:*296–301.

25. Cerny WL, Mangold KA, and Scarpelli DG. Activation of K-ras during N-nitrosobis(2-oxopropyl)amine induced pancreatic carcinogenesis. Proc Am Assoc Cancer Res 1991; *32:*138.

26. Ushijima T, Tsutsumi M, Sakai R, Ishizaka Y, Takaku F, Konishi Y, et al. Ki-ras activation in pancreatic carcinomas of Syrian hamsters induced by *N*-nitrosobis(2-hydroxypropyl)amine. Jpn J Cancer Res 1991; *82:*965–968.

27. Chang KW, Laconi S, Mangold KA, Hubchak S, and Scarpelli DG. Multiple genetic alterations in hamster pancreatic ductal adenocarcinomas. Cancer Res 1995; *55:*2560–2568.

28. Tsutsumi M, Kondoh S, Noguchi O, Horiguchi K, Kobayashi E, Okita S, et al. K-ras gene mutation in early ductal lesions induced in a rapid production model for pancreatic carcinomas in Syrian hamsters. Jpn J Cancer Res 1993; *84:*1101–1105.

29. Ornitz DM, Hammer RE, Messing A, Palmiter RD, and Brinster RL. Pancreatic neoplasia induced by SV40 T antigen expression in acinar cells of transgenic mice. Science 1987; *238:*188–193.

30. Terhune PG, Heffess C, and Longnecker DS. Human pancreatic acinar cell carcinomas contain only wild-type c-K-ras codons 12, 13 and 61. Mol Carcinog 1994; *10:*110–114.

31. Schaeffer BK, Zurlo J, and Longnecker DS. Activation of c-K-ras not detectable in adenomas or adenocarcinomas arising in rat pancreas. Mol Carcinog 1990; *3:*165–170.

32. van Kranen HJ, Vermeulen E, Schoren L, Bax J, Woutersen RA, van Iersel P, van Kreijl CF, and Scherer E. Activation of c-K-ras is frequent in pancreatic carcinomas of Syrian hamsters, but is absent in pancreatic tumors of rats. Carcinogenesis 1991; *12:*1477–1482.

33. Schaeffer BK, Terhune PG, and Longnecker DS. Pancreatic carcinomas of acinar and mixed acinar/ductal phenotypes in Ela-1-myc transgenic mice do not contain c-K-ras mutations. Am J Pathol 1994; *145:*696–701.

34. Kuhlmann ET, Terhune PG, and Longnecker DS. Evaluation of c-K-*ras* in pancreatic carcinomas from Ela-1-SV40T transgenic mice. Carcinogenesis 1993; *14:*2649–2651.

35. Okita S, Tsutsumi M, Onji M, and Konishi Y. p53 mutation without allelic loss and absence of mdm-2 amplification in a transplantable hamster pancreatic ductal adenocarcinoma and derived cell lines but not primary ductal adenocarcinomas in hamsters. Mol Carcin 1995; *13:*266–271.

36. Chang KW, Mangold KA, Hubchak S, Laconi S, and Scarpelli DG. Genomic p53 mutation in a chemically induced hamster pancreatic ductal adenocarcinoma. Cancer Res 1994; *54:*3878–3883.

37. Terhune PG and Longnecker DS. Do oncogene and tumor suppressor gene abnormalities vary with type of carcinoma of the pancreas? J Hep Bil Pancr Surg 1995; *2:*1–7.

38. Kruse F, Rose SD, Swift GH, Hammer RE, and MacDonald RJ. An endocrine-specific element is an integral component of an exocrine-specific pancreatic enhancer. Genes Dev 1993; *7:*774–786.

39. Bell RH, Jr, Memoli VA, and Longnecker DS. Hyperplasia and tumors of the islets of Langerhans in mice bearing an elastase I-SV40 T-antigen fusion gene. Carcinogenesis 1990; *11:*1393–1398.

40. Glasner S, Memoli V, and Longnecker DS. Characterization of the ELSV transgenic mouse model of pancreatic carcinoma: histologic type of large and small tumors. Am J Pathol 1992; *140:*1237–1245.

41. Sandgren EP, Quaife CJ, Paulovich AG, Palmiter RD, and Brinster RL. Pancreatic tumor pathogenesis reflects the causative genetic lesion. Proc Natl Acad Sci USA 1991; *88:*93–97.

42. Visser CJ, Bruggink AH, Korc M, Kobrin MS, de Weger RA, Seifert-Bock I, et al. Overexpression of transforming growth factor-alpha and epidermal growth factor receptor, but not epidermal growth factor, in exocrine pancreatic tumours in hamsters. Carcinogenesis 1996; *17:*779–785.

43. Visser CJ, Woutersen RA, Bruggink AH, van Garderen-Hoetmer A, Seifert-Bock I, Tilanus MG, and de Weger RA. Transforming growth factor-alpha and epidermal growth factor expression in the exocrine pancreas of azaserine-treated rats: modulation by cholecystokinin or a low fat, high fiber (caloric restricted) diet. Carcinogenesis 1995; *16:*2075–2082.

44. Sandgren EP, Luetteke NC, Palmiter RD, Brinster RL, and Lee DC. Overexpression of TGF alpha in transgenic mice: induction of epithelial hyperplasia, pancreatic metaplasia, and carcinoma of the breast. Cell 1990; *61:*1121–1135.

45. Sandgren EP, Luetteke NC, Qiu TH, Palmiter RD, Brinster RL, and Lee DC. Transforming growth factor alpha dramatically enhances oncogene-induced carcinogenesis in transgenic mouse pancreas and liver. Mol Cell Biol 1993; *13:*320–330.

46. Bockman DE. Cells of origin of pancreatic cancer: experimental animal tumors related to human pancreas. Cancer 1981; *47:*1528–1534.

47. Pour PM and Kazakoff K. Stimulation of islet cell proliferation enhances pancratic ductal carcinogenesis in the hamster model. Am J Pathol 1996; *149:*1017–1025.

48. Longnecker DS, Roebuck BD, Kuhlmann ET, and Curphey TJ. Induction of pancreatic carcinomas in rats with N-nitroso(2-hydroxypropyl)(2-oxopropyl)amine: histopathology. J Natl Cancer Inst 1985; *74:*209–217.

49. Longnecker DS, Curphey TJ, Kuhlmann ET, and Schaeffer BK. Experimental induction of pancreatic carcinoma in the hamster with N^δ-(*N*-methyl-*N*-nitrosocarbamoyl) -L-ornithine. J Natl Cancer Inst 1983; *71:*1327–1336.

50. Longnecker DS, Curphey TJ, Lilja HS, French JI, and Daniel DS. Carcinogenicity in rats of the nitrosourea amino acid N^δ-(*N*-methyl-*N*-nitrosocarbamoyl)-L-orithine. J Env Path Toxicol 1980; *4:*117–129.

51. Longnecker DS, Kato Y, Konishi Y, Freeman D, Glasner S, Memoli VA, et al. Comparison of histologic type and stage of exocrine pancreatic neoplasms from surgical series in Europe, Japan and the United States. In: Beger H, Büchler M, and Schoenberg MH. (eds), Cancer of the pancreas: molecular biology, progress in diagnosis and treatment, Springer-Verlag, Heidelberg, 1996; pp. 47–54.

52. Longnecker DS, Kuhlmann ET, and Freeman DH, Jr. Characterization of the elastase-1 SV40 T-antigen mouse model of pancreatic carcinoma: effects of sex and diet. Cancer Res 1990; *50:*7552–7554.

53. Roebuck BD, Yager JD, Jr. Longnecker DS, and Wilpone SA. Promotion by unsaturated fat of azaserine-induced pancreatic carcinogenesis in the rat. Cancer Res 1981; *41:*3961–3966.

54. Birt DF, Patil K, and Pour PM. Comparative studies on the effects of semipurified and commercial diet on the longevity and spontaneous and induced lesions in the Syrian Golden Hamster. Nutr Cancer 1985; *7:*167–177.

55. Appel MJ and Woutersen RA. Effects of dietary fish oil (MaxEPA) on *N*-nitrosobis(2-oxopropyl)amine (BOP)-induced pancreatic carcinogenesis in hamsters. Cancer Lett 1995; *94:*179–189.

56. Lhoste EF, Roebuck BD, and Longnecker DS. Stimulation of the growth of azaserine-induced nodules in the rat pancreas by dietary camostate (FOY-305). Carcinogenesis 1988; *9:*901–906.

57. Spannagel AW, Green GM, Guan D, Liddle RA, Faull K, and Reeve J., Jr, Purification and characterization of a luminal cholecystokinin-releasing factor from rat intestinal secretion. Proc Natl Acad Sci USA, 1996; *93:*4415–4420.

58. Bell RH, Kuhlmann ET, Jensen RT, and Longnecker DS. Overexpression of cholecystokinin receptors in azaserine-induced neoplasms of the rat pancreas. Cancer Res 1992; *52:*3295–3299.

59. Povoski SP, Zhou W, Longnecker DS, Roebuck BD, and Bell RH, Jr. Stimulation of growth of azaserine-induced putative preneoplastic lesions in rat pancreas is mediated specifically by way of cholecystokinin-A receptors. Cancer Res 1993; *53:*3925–3929.

60. Kennedy AR. Prevention of carcinogenesis by protease inhibitors. Cancer Res 1994; *54(Suppl):*1999s–2005s.

61. Longnecker DS, Kuhlmann ET, and Curphey TJ. Divergent effects of retinoids on pancreatic and liver carcinogenesis in azaserine-treated rats. Cancer Res 1983; *43:*3219–3225.

62. Clapper ML, Wood M, Leahy K, Lang D, Miknyoczki S, and Ruggeri BA. Chemopreventive activity of Oltipraz against *N*-nitrosobis(2-oxopropyl)amine (BOP)-induced ductal pancreatic carcinoma development and effects on survival of Syrian golden hamsters. Carcinogenesis 1995; *16:*2159–2165.

63. Appel MJ, van Garderen-Hoetmer A, and Woutersen RA. Lack of inhibitory effects of beta-carotene, vitamin C, vitamin E and selenium on development of ductular adenocarcinomas in exocrine pancreas of hamsters. Cancer Lett 1996; *103:*157–162.

64. Longnecker DS. Experimental pancreatic cancer: role of species, sex and diet. Bull Cancer 1990; *77:*27–37.

65. Lhoste EF, Roebuck BD, Brinck-Johnsen T, and Longnecker DS. Effects of castration and hormone replacement on azaserine-induced pancreatic carcinogenesis in male and female Fischer rats. Carcinogenesis 1987; *8:*699–703.

66. Visser CJ, Meijers M, van Garderen-Hoetmer A, Klijn JG, Foekens JA, and Woutersen RA. Effects of aminoglutethimide, alone and in combination with surgical castration, on pancreatic carcinogenesis in rats and hamsters. Int J Cancer 1995; *63:*732–737.

67. Szepeshazi K, Schally AV, Cai RZ, Radulovic S, Milovanovic S, and Szoke B. Inhibitory effect of bombesin/gastrin-releasing peptide antagonist RC-3095 and high dose of somatostatin analogue RC-160 on nitrosamine-induced pancreatic cancers in hamsters. Cancer Res 1991; *51:*5980–5986.

68. Szepeshazi K, Halmos G, Groot K, and Schally AV. Combination treatment of nitrosamine-induced pancreatic cancers in hamsters with analogs of LH-RH and a bombesin/GRP antagonist. Int J Pancreatol 1994; *16:*141–149.

69. Qin Y, Ertl T, Cai RZ, Halmos G, and Schally AV. Inhibitory effect of bombesin receptor antagonist RC-3095 on the growth of human pancreatic cancer cells in vivo and in vitro. Cancer Res 1994; *54:*1035–1041.

70. Douglas BR, Woutersen RA, Jansen JBMJ, de Jong AJL, Rovati LC, and Lamers CBHW. Modulation by CR-1409 (Lorglumide), a cholecystokinin receptor antagonist, of trypsin inhibitor-enhanced growth of azaserine-induced putative preneoplastic lesions in rat pancreas. Cancer Res 1989; *49:*2438–2441.

71. Lhoste EF, and Longnecker DS. Effect of bombesin and caerulein on early stages of carcinogenesis induced by azaserine in the rat pancreas. Cancer Res 1987; *47:*3273–3277.

72. Scorsone KA, Zhou, Y-Z, Butel JS, and Slagle BL. p53 Mutations cluster at codon 249 in hepatitis B virus-positive hepatocellular carcinomas from China. Cancer Res 1992; *52:*1635–1638.

73. Levison DA, Morgan RGH, Brimacombe JS, Hopwood D, Coghill G, and Wormsley KG. Carcinogenic effects of di(2-hydroxypropyl)nitrosamine (DHPN) in male Wistar rats: promotion of pancreatic cancer by a raw soya flour diet. Scand J Gastroenterol 1979; *14:*217–224.

74. Reddy JK and Rao MS. Transplantable adenocarcinoma in inbred guinea pigs induced by N-methyl-N-nitrosourea. Cancer Res 1975; *35:*2269–2277.

75. Furukawa F, Sato H, Imaida K, Toyoda K, Imazawa T, Takahashi M, and Hayashi Y. Induction of pancreatic tumors in male Syrian golden hamsters by intraperitoneal *N*-methyl-*N*-nitrosourea injection. Pancreas 1992; *7:*153–158.

76. Rivenson A, Hoffmann D, Prokopczyk B, Amin S, and Hecht SS. Induction of lung and exocrine pancreas tumors in F344 rats by tobacco-specific and areca-derived N-nitrosamines. Cancer Res 1988; *48:*6912–1917.

77. Pour PM. and Rivenson A. Induction of a mixed ductal-squamous-islet cell carcinoma in a rat treated with a tobacco-specific carcinogen. Am J Pathol 1989; *134:*627–631.

5

Role for Transforming Growth Factor-β

Clues from Other Cancers

Leslie I. Gold, Ph.D and Trilok Parekh, Ph.D.

THE ROLE FOR TRANSFORMING
GROWTH FACTOR-B IN ONCOGENESIS

Transforming growth factor-βs (TGF-β) are a family of proteins that regulate cell growth (reviews in refs. *1–4*). These proteins are one of the only endogenous inhibitors of the growth of cells and since uncontrolled cell proliferation is the hallmark of cancer, our laboratory has been intrigued by and dedicated to understanding the role for TGF-βs in neoplastic development and cancer progression. Our first approach was to determine the level of TGF-β mRNA and protein expression in a variety of cancers, in vivo, and to correlate this information with disease stage and survival. Since TGF-βs are natural inhibitors of growth, we postulated that there may be a loss or downregulation of TGF-β in cancer cells, thereby permitting their growth. However, on the contrary, we and others have generally found a marked increase in the expression of TGF-β isoform mRNA and protein in cancers of epithelial (ectodermal/endodermal), neuroectodermal, and mesenchymal origin, including malignancies of the pancreas, colon, stomach, endometrium, breast, brain, prostate, and bone *(11–21,84,147–149,169, 170,228,252–255)*. Furthermore, in most of these cancers high expression correlated with more advanced stages of malignancy and decreased survival. Therefore, it was hypothesized that the increased expression of TGF-β represents a loss in the growth inhibitory response to TGF-β and that understanding the molecular events associated with the escape of tumor cells from TGF-β regulation will provide insights into mechanisms underlying oncogenic transformation. Indeed, tumor cells in culture (i.e., colon carcinoma and glioblastoma multiforme [GBM]) have demonstrated a progressive loss of the growth inhibitory response to TGF-β that varies directly with the malignant stage of the original tumor, and the most aggressive forms actually show autocrine and/or paracrine growth stimulation by TGF-β. In addition, since TGF-βs are both angiogenic

Table 1
Expression of TGF-β Isoforms in Various Human Cancers

Pancreatic cancer *(16)*
   Predominantly autocrine mode of action
   TGF-β2 associated with advance tumor stage
   High expression of TGF-β isoforms correlates with decreased survival
Colon cancer *(17, 18, 149)*
   Intense immunoreactivity for TGF-β1 correlates with decreased survival
   High level of expression of TGF-β1 was either maintained or increased at metastatic sites
   Precancerous adenomatous polyps show reversed localization of TGF-β1 and TGF-β3,
      proliferating, and apoptotic cells, compared to normals
Gastric cancer *(20)*
   Increase immunoreactivity for all three TGF-β isoforms in carcinoma cells
   Increase mRNA expression for TGF-β1 and TGF-β3 in cancerous tissue
   Increase in collagen 1α mRNA in scirrhous cancer: TGF-βs may induce the fibrotic
      response
Endometrial cancer *(14)*
   Marked increase in TGF-β1 and TGF-β3 immunoreactivity in the glandular epithelial cells
      in complex hyperplasia and carcinoma
   Marked increase in mRNA of all TGF-β isoforms in the stromal cells in complex
      hyperplasia and carcinoma
   Switch from paracrine/autocrine to predominantly paracrine mode of TGF-β action (i.e.,
      stromal cells express increased mRNA and glandular cells show increased protein)
   Loss of stromal/epithelial interaction; glandular cells may not respond to TGF-β made by
      stromal cells
Breast cancer *(15)*
   Intense immunoreactivity for TGF-β1 correlates with progression
Gliomas *(21)*
   Predominantly autocrine mode of action
   TGF-β1 is a marker for carcinogenesis
   Intense immunoreactivity for TGF-β isoforms correlates with short-term survival in GBM
Osteosarcomas *(19)*
   High expression of TGF-β3 in tumor cells correlates with disease progression

and immunosuppressive, the increased amount of TGF-β present in tumors provides an additional selective advantage for tumor cell growth. The link between cancer development and specific genetic alterations leads to the idea that this damage may occur in genes that effect the ability of TGF-β to regulate cell growth. In the past two years, information has been accumulating that shows specific (genetic) defects in TGF-β receptors, TGF-β regulated cell cycle proteins, and TGF-β-related signal transduction/gene activation have all contributed to neoplastic transformation and progression. This chapter will provide background information on TGF-β and update the status of our knowledge of the role for TGF-β in the particular cancers that we have studied (presented in Table 1).

THE TGF-β FAMILY, STRUCTURE, AND FUNCTIONS

TGF-βs are part of a family of proteins that regulate cell growth, differentiation, and morphogenesis (more than 25 to date); they share seven conserved cyteines *(1–6)*. Included in this group of proteins are the bone morphogenetic proteins (BMPs), activins/inhibins, and mullerian inhibitory substance (MIS). There are five members of the immediate TGF-β family (TGF-β1–5) and three mammalian isoforms (TGF-β1–3) that possess 76–80% amino acid identity and nine conserved cysteines. Crystallography studies of the mature form of TGF-β2 indicated that the structure conforms to a cystine knot motif that is also characteristic of the TGF-β family and two other growth factors, nerve growth factor (NGF) and platelet-derived growth factor (PDGF), not of the TGF-β family, and sharing only 10% amino acid identity *(7,8)*. The knot is composed of six cystines joined together by three intrachain disulfide bonds that stabilize several β-sheet strands. One free cysteine forms an interchain disulfide bond with an identical monomeric chain to create the mature dimer. Whereas the genes for each TGF-β isoform are located on different chromosomes, each isoform is either completely or closely conserved within mammalian species, suggesting that they were derived by gene duplication. The evolutionary persistence of the three isoforms, and the fact that they generally have overlapping functions in vitro, originally spurred our laboratory to explore whether they may possess different functions in vivo. Indeed, we and others have found that TGF-β isoforms are differentially expressed throughout the processes of embryogenesis *(3,9,10)*, carcinogenesis *(11–21)*, inflammation and tissue repair *(22–36)*, and most recently, cranial development *(37,38)*. Since the 5′ promoter regions of each TGF-β gene contain different response elements *(39,40)*, the dynamic temporal and spatial expression of these proteins during physiological processes is consistent with differential and complex gene regulation. Interestingly, the potency of each TGF-β isoform in different in vitro assays can vary as much as 100-fold. For example, in growth inhibition assays, TGF-β3 is 50-fold more potent than TGF-β1 or TGF-β2 on epithelial cells *(41*; unpublished observations) and TGF-β2 is 100 times less potent than TGF-β1 and TGF-β3 on vascular endothelial cells and hematopoietic progenitor cells *(42)*. Moreover, only TGF-β2 is involved in mesoderm induction *(43)*. These differences may also be caused by different receptors on various cell types. TGF-βs are potent chemoattractants for immune cells, fibroblasts, smooth muscle cells, and certain tumor cells *(44–47)*. They also are strong inducers of extracellular matrix proteins, including collagens, fibronectin, proteoglycans, laminin, vitronectin, and tenascin, and they stimulate the production of protease inhibitors, such as plasminogen activator inhibitor (PAI-1) and tissue inhibitor of metalloproteinase (TIMP), that prevent the enzymatic breakdown of matrices *(1–4,48–50)*; all are important in inflammation, tissue repair, and angiogenesis. However, dysregulation of these functions is associated with scarring, fibrotic disease, and vascular stenosis *(51–53)* concomitant with increased expression of TGF-β mRNA and proteins. TGF-βs also increase the expression of intergrins, cell surface heterodimeric cell surface receptors that regulate adhesion and migration of cells on matrices and cell:cell adhesion *(1–4,54,55)*. In humans, a major source of TGF-β1 is the α granules of platelets (for delivery after tissue injury), and bone contains abundant amounts of all three isoforms *(56,57)*. Finally, TGF-β isoforms are auto- and crossinductive; thus, their presence is self-perpetuating *(39)*. TGF-βs utilize both paracrine (made by one cell type and stimulating the function of another cell type) and autocrine (made and used by the identical cell) mechanisms of action.

ACTIVATION OF TGF-B IS REQUIRED FOR FUNCTION

TGF-βs are secreted as latent precursor molecules (LTGF-β) that require activation into a mature form to enable receptor binding and subsequent activation of signal transduction pathways. TGF-β latency is a critical step in the physiological regulation of its growth inhibitory activity (reviews in refs. *6,58*). Thus, an important point is whether tumor cells are able to activate TGF-β or have access to activated protein to inhibit their growth. The latent precursor molecules are between 390 and 414 amino acids and contain an amino-terminal hydrophobic signal peptide region (for translocation to the plasma membrane to undergo exocytosis), the latent-associated peptide (LAP) region of 249 residues, and the C-terminal potentially bioactive mature region, which contains 112 amino acids per monomer. The latent precursor is secreted as an electrostatically bound complex. Each monomeric chain is precleaved intracellularly at dibasic residues located between the LAP and mature regions and is joined together as a dimer by two disulfide bonds, one each in the LAP and mature regions. The LAP portion assists in folding the bioactive domain during synthesis and undergoes mannose-6-phosphate N-linked glycoslyation, which aids in secretion of the precursor and may also prevent its activation. In vitro, extreme pH or heat activates the latent molecule causing the release of the 25 kDa dimer (2 × 12.5 kDa monomers). However, in vivo activation of TGF-β isoforms is not well understood. It has been proposed that a conformational change induced by cleavage of the LAP by various proteases is the physiological means for release of the bioactive dimer. Proteases shown to at least partially activate TGF-β include plasmin, thrombin, plasma transglutaminase, endoglycosidase *(58)*, and retinoic acid, via plasmin release *(59)*. The fact that only a small percent of total available latent TGF-β is activated in any one in vitro assay indicates that many mechanisms are involved and that activation is cell-type specific. Since TGF-β isoforms only share 35% amino-acid homology in the LAP regions, conformational differences may dictate that each TGF-β isoform undergoes differential activation. Thrombospondin also activates TGF-β through a specific binding interaction between these proteins *(60)*. Cocultures of bovine smooth muscle cells and endothelial cells indicated that heterotypic cell surface contact was required for activation *(61,62)*. These studies and others showed that latent TGF-β binds to the insulin-like growth factor II receptor/mannose-6-phosphate receptor on the endothelial cells and regenerating hepatocytes and may be targeted to lysosomes for activation *(63,64)*. However, other cells that express these receptors fail to activate LTGF-β. Finally, the LTGF-β1 is usually secreted covalently bound via the LAP region to another protein, the LTGF-β-binding protein (LTBP) *(65–68)*, which is important in assembly and secretion of LTGF-β1 *(67)* and serves to bind LTGF-β to extracellular matrices as a requirement for proteolytic activation *(68)*. The presence of LTBP was shown to be lost in malignant prostatic tissue compared to benign tissue *(69)* and may indicate its role in normal growth regulation. Two matrix proteoglycans, decorin and biglycan, bind TGF-βs for retention in extracellular matrices and may also regulate TGF-β availability *(51,52,70)*.

TGF-β REGULATION THROUGH RECEPTOR BINDING

Since signal transducing receptors were shown to be present on virtually every mammalian and avian cell type in culture, including transformed cells (except retinoblastoma cells), aberrant receptor expression or loss of receptors was not originally considered a means of loss of responsiveness to growth control by TGF-β *(1–5)*. However, most recently, exciting discoveries have elucidated mutations in TGF-β receptors that are associated with loss of growth inhibition in a number of malignancies described below. Three distinct receptors that bind all TGF-βs, termed type I (RI) (50–60 kDa), type II (RII) (75–85 kDa), and type III (RIII/betaglycan) (280 kDa), have been identified in a variety of cells *(5,71,72)*. At least nine other cell-surface-binding proteins have also been demonstrated. RI and RII are transmembrane-signal-transducing receptors that contain serine/threonine kinase cytoplasmic domains. Both RI and RII kinase domains share 40% homology with each other and with other type 1 and type II receptors having specificity for other TGF-β family members (e.g., activins, BMPs) *(5)*. The type III receptor has a core protein of 110–139 kDa adorned with heparin sulfate and chondroitin sulfate side chains. RIII is nonsignaling and serves to concentrate TGF-β ligand on the surface of cells and to present TGF-β1–3 to the signaling receptors. RIII can also be released from cells and act as a soluble inhibitor of TGF-βs and regulate its activity *(73)*. Using receptor negative mutants, it has been shown that RI and RII are required to cooperate to function in the following manner, as depicted in Fig. 1: RII is a constitutively active kinase, which is recognized by RI following ligand binding to RII *(72)*. Subsequently, RI is recruited into the complex and phosphorylated by RII. This event causes RI to initiate signal-transducing pathways. Simply stated, RII binds to ligand and RI transmits the signal function (to downstream substrates); RI will not bind ligand without the presence of RII (RI/RII heterodimeric complex binds TGF-β1: Kd $\sim 10-11\,M$ *(74)*). TGF-β receptors discriminate between the TGF-β isoforms and bind these ligands with different affinities *(75,76)*. For example, whereas TGF-β1 and TGF-β3 will bind RII, TGF-β2 requires RIII for presentation to the signaling receptors (RIII binds TGF-β1–3: Kd $=10-10\,M$) *(1)*. Thus, within these defined parameters, loss of RIII would block TGF-β2-initiated function, and loss of either RI or RII would prevent all TGF-βs from functional response. The cellular distribution of RIII is more limited than RI and RII and is absent from endothelial cells, myoblasts, and hematopoietic cells *(1,3,77)*, which, accordingly, do not respond to TGF-β2 *(42)*. Endoglin, another homodimeric cell surface glycoprotein that complexes with RI and RII *(78)*, only binds TGF-β1 and TGF-β3 and is found on endothelial cells, macrophages, and stromal cells *(79,80)*. In the context of malignant cell growth, the main function of the TGF-β receptors is to transduce signals that maintain the nonproliferative state of the cell in G1. Whereas pathways for receptor-mediated signal transduction for transcription of genes induced by mitogens, such as EGF and PDGF (tyrosine kinases), involve a cascade of numerous substrates (e.g., protein kinases and phosphatases), the proteins and pathways involved in transmitting signals from TGF-β receptors (e.g., specific substrates for ser/thr kinases) appear to be less complex. Most recently, the MAD-related, MADR2 (MAD is mothers against DPP [DPP is decapentaplegic protein, part of the TGF-β superfamily that regulates drosophila morphogenesis]) has been specifically associated with TGF-β signaling. The MAD family of proteins, also known as Smad (Smad 1,2,3, and 5), re-

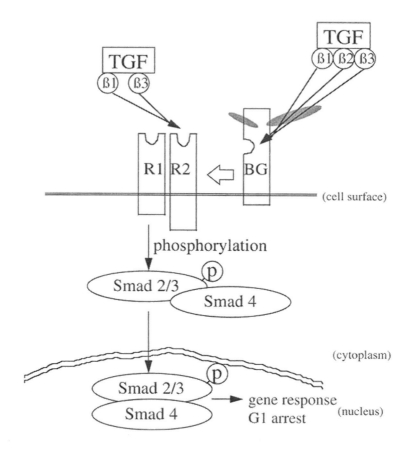

Fig. 1. Proposed TGF-β isoform signaling receptor complex. RI and RII have serine/threonine kinase (catalyze phosphorylation of proteins) cytoplasmic domains and are required to cooperate to elicit TGF-β functions in the following way. RII is a constitutively active kinase that binds the ligands TGF-β1 or TGF-β3. Following ligand binding, RI is sequestered into the complex and is phosphorylated by RII. Subsequently, RI sends downstream signals for gene activation (through phosphorylation events) that directly phosphorylates MADR2/Smad2, which forms a complex with DPC4/Smad4. The complex enters the nucleus and acts as a transcriptional activator of genes involved in TGF-β function (growth inhibition) *(72,83,256–260)*. RIII, a proteoglycan, is termed betaglycan (BG) and serves to concentrate TGF-β isoforms on the cell surface and present these ligands to RII. TGF-β2 will not bind RII without prior association with RIII. RIII also acts as a soluble inhibitor of TGF-β isoforms, thereby preventing TGF-β activity *(73)*. The shaded elipse represents glycosaminoglycan chains. Diagram modified from ref. *3*.

spond to ser/thr kinase receptors for the TGF-β family, including BMPs, activins, and DPP *(81,82,256–258)*. It was originally presumed that there are substrates downstream from RI that transduce the signal to MADR2/Smad2. However, it has been demonstrated that TGF-β RI directly interacts with and phosphorylates MADR2/Smad2 at C-terminal serines (SSXS motif), causing it to translocate and accumulate in the nucleus (Fig. 1) *(83)*. Similarly, BMP specifically induces a BMP receptor kinase to directly phosphorylate MADR1/Smad1, causing its accumulation in the nucleus *(257,259)* (*see* Fig. 1). Apparently, Smad4 is a universal ("common") component of the signaling pathway of the TGF-β family. Smad1, activated by BMPs, and Smad2 and Smad3, activated by TGF-β and activin, form a heteromeric complex with Smad4 following phosphorylation with these respective ligands *(256)*. Recently, it was shown that activated MAD, the mediator of DPP signaling *(Drosophila)*, interacts with DNA-binding proteins and binds to target gene enhancers through a sequence-specific DNA-binding region in its N-terminal *(250)*. Therefore, the MAD/Smad proteins provide a direct link between the respective receptor kinase activity (type I) and gene transcription, that initiates function *(256–258)*. Interestingly, the Smad7 protein can associate with TGF-β RI kinase domain and antagonize TGF-β signaling *(251)*. Smad4/MADR4, the "common" Smad/MAD is the protein product of the DPC4 tumor suppressor gene found Deleted in Pancreatic Cancer at a rate of 90% *(130)*.

MECHANISMS OF TGF-β REGULATION
OF CELL GROWTH THROUGH EFFECTS ON THE CELL CYCLE

TGF-β directly induces growth arrest in most epithelial cells, including carcinomas in culture, endothelial cells, neuroectodermal cells, hepatocytes, lymphocytes, and myeloid cells (review in refs. *1–4,84*). Conversely, TGF-β is generally mitogenic to mesenchymally derived cells through the induction of mitogenic growth factors, such as PDGF *(86)*. Although TGF-β induces cell-cycle arrest by blocking cells in late G1 of the cell cycle (reviewed in ref. *85*), pathways/mechanisms for this arrest are cell-type specific. To review the cell cycle: cells resting in G0 (withdrawn from the cell cycle) are brought into the G1 phase by extracellular signals, such as adhesion-associated events *(87,88)*. At this point, the cell is susceptible to mitogenic signals (e.g., growth factors) and will move on to S-phase (DNA synthetic or replication stage), followed by a shorter G2 (rest just prior to division), and finally, M (mitotic phase consisting of prophase-anaphase). G1 progression to S is blocked by TGF-β late in G1, 2 h before cells are committed to enter S-phase and after this time TGF-β can no longer exert its antiproliferative effect *(2,3,89,* and reviewed in ref. *90)*. Cancer cells are refractory to growth arrest and remain in the cell cycle (reviewed in ref. *91*). As depicted in Fig. 2, each phase of the cell cycle is controlled by specific cyclins and their respective kinases, cyclin-dependent kinases (CDKs): In early G1-cyclin D (1–3) couples with CDK6 and CDK4; in late G1 = cyclin E and CDK2; S phase=cyclin A and CDK2; G2/M=cyclin B and CDK1 [CDC2] *(97)*. Progression through the cell cycle involves the phosphorylation of the retinoblastoma tumor suppressor gene product pRB, by D and E cyclin:CDK-respective kinase activities (cyclins bind to the "large pocket" of RB and other like proteins, such as p130 and p107) *(85,90–92)*. The absence of tumor suppressor genes promotes malignant growth; the loss of RB function resulting from mutation or deletion of both alleles leads to oncogenic transformation that can be reverted by introducing a normal RB gene into a cell (reviewed in ref. *93*). The formation of CDK/cyclin complexes is regulated by the cyclin-activating kinase, CAK *(91)*. Accordingly, cell cycle arrest is associated with inhibition of phosphorylation of pRB (hypophosphorylated) and a decrease in G1 cyclins and CDKs (reviewed in refs. *85,90–92,94)*.

The activation of genes that are associated with cell cycle progression is mainly related to two proteins: the transcription family of E2F factors and the protooncogene c-*myc*. Hypophosphorylated pRB binds to a subset of E2F complexes that are released

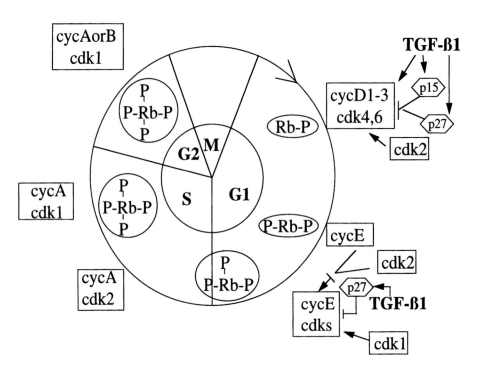

Fig. 2. TGF-β effects on the cell cycle. Growth inhibition is achieved by preventing phosphorylation of RB. The circle depicts the phases of the cell cycle. Progression through the cell cycle is controlled by the cyclins (cyc) and cyclin-dependent kinases (cdks) that are specific for each phase of the cell cycle. The cyclin/cdk complex has kinase activity and phosphorylates (P) RB, causing progression from G1 to S phase. TGF-β induces the cyclin-dependent kinase inhibitors (CKIs) p15 and p27, which bind to the cyclin/cdks, preventing phosphorylation of RB and thereby arresting cells in G1. In addition, TGF-β inhibits the expression of cyclins and cdks. As discussed, mutations have been discovered in many of these cell-cycle proteins in cancer, thereby dedicating the cell to uncontrolled proliferation (reviewed in ref. *91*).

following pRB phosphorylation *(85,90,93,95)*. The E2F complexes transactivate target genes thus initiated by the cyclin D-dependent kinases and subsequently by the cyclin E:CDK2 complex, causing transition onto S-phase *(91)*. In certain cells, including keratinocytes, TGF-β1 inhibits the transcription of c-*myc* mRNA concomitant with growth inhibition (reviewed in refs. *90,96,97*). Since the c-*myc* promoter contains E2F-binding sites, the release of E2F by pRB in its hyperhosphorylated state causes transactivation of c-*myc*. It should be noted, however, that both the dependency of TGF-β-induced growth inhibition on decreased levels of c-*myc* and/or on pRB is dissociated in certain experiments *(98)*, indicating that other pathways exist. In addition to the rapid (within 30 min) downregulation of c-*myc* transcription in response to TGF-β, the early response genes/nuclear transcription factors, c-*jun, jun*B, and c-*fos* are upregulated *(39,99,100)*. It has recently been shown that cell-cycle arrest by TGF-β is also mediated by induction of cyclin-dependent kinase inhibitors (CKIs) that bind to the cyclin:CDK complexes and inhibit their ability to phosphorylate pRB, thus maintaining cells in G1. There are two families of mammalian CKIs: the ink4 group (includes: p15, p16, p18, p19), which specifically interferes with cyclin D binding to CDK4 and CDK6, and the kip/cip proteins (includes: p27, p21, p57), which inhibit the cyclins A,D,E and their respective CDKs *(91,101)*. It was found that TGF-β specifically induces the expression of the CKIs, p15 (by 30-fold in keratinocytes), p21, and p27 *(101–104)*. The mechanism involved in TGF-β growth inhibition through the action of CKIs in certain epithelial cells has been traced. P15 induces the release of p27 from the cyclin D complexes so that it can subsequently bind cyclin E:CDK2, preventing progression to S *(94,101)*. Therefore, p27 is recovered complexed with cyclin E:CDK2 in TGF-β-treated and contact-inhibited growth arrested cells, but not proliferating cells *(103)*. In summary, TGF-β acts to arrest cell growth through two interdependent mechanisms (reviewed in refs. *105*): by inhibiting the activity and expression of cyclin:CDK expression and/or cyclin/CDK complex formation and thus, kinase activity, and by inhibiting CDK activity through the induction of CKIs (p15, p21, p27), finally leading to the inhibition of pRB phosphorylation, which sequesters E2F factors preventing their transactivation of genes involved in DNA synthesis.

Aberrant Cell-Cycle Genes/Proteins Abrogate TGF-β Mediated Growth Inhibition in Human Cancers

As suspected, studies have been rapidly surfacing that show the lack of responsiveness of tumor cells to TGF-β-induced growth arrest, undoubtedly important in the process of oncogenic transformation, results from dysregulation of proteins that control the cell cycle, including deletions and mutations in corresponding genes and degradation of these proteins. These new and interesting findings will be described below as they relate to the individual cancers discussed herein. The genes encoding cyclin D1 (on chromosome 11q13) and CDK4 have been shown to be overexpressed in many human cancers (e.g., in 43% of squamous cell carcinomas, 34% esophageal carcinomas) as a result of gene amplification and translocations *(105–107)*. Homozygous deletions of the CKI, p15, occur at a rate of 55% in gliomas and mesotheliomas, and mutations and deletions of p15 and p16 (Ink4a and b) are frequently associated with pancreatic and head and neck carcinomas *(91, and reviewed in refs. 106–109)*, the consequence of which is lack of inhibition of CDK activity and uncontrolled phosphorylation of pRB. Another mode of loss of tumor suppressor function of p15 and p16 is through hypermethylation of specific motifs in the promoter regions, resulting in transcriptional inactivation of these genes *(110)*. In addition to retinoblastoma of childhood resulting from defects in the RB gene, numerous adult cancers show genetic abnormalities that target the RB gene (specifically sarcomas and osteosarcomas) *(106)*. In support of the role for the CKI, p27, in TGF-β-mediated growth arrest in G1, overexpression of p27 has been shown to block cells in G1 *(111,112)*; p27 is most abundant in G0 of the cell cycle *(91)*. In addition, targeted deletion of the p27 gene (gene knockout) in mice showed 100% occurrence of pituitary tumors and multiple organ hyperplasia *(113,114)*. It is interesting to note that the oncogenic viral proteins, E1A of the adenovirus, SV40 large T antigen, and E7 of the Human Papilloma virus, can inactivate p27 by dissociating it from cyclin-cdk complexes *(115)*. Both the level of p27 gene expression and its integrity are unaltered in cancers *(116,117)*. However, the levels of p27 are under posttranslational control *(118,119)* and an exciting report indicated that levels of p27 protein are controlled by degradation of the protein following catalyzed ubiquitination and degradation in proteasomes *(120)*. The amount of other proteins, including cell cycle proteins (cyclins A and B), are regulated by the ubiquitin-proteasome pathway *(121,122)*. Increased degradation of p27 through the ubiquitin-proteasome pathway is an exciting novel mechanism to further investigate as a means for tumor cell escape from growth control by TGF-β.

TGF-β-RELATED MECHANISMS OF LOSS OF GROWTH REGULATION IN SPECIFIC HUMAN CANCERS

Pancreatic Cancer

We were most interested in understanding a possible role for TGF-β isoforms in pancreatic cancer since this cancer is one of the most highly aggressive and rapidly progressing cancers and is unresponsive to common modes of therapy; the 5-yr survival rate is 0.4% after resection (15–20% have resectable tumors at time of diagnosis) *(123,124)*. Baldwin and Korc have shown that TGF-β1 inhibits the growth of pancreatic carcinoma cell lines by 25–50%, which is concomitant with a dose-dependent increase in mRNA levels for TGF-β1, but not for TGF-β2 or TGF-β3 *(125)*. A direct correlation between high levels of the TGF-β RI (ALK-5 type) and sensitivity to TGF-β growth inhibitory activity was observed in pancreatic cell lines, especially the COLO 357 cell line *(126)*. Another cell line, lacking RII (MIA PaCa-2), was completely growth-resistant to TGF-β. In the normal human pancreas, TGF-β1,β2, and β3 isoform mRNA and protein were present in both the endocrine and exocrine compartments *(127)*. Whereas TGF-β2 and TGF-β3 immunoreactivity was more intense in islets, TGF-β1 protein expression was present in a larger number of acinar cells, and the same intensity of immunostaining for all three isoforms was observed in ductal cells. In a study of 60 patients with pancreatic cancer (representing grades 1–4 and stage I–IV disease), Friess et al. have shown an increase in immunoreactivity for TGF-β1, TGF-β2, and TGF-β3 in 47, 42, and 40% of tumors, respectively ($p \leq 0.001$) *(16)*. Northern blot analysis of tissues from five normal and six pancreatic carcinoma tissues indicated a statistically significant 11-, 7-, and 9-fold increase in TGF-β1, TGF-β2, and TGF-β3 mRNA, respectively. Following analysis by *in situ* hybridization, the mRNA for each TGF-β isoform was shown to be present in increased amounts in approx 30% of the cancer cells. Colocalization of the protein and mRNA in both the normal and malignant tissues indicated that TGF-β predominantly acts by an autocrine mechanism in the pancreas. Additionally, tissue adjacent to the tumors showed increased immunoreactivity demonstrating a paracrine effect of the tumor on the normal tissue. A major finding from these studies was derived from Kaplan-Meier plots of postoperative survival time, which indicated that pancreatic cancer specimens demonstrating little to no immunoreactivity for TGF-β was associated with increased survival time (Table 1). Only the expression of the TGF-β2 isoform correlated with advanced tumor stage, indicating that the presence of the TGF-β2 isoform may be a marker for progression in pancreatic cancer. In a subsequent study, it was found that the mRNA for the type II receptor for TGF-βs (RII) was upregulated 4.6-fold in human pancreatic adenocarcinoma tissue compared to normal pancreatic tissue; expression was specifically localized to the cancer cells *(128)*. In contrast, RIII mRNA levels were unaltered, and the message was localized to the stroma surrounding the tumor and a few cancer cells. More recently, a clearer understanding of at least one mechanism by which pancreatic adenocarcinoma cells escape growth control was shown *(126)*. Although the levels of the TGF-β1 RI mRNA (also referred to as ALK-5 [activin-like kinase 5], which only binds to TGF-β ligands) *(5)* and another RI (ALK-2, which binds both activin and TGF-β) were elevated by 6.8- and 9-fold, respectively, the expression of ALK-5/RI protein, as determined by immunohistochemistry, was extremely faint in the cancer cells; RII immunostaining was intense. In contrast, ductal cells adjacent to the cancer cells showed the opposite immunostaining pattern: ALK-5/RI was strong and RII was weak. Since, as explained above, RI and RII cooperate to transduce TGF-β function and RI transmits the intracellular downstream signals, the lack of RI on the pancreatic tumor cells may explain, in part, why these cells do not respond to the growth inhibitory effects of TGF-β. The increased amount of RII observed in these cells would be ineffective since presumably these cells would bind TGF-β ligand, but not be able to undergo the necessary signaling events to confer growth inhibition. Furthermore, the fact that the mRNA was increased in tumor cells that showed lack of RI protein suggests that aberrant RI expression may be hampered posttranscriptionally (e.g., message degradation).

Certain recent advances have provided further explanations for the lack of growth control by TGF-β. In an analysis of 19 different pancreatic cell lines and three xenografts of these cells, 46% were shown to have homozygous deletions of both the p15 and p16 genes *(129)*. Loss of p16 transcripts was found in 53%, and 63% had mutations in the p16 gene that led to loss of p16 protein expression. Another very recent exciting discovery showed a direct link between mutations in the DPC4 gene with pancreatic cancer *(82, 130)*. DPC4 (Deleted in Pancreatic Cancer) is part of the MAD family of newly discovered transcription factors that transduce receptor signaling by the TGF-β related proteins *(see* Fig. 1*)*. Loss of heterozygosity (LOH) occurs when a somatic mutation occurs at one allele and the second allele is lost through deletion. Many tumor suppressor genes have been found by mapping mutations showing a high degree of LOH. Approximately 90% of human pancreatic carcinomas demonstrate allelic loss at chromosome 18q. Both homozygous deletions and inactivating mutations were localized to the DPC4 locus at chromosome 18q21.1 in 25/84 and 6/27 (in those that did not have homozygous deletions) pancreatic cancers, respectively *(130)*. Although the ligand involved in DPC4 signaling remains unknown, but may be a member of the TGF-β superfamily involved in growth control of pancreatic cells, the mutations for MADR1 (responds to BMP), MAD (*Drosophila* morphogenesis), and DPC4 are in the conserved carboxyl terminal domain, which contains gene transactivating activity. The fact that both MADR2/Smad2 (responds to TGF-β signaling) and DPC4/Smad4 lie in close proximity on chromosome 18q21 (same cytogenetic band) has led Eppert et al. to propose that DPC4 and TGF-β may cooperate to function in control of proliferation *(82)*. LOH at 18q21 has been found in numerous human cancers, including osteosarcomas and colorectal cancers *(131–133)*. However, it appears that mutations in MADR2/Smad2 particularly favor the gastrointestinal tract. In summary, within the past 2 yr, significant advances with respect to failure of TGF-β-related mechanisms that may contribute to the development of pancreatic cancers have emerged. We have seen decreased expression of the signaling TGF-β RI, mutations or deletions in the TGF-β-induced cyclin-dependent kinase inhibitors (CKIs), p15 and p16, critical to maintaining the differentiated quiescent state of cells, and finally, inactivating mutations in a TGF-β-family-related "common" signal transducing protein, DPC4 (Smad4). Therefore, in pancreatic cancer, insults have been sustained in every aspect involved in transmission of TGF-β growth inhibitory function.

Colon Cancer

TGF-β is a potent inhibitor of the growth of intestinal epithelial cells and cell lines in vitro *(134,135)* and regulates cell turnover through autocrine and paracrine mechanisms *(136)*. TGF-β isoform mRNA and protein expression progressively increases ascending the tip of the villi in the normal small intestine and colon *(137)*, and paneth cells of the lower crypt were found to contain protein but not to synthesize TGF-β1 mRNA *(138)*. Since TGF-β is present in the terminally differentiated cells of the villus tips, these proteins may be integral in promoting and maintaining the differentiated state of intestinal epithelial cells. Consistent with this localization of TGF-β protein in the normal intestine, cell proliferation occurs in the crypt base and apoptosis (programmed cell death) occurs near the luminal surface, at the villus tip *(18, 139)*. To follow programmed differentiation that culminates in senescence and programmed cell death, the cells migrate from the proliferative compartment up the crypt and onto the villus tip putatively, under the influence of the autocrine and paracrine growth inhibitory and apoptosis-inducing effect of TGF-β *(140)*. Conversion of human colonic adenoma to carcinoma cells was accompanied by a reduced growth inhibitory response to TGF-β *(141)*, and 11 out of 13 subclones of a metastatic colon carcinoma cell line were growth-stimulated by TGF-β1 *(142)*. Similarly, primary cultures derived from poorly differentiated primary site and metastatic colon cancers were growth stimulated by TGF-β1 and were invasive in vitro and in highly tumorigenic in athymic mice *(143)*. Both neutralizing antibody to TGF-β1 and an antisense construct to TGF-β1 blocked cell growth, invasion, and tumorigenicity *(143,144)*. Thus, a switch from being growth inhibited to growth stimulated by TGF-β appears to be a consequence of tumor progression in colon cancer. With this alteration in growth response to TGF-β, alternative signal transducing pathways have been found in colon cancer cell lines responding to TGF-β by autocrine-negative compared to autocrine-positive growth regulation *(145)*. In another study, TGF-β1 inhibited the growth of colon carcinoma cells in vivo. Wu et al. inhibited the transcription of endogenous TGF-β1 in the FET colon cancer cell lines with an antisense TGF-β1 expression vector and demonstrated that the cloning efficiency increased fourfold, and also that the tumorigenicity of these cells was increased following injection into nude mice *(146)*.

To try to clarify the role for TGF-βs in human colon cancer, we performed in vivo studies that evaluated 34 colorectal carcinoma specimens with accompanying documentation of disease recurrence status *(17)*. The population was separated into two groups: cancer-free and recurrent disease. In each group, 94% were node-positive with similar numbers of positive nodes per patient. Following immunohistochemical analysis, the patients were grouped into intense vs low immunoreactivity. Kaplan-Meier plots of disease-free survival related to immunostaining intensity indicated a significant correlation of intense immunostaining for TGF-β1 with disease progression to metastatic disease ($p \leq 0.0013$). This result was independent of nodal status and the degree of differentiation of the primary tumor. These patients had a mean recurrence time of 27 mo compared to a mean follow-up time over twice as long in the group that did not recur. In this study, the colon cancers expressing high levels of TGF-β1 were 18 times more likely to recur at distant metastases than those having low levels (Table 1). Interestingly, TGF-β2 and TGF-β3 intensity of immunoreactivity did not correlate with disease progression. Corroborating our results, a more recent study found a 2.5-fold increase in the level of TGF-β1 mRNA, increased immunostaining for TGF-β1, and sevenfold elevated plasma level of TGF-β1 in colorectal cancer patients compared to normal controls (147). Again, this overexpression of TGF-β1 correlated with disease progression. Another study found intense immunoreactivity for TGF-β1 in advanced Dukes's stage colorectal tumors, with a poor prognosis, that was associated with decreased survival (148). To determine whether high levels of TGF-β1 were maintained in colon cancers that had metastasized, we performed a follow-up study to analyze TGF-β1 levels in paired primary site and metastatic tumor tissue, using immunohistochemistry (of 38 node-negative, 33 node-positive, 14 metastases) and Western blot analysis (for primary sites and liver metastases) (149). In 60% of the cases examined, higher expression of TGF-β1 was observed in colon cancer cells invading local lymph nodes or metastasizing to the liver than in the primary site. In 25% of the cases, the high levels of TGF-β1 at the primary site were maintained in the cancer cells invading the local lymph nodes and/or the liver. Thus, a total of 85% of colon cancers expressed high levels of TGF-β1 at metastatic sites. Both the 55-kDa latent form and 25-kDa active dimer were illustrated by Western blot analysis. Since TGF-β1 has been shown to increase the expression of PDGF-B chain in invasive and undifferentiated, but not differentiated, colon carcinoma cells and since PDGF-B is elevated in human colon cancers showing increased angiogenesis (150), the high level of TGF-β1 in metastatic colon cancer cells may confer both a selective autocrine growth advantage and increase angiogenesis. Taken together, the high expression of TGF-β1 in colorectal carcinomas may be an independent prognostic marker for poor survival and should be helpful in determining patients who may benefit from more aggressive adjuvant therapy.

Colon adenocarcinoma develops by progression from normal colonic epithelium to abnormal mucosa, on to benign neoplastic adenomatous polyps, that further become dysplastic and finally, malignant (151). Both increased proliferation as well decreased apoptosis contribute to adenoma formation (152,153). More recently, we performed another study to assess the role of TGF-β in the development of malignant lesions from adenomatous polyps (18). The normal distribution of TGF-β as well as the cells undergoing proliferation and apoptosis was strikingly reversed in the polyps compared to the normal mucosa: increased numbers of proliferating cells were observed in the villus tip (luminal surface) and TGF-β isoforms were found mainly in the crypt. We concluded that normal cell migration toward the lumen has been reversed in the polyps such that colonocytes migrate inward toward the polyp base, rather than upward toward the tip. How and when the reversal occurs is not clear. However, loss of TGF-β-related regulated growth associated with maintenance of the state of differentiation and normal architecture of villus may be critical. Interestingly, the CK1, p27[kip1], colocalized with TGF-β in the normal human intestine but was either low or completely lost in colorectal cancers (154). In 149 patients studied, reduction or loss of p27[kip1] expression was found to be an independent negative prognostic marker, especially for stage II tumors (lack of p27[kip1] correlated with a 2.9 risk ratio of death). Patients that expressed p27[kip1] had a median survival of 151 mo compared with those who lacked p27[kip1], with a median survival of 69 mo. Tumor tissue that did not express p27[kip1] also displayed enhanced proteolytic activity specific for exogenously added recombinant p27[kip1] to lysates, which was degraded in a proteasome-dependent manner *(120)*. These results are the first to implicate that tumor cells may escape growth regulation by increasing degradation of p27[kip1]. Whereas there is no direct corelation between TGF-β and p27[kip1] degradation, p27[kip1] is a protein that is induced by TGF-β that, in turn, maintains the quiescent state of cells (discussed above/cell cycle). Amplification of cyclin D2 and cyclin E genes (in 2/47 cases), leading to overexpression of both the mRNA and protein, was also found in a subset of colorectal cancers; this would promote transition through G1 and onto the S-phase of the cell cycle *(155)*.

Microsatellite (genetic) instability is characterized by sequences of simple repetitive DNA at microsatellite loci that frequently undergo deletion and insertion. Mutations and deletions can be determined by genetic analyses with probes specific for these regions of DNA. Mutations in microsatellite DNA, referred to as replication errors (RER+) are prevalent in many cancers *(156)*. In addition to the sequential accumulation of multiple mutations of oncogenes and tumor suppressor genes in carcinogenesis, RER+ is a characteristic phenotype of cancers found in HNPCC (hereditary nonpolyposis colorectal cancer) a familial cancer syndrome, exhibiting a high incidence in colon *(157,158)*, endometrial *(159)*, and gastric cancers *(160)*. In addition, replication errors in the form of somatic mutations were found at different microsatellite loci in nonfamilial colorectal cancer *(161)*. The first indication that loss of TGFβ RII receptor may be linked to the development of cancer and escape from TGF-β-mediated growth control was demonstrated in colon cancer cell lines with high rates of microsatellite instability (RER+) and in xenografts of colon cancer tissue, also RER+, implanted into athymic mice *(162)*. Three different (somatic) frameshift mutations (and resultant protein truncation) were found within a 10-bp polyadenine repeat of the RII coding region in the RER+ samples, which was accompanied by decreased RII transcripts and complete loss of RII cell surface receptors *(162,163)*. In two subsequent studies, the correlation of mutations in RII with RER+ was shown to be at the rate of 71% in 25 HNPCC patients and at 90% in another study (100/111), again, specifically in the polyadenine region of RII (RER+) *(164,165)*. Thus, in these studies, tumor progression was related to a defect in DNA repair enzymes, which was linked to mutations in a small region of repeat sequences (vulnerable to RER+-associated mechanisms of mutation) in the TGF-β RII. In addition, four missense inactivating mutations in the MADR2 gene were recently disclosed in colorectal carcinoma *(82)*. Since inactivation of TGF-β RII and MADR2 is a mechanism by which human colon cancer cells lose growth inhibitory responsiveness to TGF-β, these two genes can also be considered as tumor suppressor genes.

Gastric Cancer

Gastric cancer is a major cause of morbidity and mortality worldwide *(166)*. Certain tissue changes representing sequential steps toward the development of gastric malignancies are noted. These include superficial gastritis, chronic atrophic gastritis (of glands), small intestinal metaplasia, colonic metaplasia and dysplasia *(166,167)*, pernicious anemia, *Helicobacter pylori* infection, Menetriers disease, adenomatous polyps, Barrett's esophagus, and ingestion of carcinogens *(168)*. There is a 30–40% 5-yr survival rate following curative total gastrectomy; however, it is <20% overall. Elevated levels of TGF-β1 were reported in human gastric cancer; this increase was suggested to have a causative role in scirrhous gastric cancer *(169,170)*. To determine the distribution of TGF-β isoforms in the normal stomach compared to gastric carcinoma, we analyzed four normal mucosal samples, 12 normal mucosal samples adjacent to tumors, and 12 gastric carcinomas (intestinal-type) for TGF-β mRNA and protein expression, by Northern blot analysis and immunohistochemistry, respectively *(20)*. There was a remarkable nonoverlapping differential distribution of each TGF-β isoform in normal stomach. TGF-β1 was localized in the cytoplasm of the acid-secreting parietal cells, which are distributed along the length of the glands but most numerous in isthmus (middle) region. TGF-β1 was also present in some surface mucus-secreting glands, which cover the entire luminal surface of the stomach and line the gastric pits *(171)*. In contrast, TGF-β2 immunoreactivity was exclusively confined to the pepsin-secreting chief cells, located toward the base of the gastric glands. TGF-β3 was present in mucus, parietal, and chief cells. Since these cell types of the gastric mucosa perform specific functions, it is possible that each TGF-β isoform may have different functions in the stomach. The gastric cancers showed intense immunoreactivity for all three TGF-β isoforms and a 4.8- ($p < 0.001$) and 6-fold ($p < 0.003$) increase in the synthesis of TGF-β mRNA compared to normal gastric tissue, for TGF-β1 and TGF-β3, respectively. TGF-β2 mRNA levels were comparable between the normal and cancerous tissue. In addition, a 10-fold increase in collagen type 1α mRNA was observed in gastric cancer. This is of interest since TGF-β1 has been shown to promote extensive fibrosis in the cancer stroma and granulation tissue in scirrhous gastric cancer by stimulating collagen deposition by fibroblasts, which contract the collagenous stroma leading to a disorder referred to as "linitis plastica" *(170,172,173)*. In this study, collagen type Iα, TGF-β1, and TGF-β3 mRNA were highest in the poorly differentiated partly scirrhous type of gastric cancer, also indicating that the high levels of TGF-βs produced by the malignant cells may lead to the fibrotic phenotype of this specific cancer.

TGF-β inhibits the growth of gastric epithelial cells in culture *(174)*. TGF-β1 mRNA was present in 12 gastric cancer cell lines; however, RI and RII mRNA was not expressed in 6/12 of them *(175)*. The presence of RI and RII conferred TGF-β-induced apoptosis in these lines. Thus, absence of TGF-β receptors in gastric cancers may eliminate normal apoptosis necessary for cell renewal. Whereas growth stimulation of the poorly differentiated adenocarcinomas has not been reported, it is likely, as shown in colon cancers, that the overexpression of TGF-β isoforms in gastric cancer represents a breakdown in the growth inhibitory response to TGF-βs and that the excessive amounts of TGF-β present is both angiogenic and immunosuppressive. Alterations in the expression of several oncogenes and tumor suppressor genes have been demonstrated in gastric cancers *(176)*. As shown in colon cancers, the RER+ phenotype is highly associated with the familial cancer syndrome HNPCC *(160)*. Following the original report that indicated that mutations in the TGF-β RII was connected with a defect in mismatch repair enzymes, loss of TGF-β receptors, and loss of growth inhibitory control by TGF-β, a subsequent study similarly showed the identical frameshift mutation occurring at a rate of 71% in RER+ gastric cancers *(163)*. Thus, the TGF-β RII is a target for mutation (inactivation) in mismatch repair-deficient gastric tumors. However, another study did not find mutations in RII associated with RER+ gastric cancers *(177)*. Overexpression of cyclin E was found in gastric carcinomas *(91,106)*, which would promote transition to S-phase.

Endometrial Hyperplasia and Carcinoma

Endometrial cancer is the most common gynecological malignancy and ranks as the fourth most common among women in the United States (39,000/yr); 75% occur in perimenopausal and postmenopausal women (review in refs. *178–181*). In endometrial carcinoma, hyperplasia of the glandular epithelium (especially with cytologic atypia) precedes carcinoma *(179–182)*, providing an excellent model to study the changes in response to TGF-β that accompany tumorigenesis and progression. In fact, tissue specimens from endometrial carcinoma often represent a histopathological spectrum ranging from normal to malignant tissue and including both simple and complex hyperplasia *(183)*. A major cause of endometrial hyperplasia is chronic stimulation of the endometrium by estrogen in the absence of progesterone (e.g., anovulation, unopposed estrogen therapy [ERT]) *(180,182–185)*. The glandular epithelial cells that give rise to endometrial carcinoma respond to estrogen with increased proliferative activity. Many studies have shown that after 10–15 yr of therapeutic doses of estrogen the risk for endometrial cancer increases by 10-fold *(182)*. A more recent concern is that there is a 7.5-fold risk in the development of endometrial cancer in patients receiving the antiestrogen, Tamoxifen (Tam), for estrogen receptor (ER)-responsive breast tumors (reviewed in refs. *186,187*). Tam has opposite effects in these two tissues because of activation of different tissue-specific response elements by the ERs complexed with the steroids *(188)*. Conversely, progestins are used therapeutically to induce regression of endometrial carcinoma *(178,179,182)*. We were interested in studying the expression of TGF-β isoforms in the endometrium since it is a target organ for autocrine, paracrine, and endocrine regulation of proliferation, differentiation, and angiogenesis and is highly active in these processes. Tissue specimens from 70 patients representing normal, hyperplastic (simple and complex), and carcinomatous endometrium were analyzed in the laboratory *(11)*. The endometrium consists mainly of glandular epithelial cells and stromal cells. In the normal endometrium, immunoreactivity for TGF-β isoforms is localized differentially. TGF-β1 and TGF-β3 is present in both the glands and stroma and TGF-β2 is more intense in the stroma *(11)*. Expression of TGF-βs is increased in the secretory compared to the proliferative phase of the menstrual cycle, indicating possible steroidal regulation of TGF-β. The glandular epithelium demonstrated a statistically progressive increase in TGF-β isoform immunoreactivity from normal to simple hyperplasia and on to complex hyperplasia, with no further increase in adenocarcinoma. In contrast, the stromal element was unchanged. In comparison with proliferative endometrium, there was a 5.1-, 3.4-, and 2.6-fold increase in TGF-β1, TGF-β2, and TGF-β3 immunoreactivity, respectively ($p \leq 0.001$) in complex hyperplasia (Fig. 3A [normal] and 3B [complex hyperplasia]). In contrast, by *in situ* hybridization using isoform-specific riboprobes, a progressive increase in mRNA levels for all three TGF-β isoforms that varied directly with disease severity was observed in the stromal cell constituent. These results suggested that there may be a switch from an autocrine, in the normal endometrium, to a paracrine mechanism of action in the pathological endometrium (Table 1). The marked increase in TGF-β immunoreactive protein and mRNA in complex hyperplasia suggested that TGF-βs play a role in the regulation of endometrial growth and in the development of hyperplasia. Moreover, in this preneoplastic disease events have already occurred that may have caused the glandular epithelium not to respond to TGF-β as a growth inhibitor.

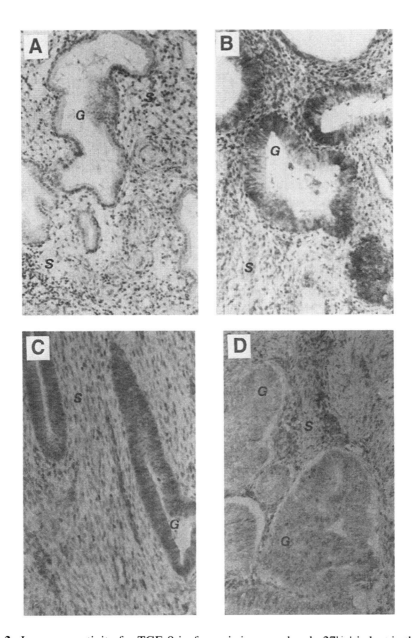

Fig. 3. Immunoreactivity for TGF-β isoforms is increased and p27[kip1] is lost in the glands of patients with endometrial hyperplasia and carcinoma. Paraffin sections were treated with primary antibody, followed by peroxidase-labeled secondary antibody. The color was developed with DAB as substrate. **(A, B)** Rabbit anti-TGF-β3: Intense immunoreactivity for TGF-β3 can be observed in the glands (G) of complex hyperplasia in (B) compared to little to no immunostaining in the glands of normal secretory endometrium in (A). The stromal (S) cells are moderately immunoreactive in both normal and hyperplastic endometrium (from ref. *11*). **(C,D)** Mouse (monoclonal) antibody to p27[kip1] (a cyclin-dependent kinase inhibitor [CKI]). P27[kip1] is normally induced by TGF-β and prevents cells from entering DNA synthesis (S phase) by binding to cyclin E/cdk2 and preventing pRB phosphorylation. This blocks cells late in G1. As shown in (C) in the normal endometrium, p27 levels are high in the glands. However, the glands of a differentiated adenocarcinoma have completely lost immunoreactivity for p27, as shown in (D). This may be caused by excessive degradation of p27 in proteasomes *(120)*. Cancer cells may have increased degradation of p27 *(154)*, which may aid their escape from negative growth control (by TGF-β).

Hormonal responses in target organs have been shown to be mediated by growth factors (reviewed in refs. *188,190*). Since, as described above, endometrial carcinoma is etiologically related to estrogen stimulation and ameliorated by progestins, this malignancy is ideal for studying the effects of gonadal steroids on TGF-β mediated/related growth control and its role in neoplastic progression. The development, growth, and differentiation of the endometrium and other hormone-responsive organs is dependent on a strong collaboration between its constituent stromal and epithelial cells *(191)*. Hormonal effects on epithelial cells are often elicited through stromal hormone receptors via paracrine mechanisms (shown for mammary, prostate, and endometrium) (reviewed in refs. *189,192*). In proof, using human endometrial explants, we have previously shown that progesterone induces stromal cells to secrete TGF-β that subsequently acts on the glandular epithelial cells to reduce the levels of the metalloproteinase matrylisin, a necessary event associated with the secretory phase of the menstrual cycle *(193)*. Our more recent studies are therefore directed toward determining cellular mechanisms involved in the loss of cellular growth inhibitory response to TGF-β and the role for stomal/epithelial interactions and steroid-induced effects in the regulation of this response.

In the past, cell lines derived from endometrial carcinoma have been employed to study their growth response to TGF-β and they have shown inhibitory, refractory, and stimulatory growth profiles *(194–196)*. Since results utilizing cell lines cannot reliably be employed as physiological paradigms, we have examined the effects of TGF-β in primary cultures (90% pure) of glandular epithelial cells derived from endometrial carcinoma tissue compared to normal tissue. Exogneously added TGF-β1 inhibited the growth of normal endometrial glandular cells by 20–50%, whereas the growth of endometrial carcinoma cells were not growth inhibited ($n = 10$ of each; *262*). In addition, by Northern blot hybridization using ^{32}P-UTP riboprobes, the glandular epithelial cells from two patients exhibited a smaller mRNA TGF-β RII species. In one of these patients, we discovered an adenine deletion in a poly A region of the 5' half of the TGF-β RII mRNA in 50% of the cloned mRNA (3/6), indicating that a (somatic) frame shift mutation had ocurred and also explaining the loss of the TGF-β growth inhibitory response in these cells. Accordingly, by immunohistochemical analysis, a loss of RI and RII was demonstrated in the corresponding tumor tissue. In another report, out of eight RER+ endometrial carcinoma tissues screened for mutations in the TGF-β RII, one patient showed a deletion that inactivates RII through a frameshift mutation *(164)*. This mutation was not found in corresponding normal cells, indicating that a somatic mutation had occurred. In contrast, another study only found mutations in the TGF-β RII in 17% in RER+ endometrial carcinoma cell lines and tumor tissues compared to mutations found in 71% in RER+ gastric cancers *(163)*.

The CKI p27 is regulated by TGF-β and is important in maintaining cells in G_0. Since p27 was not found to have mutations or deletions in the gene, or to be regulated at the level of transcription (described above/cell cycle) *(118,119)*, we and others have investigated possible differences between tumor and normal cells at the level of protein expression *(154,197)*. By immunohistochemistry, six endometrial carcinoma tissue specimens showed a nearly complete loss of p27 compared to normals (Fig. 1C [normal] and 1D [carcinoma]). This is contrasted with the overexpression of TGF-β3 in complex hyperplasia, shown in Fig. 1B, compared to normal tissue, shown in Fig. 1A.

Therefore, interestingly, concomitant with the aberrant overexpression of TGF-β in complex hyperplasia is the loss of p27 from the carcinoma cells. In addition, immunostaining for p27 was slightly higher in an area of complex hyperplasia compared to regions of adenocarcinoma. These results indicate a progressive loss of p27 with increasing lesion severity. Therefore, another mechanism by which endometrial cells may escape TGF-β-related growth regulation is by reduction of p27, most likely through ubiquitin-mediated degradation in proteasomes; this is currently under investigation *(120)*.

In preliminary studies, Northern blot analyses performed in our laboratory have shown that primary cultures of endometrial stromal and glandular cells from patients with endometrial cancer displayed an altered expression of TGF-β mRNA and receptors compared to normal stromal cells in response to different gonadal steroids (i.e., estrogen, progestins, Tam) *(261,262)*. For example, TGF-β1 mRNA was induced by progesterone in normal stromal cells but the stromal cells from the cancer patients lost this response and now responded to estrogen with increased expression of TGF-β1 mRNA *(261,262)*. Similarly, an increase in TGF-β RI, RII, and RIII mRNA was observed in response to combined estrogen and progesterone and Tam decreased the mRNA levels. However, TGF-β receptor mRNA levels in the stromal cells derived from malignant endometrial tissue were completely refractory to the steroids tested (*n* = 6). These studies suggest that the development of endometrial carcinoma may be related to loss of hormonal regulation of both TGF-β ligand and receptors, and further implicate the involvement of the interaction between steroids and growth factors in this estrogen-driven carcinoma and, most likely, in in other hormonally regulated cancers. Furthermore, the aberrant behavior of the stromal cells in a cancer of epithelial origin suggests that a breakdown in epithelial/stromal interactions may play a role in the pathogenesis of endometrial carcinoma.

Breast Cancer

Normal mammary epithelial cells and both estrogen receptor (ER)-positive and negative human breast cancer cells, in vitro, express TGF-β1 mRNA and protein and are growth inhibited by the addition of picomolar concentrations of TGF-β *(198–201)*. Growth inhibition of breast cancer cells can be induced by triphenylethylene antiestrogens, such as Tam, synthetic progestins, and retinoids, and is directly related to the induction of TGF-β (reviewed in ref. *202*), as shown by the following studies: The addition of inhibitory concentrations of antiestrogen to the ER-positive breast carcinoma cell line MCF-7 and the ER-negative breast cancer cell line MDA-231 induced an increase in the secretion of TGF-β1 protein and growth inhibitory activity *(199)*, and an increase in TGF-β1 mRNA *(203,204)*. Furthermore, in other ER-positive and ER-negative breast cancer cell lines, Tam caused a dose and time-dependent blockade in G1/G0 and induced apoptosis that was abolished by neutralizing antibody to TGF-β, thus proving that these responses were mediated solely by TGF-β. Moreover, these studies elucidated that the mechanism by which antiestrogens act as therapeutic agents in breast cancer, in vivo, is through TGF-β-mediated growth inhibition of breast cancer cells. It was reasoned that Tam may have a direct effect on TGF-β mRNA transcription since the response was not be mediated by the ER (in ER-negative breast cancer cells). In a separate study, Tam was shown not to induce TGF-β1 transcription in

MCF-7 cells, but to cause an increase in TGF-β1 by a posttranscriptional mechanism. However, TGF-β1 directly induced the transcription of TGF-β2; TGF-β2 was therefore considered a marker of Tam action *(205)*. In a study of 37 patients with ER-positive breast cancer, Tam treatment did not alter TGF-β1 or TGF-β3 protein expression but, in agreement with the study using MCF-7 cells, did augment TGF-β2 expression. Interestingly, the increase in TGF-β2 expression in 11/15 tumors also correlated with improvement-related therapy, which was not present in nonresponders *(206)*. High plasma levels of TGF-β2 during Tam therapy similarly reflected response to therapy *(205)*. In contrast to these studies, high expression of TGF-β has been shown to have deleterious effects. In vitro, constitutively high levels of TGF-β1 were secreted by estrogen-independent highly tumorigenic breast cancer cells *(207)*, indicating a possible lesion in the TGF-β response loop. Additionally, it has been shown that TGF-β1 mRNA was increased in transformed compared to normal breast epithelial cells *(208)* and the expression of TGF-β1 was shown to be associated with increased metastatic potential of mammary tumor cells *(209)*. MCF-7 cells, overexpressing TGF-β1 mRNA and protein through transfection (> 10-fold), showed 100% tumor formation following injection into ovariectomized athymic (nude) mice; the parent cells only formed tumors after estrogen supplementation *(210)*. Confirmation of higher levels of TGF-β1 in the tumors of the transfected cells than of the parent cell line was shown immunohistochemically. To further complicate the role of TGF-βs in breast cancer, another study using transgenic mice that were genetically engineered to secrete TGF-β1 in its active form did not form spontaneous tumors. However, mammary duct development was inhibited but not alveolar outgrowth during pregnancy *(211)*.

Apart from studies employing cells in culture and in vivo studies employing strains of mice and genetically manipulated cells, we studied 30 breast cancer specimens for intensity of TGF-β isoform immunostaining; this information was related to tumor recurrence, progression, or last follow-up (time) *(15)*. In benign breast tissue, TGF-β1 immunoreactivity was observed in ductal epithelium, TGF-β2 primarily in stromal fibroblasts and the luminal surfaces of ducts, and TGF-β3 in stromal fibroblasts and myoepithelial cells surrounding the glandular epithelial cells. In contrast, the breast carcinomas showed greater variability in the intensity of immunostaining for all TGF-β isoforms. The patients were divided into two groups: tumors that expressed high levels and those that contained low levels of each TGF-β isoform. Kaplan-Meier plots were generated by comparison of intensity with progression-free survival. The results indicated that TGF-β1, but not TGF-β2 or TGF-β3, was positively associated with the rate of disease progression, which was independent of age, stage, estrogen receptor status, or nodal involvement ($p = 0.009$) (Table 1).

More recent studies have elucidated mechanisms by which breast cancer cells can escape growth regulation by TGF-β leading to malignant progression. Although mutations in TGF-β RII have not been reported, as described above for pancreatic, colon, gastric, and endometrial cancers, loss or decrease in the TGF-β RII has been shown to be related to decreased sensitivity to the growth inhibitory activity of TGF-β in both ER-positive and ER-negative breast cancer cell lines *(201)*. These same cell lines were also tested for their growth inhibitory response to activin, another member of the TGF-β family shown to share a common RI (ALK-1). Interestingly, whereas ER-positive cell lines were growth inhibited by activin A, the ER-negative lines were unresponsive.

TGF-β RIIs were absent in two T47D breast cancer cell line variants shown to be resistant to TGF-β. Growth inhibition (both anchorage-dependent in monolayer and anchorage-independent in soft agar) by TGF-β1 and TGF-β2 was restored following stable transfection of RII into these cells. Consistent with these results, stable transfection of TGF-β RII into MCF-7 cells yielded clones of cells that displayed decreased malignancy by a variety of criteria: They were more sensitive to growth arrest, showed reduced clonogencity (in soft agar) and tumorigenicity (in ovariectomized athymic mice), and showed delayed tumor formation compared to clones with low levels of RII *(212)*. Thus, with signal transduction pathways for TGF-β intact, RII can rescue the malignant phenotype of breast cancer cells. However, other TGF-β-related defects have been found associated with breast cancer. The cyclin D1 gene, located on chromosome 11q13, is amplified in 13% of primary breast carcinomas (and in 43% of head and neck squamous cell carcinomas *[406]*. Interestingly, however, more than 50% of breast carcinomas overexpress cyclin D1 protein, suggesting that transcriptional or translational regulation may cause abundance of this gene product, propelling cells into a hyperproliferative state (increased phosphorylation of RB). In support of the oncogenic potential caused by overexpression of cyclin D, targeted overexpression of cyclin D1 in mammary epithelial cells led to ductal hyperproliferation and subsequent tumor formation in transgenic mice. Accordingly, mice lacking expression of D1, by targeted deletion of this gene, lacked a normal mammary proliferative response during pregnancy (in the presence of steroid hormones) *(213)*. This indicates that steroid-induced proliferation of mammary epithelium may be transduced by D1 cyclins. Conversely, cyclins D2 and D3 are not overexpressed in human cancers, possibly because of chromosomal locations that may not be amplified *(91)*. Cyclin E is also overexpressed in breast cancer *(214)*. Inactivation of p16 by gene mutation was shown in 4/4 normal breast epithelial cells that were immortalized in tissue culture but was not found in 24 primary breast carcinomas. However, loss of heterozygosity (LOH) in chromosome 9p21–22, proximal to the locus for the p16 gene, was present in 58% of these cases, indicating another possible tumor suppressor gene in this region *(215)*. This study suggests that inactivation of p16 may, in part, be responsible for adapting breast epithelial cells to culture. The absence of the cyclin-dependent kinase inhibitor protein (CKI), p27[kip1], in cancer was also demonstrated in a recent breast cancer study involving 202 patients with stage T1a,b, characterized by tumor size of 1.0 cm. In this study, low expression or loss of p27[kip1] protein in breast carcinomas was shown to be an independent prognostic marker for decreased survival, with a relative risk of death from disease of 3.1 for low expressors *(197)*. As shown for colon and endometrial cancers, breast cancer cells may reduce the levels of p27[kip1] through the ubiquitin-proteasome pathway and thus, loss of p27, important in TGF-β-related cell cycle control, may be a significant factor in the development of human breast cancer.

Gliomas

Gliomas, the most common primary brain tumor, are derived from neuroectodermal glial cells (reviewed in ref. *216*). TGF-β isoforms play a role in neural embryogenesis, by regulation of proliferation and differentiation and in neoplasia, through proliferative and immunosuppressive effects (reviewed in ref. *12*). Patients with glioblastomas are markedly immunosuppressed *(218)*. This observation led to the isolation of a "T cell suppressor factor" (TcSF) from a glioblastoma cell line, which inhibited T cell activity in vitro *(218)*. This factor was later proven to be the TGF-β2 isoform; all TGF-βs demonstrate a potent suppressive effect on many immune cells (reviewed in refs. *1,4,44*). For example, TGF-βs inhibit the activity of Natural Killer cells (NK), lymphokine-activated killer cells (LAK), tumor-infiltrating lymphocytes (TILs), antigen-specific cytotoxic lymphocytes, and the proliferative activity of many immune cells (e.g., T and B cells) *(44,217,219*, and reviewed in ref. *220)*. Specifically, TGF-β interferes with the induction of cytotoxic lymphocytes and inhibits helper T cell production of cytokines (e.g., IL-2) *(219,220)*. TGF-β induces apoptosis in T cell lines and may prevent tumor cell killing by inducing apoptosis of TILs in vivo (reviewed in ref. *219)*. The progression of lower-grade astrocytomas to a more malignant phenotype is associated with the activation of oncogenes and inactivation of tumor suppressor genes *(221)*. In addition, amplification and overexpression of growth factors, such as EGF and PDGF, causing autocrine positive regulation, occurs at high rate in gliomas *(222)*.

The present histopathological grading system of astrocytomas (graded I–IV) does not discriminate among subgroups within the classification and does not consistently correlate with survival. Based on the idea that TGF-β2 and probably TGF-β1 expression may promote tumor growth in the brain through aberrant growth control and by suppressing host defenses, we postulated that a poorer prognosis might be associated with elevated expression of TGF-β2 or one of the other isoforms. We therefore evaluated the mRNA synthesis and expression of TGF-β isoforms in graded astrocytomas *(21)*. In the normal brain, the mRNA and protein for all isoforms of TGF-β were found in neural cells of the cerebrum, oligodendrocytes, leptomeningeal cells, purkinje cells of the cerebellum, and in smooth muscle cells and endothelial cells of vessels. Whereas TGF-β2 and TGF-β3 were expressed by astrocytes, TGF-β1 was not present in these cells. However, in all astrocytomas, irrespective of pathological grade, there was an increase in the expression of all TGF-β isoforms in both tumor and "reactive" astrocytes. Thus, TGF-β1 may be a potential marker for carcinogenesis in astrocytomas (Table 1). Furthermore, tumor specimens showing increased expression of TGF-βs correlated with short term survival (<3 mo) (unpublished data). The mRNA was concordantly increased with protein expression, illustrating an autocrine mode of activity. In contrast, in primitive neuroectodermal tumors (PNETs), the poorly differentiated cells did not show immunostaining for TGF-β compared to positively immunoreactive more differentiated astrocytic cells. Gliosarcomas, composed of malignant sarcomatous and astrocytic components, showed marked expression of TGF-β isoforms in both cell constituents in all tumors examined. Normal brain adjacent to all tumor types showed increased immunoreactivity for TGF-βs, which decreased distal to the tumor, indicating a paracrine effect of TGF-β produced by the tumors on normal brain. A more recent study corroborated our results. In an animal model of gliomas, both TGF-β1 mRNA and protein were highly expressed in rat gliomas compared to lack of expression in the contralateral unaffected hemisphere. This increased expression of TGF-β1 was associated with the presence of macrophages, in the absence of detectable regression of the tumors *(223)*. In addition to showing increased expression of all three TGF-β isoforms in tissues of advanced malignant gliomas compared to benign gliosis, increased expression of RI and RII was also found *(224)*. Moreover, three glioma cell lines were refractory to the growth inhibitory effects of TGF-β although, they expressed TGF-β ligand and receptors.

In certain studies using primary cultures of resected malignant gliomas and PNETs, only latent inactive TGF-β was found in conditioned media (obviating growth inhibitory activity), whereas in other studies both glioblastoma cell lines and primary cultures produced active TGF-β1 and TGF-β2 *(12,13,225,226,228)*. Exogenously added TGF-β has been shown to inhibit normal astrocytes in culture and lower grades of both astrocytomas and PNETs *(12,13,227,228)*. As observed with colon cancer cells in vitro, there was a switch in growth response to exogenously added TGF-β1 and TGF-β2 from growth inhibition in lower grade astrocytomas to growth stimulation in higher grade astrocytomas, that also displayed increased anaplasia and karyotypic divergence *(228)*. Furthermore, whereas exogenous addition of TGF-β1 and TGF-β2 inhibited the proliferation and clonogenicity (growth in soft agar as a marker for transformation) in near diploid cultures of human medulloblastomas, neuroectodermal tumors, and ependymomas, TGF-βs were growth stimulatory to primary cultures derived from highly aggressive tumors that showed progressive anaplasia and karyotypic divergence *(13)*. Neutralizing antibodies to TGF-β caused growth stimulation in less malignant cells and growth inhibition in the poorly differentiated cells, confirming that TGF-β growth regulation is autocrine-regulated in these brain neoplasms. Recently, it was shown that exogenous TGF-β1 inhibited or stimulated glioma cell lines; however, TGF-β2 only stimulated these same cells *(229)*. Furthermore, using antisense oligodeoxynucleotide separately targeted for TGF-β1 mRNA and TGF-2 mRNA, it was determined that it was endogenously produced TGF-β2 that regulated glioma cell proliferation.

The role of TGF-β in immobilizing the immune system, obviating tumor killing, was directly shown in fluids derived from the cavities of partially removed glioblastomas. In an in vitro assay, these fluids inhibited the proliferation and antitumor cytotoxicity of LAK cells, isolated from the peripheral blood of these patients, which was ameliorated by neutralizing antibodies to TGF-β *(230)*. Antisense oligonucleotides specific for TGF-β reversed autologous T cell immunosuppression caused by the malignant gliomas, more directly indicating that the depressed systemic immune cellular response observed in patients with malignant gliomas is caused by the over production of TGF-β by the tumor *(231)*. In another experiment, transplanted rat gliosarcomas transfected with plasmids containing TGF-β antisense showed a significant number of animals surviving longer than animals containing control plasmid vectors *(232)*. Moreover, there was no evidence of residual antisense plasmid-containing tumors at transplantation sites. These antisense-containing tumor cells also possessed a three- to four-fold increase in an in vitro tumor cytotoxicity assay compared to controls. Taken together, these studies indicate that the failure of current adoptive cellular immunotherapy of malignant gliomas is related to the presence of increased amount of TGF-β locally released by the tumor. Therefore, immunotherapy for malignant gliomas should be more directed toward preventing local inactivation and apoptosis of immune cells otherwise targeted for glioma destruction *(219)*. TGF-β also contributes to the angiogenesis associated with tumors, both by its chemotactic effect on endothelial cells and by stimulating extracellular matrix proteins, including tenascin, which endothelial cells adhere and spread upon *(233,234)*. Increased expression of tenascin has been correlated with angiogenesis in brain tumors. In addition, TGF-β1 has been shown to be highly stimulatory in an in vitro assay of tumor cell migration and invasiveness *(235)*.

In search of mechanisms that are faulty in TGF-β growth regulation of gliomas, loss of TGF-β receptors (or mutations thereof) have not, as yet, been described. However, mutations and/or deletions in genes of proteins that control the cell cycle in response to TGF-β have been found. The gene encoding CDK4, located on chromosome 12q13, was shown to be amplified in gliomas *(106)*. Hypermethylation of the promoter region (5'-CpG islands) of the p15 gene, resulting in inactivation by loss of transcription, has been shown to be a specific aberration associated with gliomas and leukemias compared to other cancers *(110)*. Others have found both p15 and p16 genes homozygously deleted (no intragenic mutations were found) in glioblastoma multiforme (in primary tumors and xenograft of these tumors) but not in medulloblastomas or ependymonas *(108)*. Thus, loss of both p15 and p16 may play a role in glioblastoma tumorigenesis. In general, these studies present examples of the "classic" loss of tumor suppressor gene function, specifically of proteins that inhibit cyclin-dependent kinase activity (i.e., p15, p16) necessary for DNA synthesis in cancer pathogenesis.

Osteosarcomas

Osteosarcomas, malignant bone tumors that produce osteoid, are the most common human primary tumor of the bone, most often observed in males and in the second decade of life *(236)*. Bone is one of the most abundant sources of TGF-β isoforms *(56,57)*. Accordingly, TGF-βs are major regulators of bone formation in vivo and in vitro (reviewed in refs. *1,4,9*). Injection of TGF-β1 into the subperiosteal region of rat femurs results in stimulation of new bone, resembling embryologic bone formation and fracture repair *(237)*, and the exogenous application of TGF-β-induced repair of intramembraneous bone and of calvarial defects *(238,239)*. TGF-β isoforms induce both osteogeneic and chondrogenic bone repair by recruiting osteoblasts and osteoclasts to the injured area, increasing the proliferation of these cells and inducing their production of extracellular matrix proteins *(238* and reviewed in ref. *240)*. Previous studies showed that, in vitro, osteosarcoma cell lines produce both latent and active TGF-β, possess TGF-β receptors, respond to exogenous TGF-β by growth stimulation, and are growth-inhibited in the presence of neutralizing antibodies to TGF-β, indicating an autocrine stimulatory loop *(241)*. Because these studies indicated a possible role for TGF-β in osteosarcoma cell growth and our studies of various cancers indicated that increased expression of TGF-β isoforms correlated with disease progression and decreased patient survival, we undertook a study to determine the prevalence and distribution of TGF-β isoforms in high grade, stage 2B classical osteosarcoma of the appendicular skeleton *(19)*. Moreover, this is the first cancer studied whereby TGF-β normally stimulates cell growth of the normal cell counterpart. Twenty-five osteosarcomas classified as osteoblastic, chondroblastic, fibroblastic, telangiectatic, giant cell, or mixed were studied by immunohistochemistry and intensity compared with patient survival. The mineralized bone in normal or osteosarcoma tissue and normal nonmineralized bone showed little immunoreactivity. Interestingly, TGF-β has previously been shown to inhibit bone mineralization, and overexpression of TGF-β2 in transgenic osteoblasts resulted in an osteoporosis-like phenotype *(242)*. Moderate to intense immunostaining for one or more of the TGF-β isoforms was present in the tumor cells and slightly in the surrounding extracellular matrix of all the osteosarcomas (TGF-β1 = 44%; TGF-β2 = 23%, TGF-β3 = 56%). Tumor osteocytes embedded in woven bone were more strongly immunoreactive for all TGF-β isoforms than normal osteocytes in normal lamellar bone, and actively resorbing osteoclasts at the outer edges of pathologic bone were highly immunoreactive. Following construction of Kaplan-Meier plots of survival, there was a statistically significant decrease in disease-free survival as the intensity of immunoreactivity for TGF-β3 increased ($p < 0.006$); TGF-β1 and TGF-β2 did not show this correlation. Thus, TGF-β3 may play a role in the progression of osteosarcomas and may provide a prognostic marker for this highly malignant subgroup of bone tumors (Table 1). A high level of angiogenesis, demonstrating intense immunoreactivity for TGF-βs, was observed in the endothelial cells and perivascular muscle cells within the tumors and in the stroma surrounding 50% of tumors, depicting the angiogenic role for TGF-β in these tumors. In another study, increased immunostaining for TGF-β1 and TGF-β3 was demonstrated in Ewings sarcoma and rhabdomyosarcomas in children *(243)*. Also, in recurrent giant cell tumors of the bone, TGF-β1 and TGF-β2 mRNA was observed in osteoclast-like giant cells, neoplastic stromal cells, and osteoblasts active in forming metaplastic bone (TGF-β3 expression was not analyzed) *(244)*. Since TGF-β stimulates the growth of normal mesenchymally derived bone cells, high levels of TGF-β may provide a continuous autocrine and paracrine-positive stimulation of growth of bone tumors. In this light, constitutive activation of CDKs or loss of tumor suppressor genes may not permit osteosarcomas to leave the cell cycle for quiescence in G0, hence causing their continuous cycling/proliferation. Certainly both the angiogenic and immunosuppressant effects of abnormally high levels of TGF-β would favor tumor growth and survival. Moreover, most likely the TGF-β present in osteosarcomas is in its activated form since osteoclasts, containing a lysosomal acidic environment, are, to date, one of the only known cellular physiological activators of latent TGF-β *(245)*. In other studies, the presence of BMPs (of the TGF-β superfamily) in a subset of human osteosarcomas was correlated with a particular histological subtype, a poor response to chemotherapy, and a poor clinical outcome *(246)*. No reports of deletions of inhibitors of the cell cycle have emerged associated with osteosarcomas. However, inactivation/LOH of the tumor suppressor gene, RB, is predisposed in sarcomas and osteosarcomas *(247–249)* and recently LOH at chromosome 18q, associated with MADR2 loss of function (TGF-β receptor-induced transcription factor), was reported *(263)*.

Reflections on TGF-β in the Etiopathogenesis of Cancer

Consistent with the concept that escape from negative growth control is a critical element in neoplastic development and progression, the role for TGF-β is of distinct significance. Since TGF-β is a natural inhibitor of epithelial and neuroectodermal cells, it is most important to study the breakdown in the growth inhibitory response in carcinomas and in brain malignancies. However, as we have shown, both highly aggressive colon carcinomas and gliomas (GBMs) have switched from being autocrine growth inhibited to autocrine growth stimulated. Thus, it is apparent that these particular cells should have TGF-β receptors intact to transduce the growth-stimulatory response following TGF-β ligand binding. Moreover, new "abnormal" signal transduction pathways as well as activation of a different set of genes by different transcription factors would ostensibly accompany this opposite growth effect on cells. In light of the studies that indicate that a high percentage of gastric and colon cancers have mutations in the TGF-β RII, one would predict that these particular cells would not be able to be stimulated by TGF-β, but instead, would be refractory to any TGF-β effects. In the past two years, a plethora of exciting discoveries have not only increased our depth of understanding of mechanisms of TGF-β-related growth inhibition with respect to proteins that control the cell cycle and in signal transduction, but have also elucidated where aberrations occur in the pathway that elicits the growth inhibitory response to TGF-βs that lead to cancer. Specifically, mutations and/or altered expression/levels (genes and proteins) found in TGF-β receptors, cell cycle proteins involved in effectuating the TGF-β growth inhibitory response (i.e., CKIs), and a key transcriptional activator, MADR2, directly responsive to the TGF-β signaling receptor complex, have vastly improved our understanding of how tumor cells escape negative growth control by TGF-β. In every cancer presented herein, we have shown that often different investigators have obtained directly opposite results with respect to whether the expression, overexpression (transfection experiments), or lack of expression of TGF-β by a particular tumor cell type promotes or inhibits a more aggressive behavior and/or malignant phenotype. The complexity observed can be explained by the fact that both cell lines and primary cultures derived from cancer cells at various stages of malignancy have incurred a different set(s) of defects that contribute to the multistep process toward tumor progression. Furthermore, as explained, apart from the inherent effect on tumor cells, the high levels of TGF-β that are released by the most aggressive tumor types, including epithelial, neuroectodermal, and mesenchymally derived tumor cell types, are both highly immunosuppressive (and also originally affecting immunosurveillance) and angiogenic, favoring tumor cell growth. The eminent task is to more rigorously associate the specific defects within the pathway of the TGF-β growth inhibitory response with tumor stage, so that this new information can be useful both prognostically and in designing appropriate adjuvant therapy.

REFERENCES

1. Massague J. The transforming growth factor-β family. Annu Rev Cell Biol 1990; *6:*597–641.
2. Moses HL, Pietenpol JA, Munger K, Murphy CS, Yang EY. TGF-β regulation of epithelial cell proliferation: role of tumor suppressor genes. Princess Takamatsu Symp 1991; *22:*183–195.
3. Massague J, Cheifetz S, Laiho M, Ralph DA, Weis FMB, Zentella A. Transforming growth factor-β. In: Franks LM (ed). Cancer surveys. Tumor suppressor genes, the cell cycle and cancer vol XII, Cold Spring Harbor Laboratory, Cold Spring Harbor, NY, 1992; pp. 81–103.
4. Sporn MB, Roberts AB. TGF-β: problems and prospects. Cell Regulation 1990; *1:*875–882.
5. Kingsley DM. The TGF-β superfamily: new members, new receptors, and new genetic tests of function in different organisms. Genes Develp 1994; *8:*133–146.
6. Miyazono K, Ichijo H, Heldin C-H. Transforming growth factor-β: latent forms, binding proteins and receptors. Growth Factors 1993; *8:*11–22.
7. Daopin S, Piez KA, Ogawa Y, Davies DR. Crystal structure of transforming growth factor-β2: an unusual fold for the superfamily. Science 1992; *257:*369–373.
8. Schlunegger MP, Grutter MG. An unusual feature revealed by the crystal structure of 2.2 Å resolution of human transforming growth factor-β. Nature 1992; *358:*430–434.

9. Pelton RW, Saxena B, Jones M, Moses HL, Gold LI. Immunohistochemical localization of TGF-β1, TGF-β2, and TGF-β3 in the mouse embryo: expression patterns suggest multiple roles during embryonic development. J Cell Biol 1991; *115:*1091–1105.

10. Pelton RW, Johnson MD, Perkett EA Gold LI, Moses HL. Expression of transforming growth factor-β1, β2, and β3 mRNA and protein in the murine lung. Am J Respir Cell Mol Biol 1991; *5:*522–530.

11. Gold L, Saxena B, Mittal K, Marmor M, Goswami S, Nactigal L, Korc M, Demopoulos R. Increased expression of transforming growth factor-β isoforms and basic fibroblast growth factor in complex hyperplasia and adenocarcinoma of the endometrium: evidence for paracrine and autocrine action. Cancer Res 1994; *54:*2347–2358.

12. Johnson MD, Jennings MT, Gold LI, Moses HL Transforming growth factor-β in neural embryogenesis and neoplasia. Human Pathol 1993; *24:*457–462.

13. Jennings MT, Kaariainen BA, Gold LI, Maciunas RJ, Commers BA TGF-β1 and TGF-β2 are potential growth regulators for medulloblastomas, primitive neuroectodermal tumors and eppendymomas: evidence in support of an autocrine hypothesis. Human Pathol 1994; *25:*464–475.

14. Gold L, Korc M. Expression of transforming growth factor-β1, 2 and 3 mRNA and protein in human cancers. Dig Surg 1994; *11:*150–156.

15. Gorsch SF, Memoli VA, Stukel TA, Gold LI, Arrick BA. Immunohistochemical staining for transforming growth factor-β1 associates with disease progression in human breast cancer. Cancer Res 1992; *52:*6949–6952.

16. Friess H, Yamanka Y, Buchler M, Ebert M, Beger HG, Gold LI, Korc M. Enhanced expression of transforming growth factor β isoforms in pancreatic cancer correlates with decreased survival. Gastroenterology 1993; *105:*1846–1856.

17. Hafez MM, Gold LI, Klimstra D, Zeng Z, Zauber A, Winawer S, Cohen A, Friedman E. High levels of TGF-β1 by immunohistochemistry correlate with disease progression in human colon cancer. Cancer Epidemiol Biomarkers Prevention 1995; *4:*549–554.

18. Moss SF, Liu TC, Petrotos A, Shu T, Gold LI, Holt PR. Inward growth of colonic adenomatous polyps. Gastroenterology 1996; *111:*1425–1432.

19. Kloen P, Gebhardt MC, Perez-Atayde A, Rosenberg AS, Springfield DS, Gold LI, Mankin HJ. Expression of transforming growth factor-beta (TGF-β) isoforms in osteosarcomas: TGF-β3 is related to disease progression. Cancer 1997; *80:*2230–2239.

20. Naef M, Ishiwata T, Friess H, Buchler M, Gold LI, Korc M. Differential localization of transforming growth factor β isoforms in human gastric mucosa and over-expression in gastric carcinoma. Int J Cancer 1997; *71:*131–137.

21. Gold LI, Saxena B, Zagzag D, Miller DC, Koslow M, Brandeis L, Farmer JP. Increased expression of TGF-β isoforms by malignant gliomas. J Cell Biol 1992; *16B:*122.

22. Levine JH, Moses HL, Gold LI, Nanney LB. Spatial and temporal patterns of immunoreactive TGF-β1, β2, and β3 during excisional wound repair. Am J Pathol 1993; *143:*368–380.

23. Chegini N, Gold LI, Williams RS, Masterson BJ. Localization of transforming growth factor beta isoforms TGF-β1, TGF-β2, TGF-β3 in surgically induced pelvic adhesions in the rat. Obstet Gynecol 1994; *83:*449–454.

24. Botney MD, Bahadori LM, Gold LI. Vascular remodeling in primary hypertension: potential role for transforming growth factor-β. Am J Pathol 1994; *144:*286–295.

25. Perkett EA, Pelton RW, Meyrick B, Gold LI, Miller DA. Expression of transforming growth factor-β mRNAs and proteins in pulmonary vascular remodeling in the sheep air embolization model of pulmonary hypertension. Am J Resp Cell Mol Biol 1994; *11:*16–24.

26. McMullen H, Longaker MT, Cabrera RC, Sung JJ, Canete J, Siebert JW, Lorenz HP, Gold LI. Analysis of TGF-β1, TGF-β2, and TGF-β3 immunoreactivity during ovine wound repair. Wound Repair Regen 1995; *3:*141–156.

27. Bhadori L, Milder J, Gold LI, Botney MD. Macrophage associated TGF-β co-localizes with type 1 procollagen gene expression in atherosclerotic human pulmonary arteries. Am J Pathol 1995; *146:*1140–1149.

28. Santana A, Saxena B, Nobel NA, Gold LI, Marshall BC. Increased expression of transforming growth factor β isoforms (β1,β2,β3) in bleomycin-induced pulmonary fibrosis. Am J Resp Cell Mol Biol. 1995; *13:*34–44.

29. Shihab FS, Yamamoto T, Nast CC, Cohen AH, Nobel NA, Gold LI, Border WA. Transforming growth factor-β in acute and chronic rejection of the kidney correlates with fibrosis. J Am Soc Nephrol 1995; *6:*286–294.

30. Yamamoto T, Nobel NA, Cohen AH, Hishida A, Gold LI, Border WA. Expression of transforming growth-β isoforms in human glomerular disease. Kidney Int 1996; *49:*461–469.

31. Johnson MD, Gold LI. Distribution of transforming growth factor β in HIV-1 encephalitis. Human Pathol 1996; *27:*643–649.

32. Shankland S, Pippin J, Pichler RH, Gordon KL, Friedman S, Gold LI, Johnson RJ, Couser WG. Differential expression of transforming growth factor-β isoforms and receptors in experimental membranous nephropathy. Kidney Int 1996; *50:*116–124.

33. Meddahi A, Caruelle JP, Gold LI, Rosso V, Barritault D. New concepts in tissue repair: skin as an example. Diabetes Metab 1996; *22:*274–278.

34. Friess H, Zhao L, Riesle E, Waldemar U, Brundler A-M, Horvath L, Gold LI, Korc M, Buchler MW. Enhanced expression of TGF-βs and their receptors in human acute pancreatitis. Ann Surg 1997; in press.

35. Riesle E, Friess H, Deflorin J, Zhao L, Baczako K, Gold LI, Korc M, Buchler MW. Overexpression of TGF-βs following acute edematous pancreatitis in rats suggests a role in pancreatic regeneration, Gut, 1997; *40:*73–79.

36. McGowan SE, Jackson SK, Olson PJ, Gold LI. Influence of exogenous and endogenous transforming growth factor-β on elastin gene expression in lung fibroblasts. Am J Resp Cell Mol Biol 1997; *17:*25–35.

37. Roth DA, Gold LI, Han VK, McCarthy JG, Sung JJ, Wisoff JH, Longaker MT. Immunolocalization of transforming growth factor-β1, β2, and β3 and insulin-like growth factor-1 in premature cranial suture fusion. Plastic Reconstruct Surg 1997; *99:*300–309.

38. Roth DA, Longaker MT, McCarthy JG, McMullen HF, Gold LI. Increased immunoreactivity for TGF-β isoforms (β1, β2, and β3) during rat cranial suture fusion suggests their role in cranial suture development. J Bone Mineral Res 1997; *12:*311–321.

39. Kim SJ, Jeang KT, Glick A, Sporn MB, Roberts AB. Promoter sequences of the human transforming growth factor-β1 gene responsive to transforming growth factor-β1 autoinduction. J Biol Chem 1989; *264:*7041–7045.

40. Lafyatis R, Lechleider R, Kin SJ, Jakowlew S, Roberts AB, Sporn MB. Structural and functional characterization of the transforming growth factor-β3 promoter: a cAMP responsive element regulates basal and induced transcription. J Biol Chem 1990; *265:*19,128–19,136.

41. Graycar JL, Miller DA, Arrick BA, Lyons RM, Moses HL, Derynck R. Human transforming growth factor-β3: recombinant expression, purification, and biological activities in comparison with transforming growth factor-β1 and β2. Mol Endocrinol 1989; *3:*1977–1986.

42. Merwin JR, Newman W, Dawson LD, Tucker A, Madri JA. Vascular cells respond differentially to transforming growth factors beta1 and beta2 in vitro. Am J Pathol 1991; *138:*37–51.

43. Rosa F, Roberts AB, Danielpour D, Dart LL, Sporn MB, David IB. Mesoderm induction in amphibians: role of TGF-β2-like factors. Science 1988; *236:*783–786.

44. Wahl SM. Transforming growth factor beta (TGF-β) in inflammation: a cause and a cure. J Clin Immunol 1992; *12:*61–74.

45. Parekh T, Saxena B, Reibman J, Cronstein B, Gold LI. Neutrophil chemotaxis in response to transforming growth factor-β isoforms (TGF-β1, TGF-β2, and TGF-β3) is mediated by fibronectin. J Immunol 1994; *152*:2456–2466.

46. Koyama NT, Koshikawa N, Morisaki Y, Saito Y, Yoshida S. Bifunctional effects of transforming growth factor-β on migration of cultured rat aortic smooth muscle cells Biochem Biophys Res Commun 1990; *169*:725.

47. Postlewaite AE, Keski-Oja J, Moses HL, Kang AH. Stimulation of the chemotactic migration of human fibroblasts by transforming growth factor-beta. J Exp Med 1987; *165*:251–256.

48. Ignotz RA, Massague J. Transforming growth factor-β stimulates the expression of fibronectin and collagen and their incorporation into the extracellular matrix. J Biol Chem 1987; *261*:4337–4345.

49. Laiho M, Saksela O, Keski-Oja J. Transforming growth factor-β induction of type-1 plasminogen activator inhibitor. J Biol Chem 1987; *262*:17,467–17,474.

50. Kubota S, Fridman R, Yamada Y. Transforming growth factor-β suppresses the invasiveness of human fibrosarcoma cells in vitro by increasing expression of tissue inhibitor of metalloproteinase. Bichem Biophys Res Commun 1991; *176*:129–136.

51. Border WA, Ruoslahti E. Transforming growth factor-β in disease: the dark side of tissue repair. J Clin Invest 1992; *90*:1–7.

52. Border WA, Noble NA. Transforming growth factor-β in tissue fibrosis. N Engl J Med 1994; *331*:1286–1292.

53. Nikol S, Isner JM, Pickering JG, Kearney M, Leclerc G, Weir L. Expression of transforming growth factor-β1 is increased in human vascular restenosis lesions. J Clin Invest. 1992; *90*:1582–1592.

54. Ignotz RA, Massague J. Cell adhesion receptors as targets for transforming growth factor-β action. Cell 1987; *51*:189–197.

55. Arrick BA, Lopez AR, Elfman F, Ebner R, Damsky CH, Derynck R. Altered metabolic and adhesive properties associated with increased expression of transforming growth factor-β1. J Cell Biol 1992; *118*:715–726.

56. Assoian RK, Sporn MB. Type-beta transforming growth factor in human platelets: release during platelet degranulation and action on vascular smooth muscle cells. J Cell Biol 1986; *102*:1712–1733.

57. Seyedin SM, Thomas TC, Thompson AY, Rosen DM, Piez KA. Purification and characterization of two cartilage-inducing factors from bovine demineralized bone. Proc Natl Acad Sci USA 1985; *82*:2267–2271.

58. Flaumenhaft R, Kojima S, Abe M, Rifkin DB. Activation of latent transforming growth factor β. Adv Pharmacol 1993; *24*:51–76.

59. Nunes I, Kojima S, Rifkin DB. Effects of endogenously activated transforming growth factor-β on growth and differentiation of retinoic acid-treated HL-60 cells. Cancer Res 1996; *56*:495–499.

60. Schultz-Cherry S, Ribeiro S, Gentry L, Murphy-Ullrich JE. Thrombospondin binds and activates the small and large forms of latent transforming growth factor-β in a chemically defined system. J Biol Chem 1994; *269*:26,775–26,782.

61. Flaumenhaft R, Abe M, Sato M, Miyazono K, Harpel J, Heldin C-H, Rifkin DB. Role of the latent TGF-β binding protein in the activation of latent TGF-β by co-cultures of endothelial and smooth muscle cells. J Cell Biol 1993; *120*:995–1002.

62. Sato Y, Tsuboi R, Lyons R, Moses HL, Rifkin DB. Characterization of the activation of latent TGF-β by co-cultures of endothelial cells and pericytes or smooth muscle cells: a self regulating system. J Cell Biol 1990; *111*:757–763.

63. Sato Y, Okada F, Abe M, Tadashi S, Kuwano M, Sato S, Furuya A, Hanai N, Tamaoki T. The mechanism for the activation of latent TGF-β during co-culture of endothelial cells

and smooth muscle cells: cell-type specific targeting of latent TGF-β to smooth muscle cells. J Cell Biol 1993; *123:*1249–1254.

64. Jirtle RL, Carr BI, Scott CD. Modulation of the insulin-like growth factor II/mannose 6-phosphate receptors and transforming growth factor-beta 1 during liver regeneration. J Biol Chem 1991; *266:*22,444–22,450.

65. Miyazono KP, Hellman C, Wernstedt C, Heldin C-H. Latent high molecular weight complex of transforming growth factor-β1. Purification from human platelets and structural characterization. J Biol Chem 1988; *263:*6407–6415.

66. Taipale J, Miyazono K, Heldin C-H, Keski-Oja J. Latent transforming growth factor-β1 associates to fibroblast extracellular matrix via latent TGF-β binding protein. J Cell Biol 1994; *124:*171–181.

67. Miyazono K, Hellman U, Wenstedt C, Heldin C-H. A role of the latent TGF-β1-binding protein in the assembly and secretion of TGF-β1. EMBO J 1991; *10:*1091–1101.

68. Taipale J, Lohi J, Saarinen J, Kovanen PT, Keski-Oja J. Human mast cell chymase and leukocyte leastase release latent transforming growth factor-β1 from the extracellular matrix of cultured human epithelial and endothelial cells. J Biol Chem 1995; *270:*4689–4696.

69. Eklov S, Funa K, Nordgren H, Olofsson A, Kanzaki T, Miyazono K, Nilsson S. Lack of the latent transforming growth factor β binding protein in malignant but not benign prostatic tissue. Cancer Res 1993; *53:*3193–3197.

70. Yamaguchi Y, Mann DM, Ruoslahti E. Negative regulation of transforming growth factor-β by the proteoglycan decorin. Nature 1990; *346:*281–283.

71. Massague J. Receptors for the TGF-β family. Cell 1992; *69:*1067–1070.

72. Wrana J, Attisano L, Weisser R, Ventura F, Massague J. Mechanism of activation of TGF-β receptor. Nature 1994; *370:*341–347.

73. Lopez-Casillas F, Payne HM, Andres JL, Massague J. Betaglycan can act as a dual modulator of TGF-β access to signaling receptors: mapping of ligand binding and GAG attachment sites. J Cell Biol 1994; *124:*557–568.

74. Attisano L, Carcamo J, Ventura F, Weis FMB, Massague J, Wrana J. Identification of human activin and TGF-β type I receptors that form heteromeric kinase complexes with type II receptors. Cell 1993; *75:*671–680.

75. Cheifetz S, Hernandez H, Laiho M, ten Dijke P, Iwata KK, Massague J. Distinct transforming growth factor-β (TGF-β) receptor subsets as determinants of cellular responsiveness to three TGF-β isoforms. J Biol Chem 1990; *265:*20,533–20,538.

76. McKay K, Danielpour D. Novel 150 and 180 kDa glycoproteins that bind transforming growth factor (TGF)-β1 but not TGF-β2 are present in several cell lines. J Biol Chem 1991; *266:*9907–9911.

77. Ohta M, Greenberger JS, Anklesaria P, Bassols A, Massague J. Two forms of transforming growth factor-β distinguished by multipotential haematopoietic progenitor cells. Nature 1987; *329:*539–541.

78. Zhang H, Shaw ARE, Mak A, Letarte M. Endoglin is a component of the transforming growth factor (TGF)-β receptor complex of human pre-B leukemic cells. J Immunol 1996; *156:*565–573.

79. St. Jacques S, Cymerman U, Pece N, Letarte M. Molecular characterization and in situ localization of murine endoglin reveal that it is a transforming growth factor-β binding protein of endothelial and stromal cells. Endocrinology 1994; *34:*2645–2657.

80. Lastres P, Letamendia A, Zhang H, Rius C, Almendro N, Raab U, Lopez LA, Langa C, Fabra A, Letarte M, Bernabeu C. Endoglin modulates cellular responses to TGF-β1. J Cell Biol 1996; *133:*1109–1121.

81. Graff JM, Bansal A, Melton DA. Xenopus Mad proteins transduce distinct subsets of signals for the TGF-β superfamily. Cell 1996; *85:*479–487.

82. Eppert K, Scherer SW, Ozcelik H, Pirone R, Hoodless P, Kim H, Tsui L-C, Bapat B, Gallingerr S, Andrulis IL, Thomsen GH, Wrana JL, Attisano L. MADR2 maps to 18q21 and encodes a TGF-—regulated MAD-related protein that is functionally mutated in colorectal carcinoma. Cell 1996; *86:*543–552.

83. Macias-Silva M, Abdollah S, Hoodless P, Pirone R, Attisano L, Wrana JL. MADR is a substrate of the TGF-β receptor and its phosphorylation is required for nuclear accumulation and signaling. Cell 1996; *87:*1215–1224.

84. Filmus J, Kerbel RS. Development of resistance mechanisms to the growth-inhibitory effects of transforming growth factor-β during tumor progression. Curr Opin Oncol 1993; *5:*123–129.

85. Ewen M. The cell cycle and the retinoblastoma protein family. Cancer Metast Rev 1994; *13:*45–66.

86. Battegay EJ, Raines EW, Seifert RA, Bowen-Pope F, Ross R. TGF-β induces bimodal proliferation of connective tissue cells via complex control of and autocrine PDGF loop. Cell 1990; *63:*515–524.

87. Guadagno TM, Assoian RK. G1/S control of anchorage-independent growth in the fibroblast cell cycle. J Cell Biol 1991; *115:*1419–1425.

88. Kyu-Ho Han E, Guadagno TM, Dalton SL, Assoian RK. A cell cycle and mutational analysis of anchorage-independent growth: cell adhesion and TGF-β1 control G1/S transit specifically. J Cell Biol 1993; *1222:*461–471.

89. Laiho M, De-Caprio JA, Ludlow JW, Livingston DM, Massague J. Growth inhibition by TGF-β linked to suppression of retinoblastoma protein phosphorylation. Cell 1990; *62:*175–185.

90. Satterwhite DJ, Moses HL. Mechanisms of transforming growth factor-beta 1-induced cell cycle arrest. Invasion Metast 1994–1995; *14:*309–318.

91. Sherr CJ. Cancer cell cycles. Science 1996; *274:*1672–1677.

92. Ewen ME, Sluss HK, Sherr CJ, Matsushime H, Kato J-Y, Livingston DM. Functional interactions of the retinoblastoma protein with mammalian D-type cyclins. Cell 1993; *73:*487–497.

93. Weinberg RA. The retinoblastoma gene and gene product. In: Franks LM (ed). Cancer surveys. Tumor suppressor genes, the cell cycle and cancer, vol. XII. Cold Spring Harbor Laboratory, Cold Spring Harbor, NY, 1992; pp. 43–79.

94. Koff A, Ohtsuki M, Polyak K, Roberts J, Massague J. Negative regulation of G1 in mammalian cells: inhibition of cyclin E-dependent kinase by TGF-β. Science 1993; *260:*536–239.

95. Weintraub SJ, Prater CA, Dean DC. Retinoblastoma protein switches the E2F site from positive to negative element. Nature 1992; *358:*259–261.

96. Pietenpol JA, Holt JT, Stein RW, Moses HL. Transforming growth factor-β1 suppression of c-myc gene transcription: role in inhibition of keratinocyte proliferation. Proc Natl Acad Sci USA 1990; *87:*3758–3762.

97. Fernandez-Pol JA, Talked VD, Klos DJ, Hamilton PD. Suppression of the EGF-dependent induction of c-myc proto-oncogene expression by transforming growth factor-β in a human breast carcinoma cell line. Biochem Biophys Res Commun 1987; *144:*1197–1205.

98. Roberts PD, Kin S-J, Sporn MB. Is there a common pathway mediating growth inhibition by TGF-β and the retinoblastoma gene product. Cancer Cells 1991; *3:*19–21.

99. Laiho M, Ronnstrand L, Heino J. Control of JunB and extracellular matrix protein expression by transforming growth factor-β is independent of simian virus 40 T antigen-sensitive growth-inhibitory events. Mol Cell Biol 1991; *11:*972–978.

100. Li L, Hu JS, Olson EN. Different members of the jun photo-oncogene family exhibit distinct patterns of expression in response to type β transforming growth factor. J Biol Chem 1990; *265:*1556–1562.

101. Reynisdottir I, Polyak K, lavarone A, Massague J. Kip/cip and Ink4 cdk inhibitors cooperate to induce cell cycle arrest in response to TGF-β. Genes Devel. 1995; *9:*1831–1945.

102. Hannon GJ, Beach D. p15INK4B is a potential effector of TGF-beta-induced cell cycle arrest. Nature 1994; *371:*257–261.

103. Polayak K, Kato J, Soloman J, Sherr C, Massague J, Roberts J, Koff A. P27Kip 1, a cyclin-cdk inhibitor link transforming growth factor-β and contact inhibition to cell cycle arrest. Genes Devel 1994; *8:*9–22.

104. Datto MB, Yu Y, Wang XF. Functional analysis of the transforming growth factor beta responsive elements in the WAF/Cip1/p21 promoter. J Biol Chem 1995; *270:*28,623–28,628.

105. Hunter T, Pines J. Cyclins and cancer II: cyclin D and CDK inhibitors come of age. 1994; *79:*573–582.

106. Hall M, Peters G. Genetic alterations in cyclins, cyclin-dependent kinases, and cdk inhibitors in human cancer. Adv Cancer Res 1996; *68:*67–108.

107. Motokura T, Bloom T, Kin HG, Juppner H, Ruderman JV Kronenberg HM, Arnold A. A novel cyclin encoded by a bcl1-linked candidate oncogene. Nature 1991; *350:*512–515.

108. Jen J, Harper W, Bigner S, Papadopoulos N, Markowitz S, Willson J, Kinzler K, Vogelstein B. Deletion of p16 and p15 genes in brain tumors. Cancer Res 1994; *54:*6353–6358.

109. Elledge SJ, Harper JW. cdk inhibitors: on the threshold of checkpoints and development. Curr Opinion Cell Biol 1994; *6:*847–852.

110. Herman J, Jen J, Merio A, Baylin S. Hypermethylation-associated inactivation indicates a tumor suppressor role of p15INK4B1. Cancer Res 1996; *56:*722–727.

111. Polyak K, Lee M-H, Erdjument-Bromage H, Koff A, Roberts JM, Tempst P, Massague J. Cloning of p27kip1, a cyclin-dependent kinase inhibitor and potential mediator of extracellular antimitogenic signals. Cell 1994; *78:*59–66.

112. Toyoshima H, Hunter T. p27, a novel inhibitor of G1-cyclin-cdk protein kinase activity is related to p21. Cell 1994; *78:*67–74.

113. Kiyokawa H, Kineman RD, Manova-Todorova KO, Soares VC, Hoffman ES, Ono M, Khanam D, Hayday AC, Frohman LA, Koff A. Enhanced growth of mice lacking the cyclin-dependent kinase inhibitor function of p27kip1. Cell 1996; *85:*721–732.

114. Fero, ML, Rivkin M, Tasch M, Porter P, Carow CE, Firpo E, Polyak K, Tsai L-H, Broudy V, Perlmutter RM, Kaushansky K, Roberts JM. A syndrome of multiorgan hyperplasia with features of gigantism, tumorigenesis, and female sterility in p27kip1-deficient mice. Cell 1996; *85:*733–744.

115. Mal A, Poon RYC, Howe PH, Toyoshima H, Hunter T, Harter M. Inactivation of p27kip1 by the viral E1A oncoprotein in TGF-—treated cells. Nature 1996; *380:*262–266.

116. Kawamata N, Morosetti R, Miller CW, Park D, Spirin, KS, Nakamaki T, Takeuchi S, Hatta Y, Simpson J, Wilczynski S, Lee YY, Bartrum CR, Koefler HP. Molecular analysis of the cyclin-dependent kinase inhibitor gene p27/kip1 in human malignancies. Cancer Res 1995; *55:*2266–2269.

117. Ponce-Castaneda MV, Lee M-H, Latres E, Polyak K, Lacombe L, Montgomery K, Matthew S, Krauter K, Sheinfeld J, Massague J, Cordon-Cardo C. p27jip1: chromosomal mapping to 12p12–12p13.1 and absence of mutations in human tumors. Cancer Res. 1995; *55:*1211–1214.

118. Hengst L, Reed S. Translation control of p27kip1 accumulation during the cell cycle. Science 1996; *271:*1861–1864.

119. Millard SS, Yan JS, Nguyen H, Pagano M, Kiyokawa H, Koof A. Enhanced ribosomal association of p27kip1 mRNA is a mechanism contributing to accumulation during growth arrest. J Biol Chem 1997; 272:7093–7098.

120. Pagano M, Tam SW, Theodoras AM, Beer-Romero P, Del Sal G, Chau V, Yew PR, Draetta GF, Rolfe M. Role of the ubiquitin-proteasome pathway in regulating abundance of the cyclin-dependent kinase inhibitor p27. Science 1995; *269:*682–685.

121. Barinaga M. A new twist to the cell cycle. Science 1995; *269:*631, 632.

122. King RW, Glotzer M, Kirschner MW. Mutagenic analysis of the destruction signal of mitotic cyclin and structural characterization of ubiquitinated intermediates. Mol Biol Cell 1996; *7:*1343–1357.

123. Buchler M, Friess H, Schultheiss KH, Gebhardt CH, Muhrer KH, Winkelmann M, Wagner T, Klapdor R, Muller G, Beger HG. A randomized controlled trial of adjuvant immunotherapy (murine monoclonal antibody 494/32) in resectable pancreatic cancer. Cancer 1991; *168:*1507–1512.

124. Gudjonsson B. Cancer of the pancreas. 50 years of surgery. Cancer 1987; *60:*2284–2303.

125. Baldwin RL, Korc M. Growth inhibition of human pancreatic carcinoma cells by transforming growth factor beta-1. Growth Factors 1993; *8:*23–34.

126. Baldwin RL, Friess H, Yokoyama M, Lopez ME, Kobrin MS, Buchler MW, Korc M. Attenuated ALK-5 receptor expression in human pancreatic cancer: correlation with resistance to growth inhibition. Int J Cancer 1996; *67:*283–288.

127. Yamanaka Y, Friess H, Buchler M, Beger HG, Gold LI, Korc M. Synthesis and expression of transforming growth factor β-1, β-2, and β-3 in the endocrine and exocrine pancreas. Diabetes 1993; *42:*746–756.

128. Friess H, Yamanaka Y, Buchler M, Beger HG, Kobrin MS, Baldwin RL, Korc M. Enhanced expression of the type II transforming growth factor β receptor in human pancreatic cancer cells without alteration of type III receptor expression. Cancer Res 1993; *53:*2704–2707.

129. Nauman M, Savitskaia N, Eilert C, Schramm A, Kalthoff H, Schmiegel W. Frequent codeletion of p16/MTS1 and p15/MTS2 and genetic alterations in p16/MTS1 in pancreatic tumors. Gastroenterology 1996; *110:*1215–1224.

130. Hahn SA, Schutte M, Shamsul Hoque ATM, Moskaluk CA, da Costa LT, Rozenblum E, Weinstein CL, Fischer A, Yeo CJ, Hruban RH, Kem SE. DPC4, a candidate tumor suppressor gene at human chromosome 18q21.1. Science 1996; *271:*350–356.

131. Vogelstein B, Fearon ER, Hamilton SR, Kern SE, Preisinger AC, Leppert M, Nakamura Y, White R, Smits AMM, Bos JL. Genetic alterations during colorectal tumor development. N Engl J Med 1988; *319:*213–221.

132. Yamaguchi T, Toguchida J, Yamamuro T, Kotoura Y, Takada N, Kawaguchi N, Kaneko Y, Nakamura Y, Sasaki MS, Ushizaki K. Allelotype analysis in osteosarcomas; frequent allele loss on 3q, 13q, 17p, and 18q. Cancer Res 1992; *52:*2419–2423.

133. Fearon ER, Cho KR, Nigro JM, Kern SE, Simons JW, Ruppert JM, Hamilton SR, Preisinger AC, Thomas G, Kinzler KW, Volgestein B. Identification of a chromosome 18q gene that is altered in colorectal cancers. Science 1990; *247:*40–56.

134. Migdalska A, Molineus G, Demuynck H, Evans GS, Ruscetti F, Dexter TM. Growth inhibitory effects of transforming growth factor-beta1 in vivo. Growth Factors 1991; *4:*239–245.

135. Barnard JA, Beauchamp RD, Coffey RJ, Moses HL. Regulation of intestinal epithelial cell growth by transforming growth factor type β. Proc Natl Acad Sci USA 1989; *86:*1578–1582.

136. Dignass AU, Podolsky DK. Cytokine modulation of intestinal epithelial monolayers. Gastroenterology 1993; *105:*1323–1332.

137. Barnard JA, Warwick GJ, Gold LI. Localization of transforming growth factor β isoforms in the normal murine small intestine and colon. Gastroenterology 1993; *105:*67–73.

138. Gang Q, Babyatsky M, Gold LI, Podolsky DK, Ahnen DJ. Localization of TGF-β1 mRNA and protein in intestinal mucosa: Specific expression in the epithelium, submitted for publication.

139. Hall PA, Coates PJ, Ansari B, Hopwood W. Regulation of cell numbers in the mammalian gastrointestinal tract: the importance of apoptosis. J Cell Sci 1994; *107:*3569–3577.

140. Wang CY, Eshelman JR, Wilson JKV, Markowitz S. Both transforming growth factor-β and substrate release are inducers of apoptosis in a human colon adenoma cell line. Cancer Res 1995; *55:*5101–5105.

141. Manning AM, Williams AC, Game SM, Paraskeva C. Differential sensitivity of human colonic adenoma and carcinoma cells to transforming growth factor β (TGF-β): conversion of an adenoma cell line to a tumorigenic phenotype is accompanied by a reduced response to the inhibitory effects of TGF-β. Oncogene 1991; *6:*1471–1476.

142. Fan D, Chakrabarty S, Seid C, Bell CW, Schackert H, Morikawa K, Fidler IJ. Clonal stimulation of human colon carcinomas and human renal cell carcinomas mediated by TGF-β1. Cancer Commun 1989; *1:*117–125.

143. Hsu S, Huang F, Hafez M, Winawer S, Friedman E. Colon carcinoma cells switch their response to transforming growth factor-β1 with tumor progression. Cell Growth Differen 1994; *5:*267–275.

144. Huang F, Newman E, Kerbel R, Friedman E. TGF-β1 is an autocrine positive regulator of colon carcinoma U9 cells in vivo as shown by transfection of a TGF-β1 antisense expression plasmid. Cell Growth Differen 1995; *6:*1653–1642.

145. Yan Z, Winawer S, Friedman E. Two different signal transduction pathways can be activated by transforming growth factor β1 in epithelial cells. J Biol Chem 1994; *269:*13,231–13,237.

146. Wu S, Theodorescu D, Kerbel RS, Wilson JKV, Mulder KM, Humphrey LE, Brattain MG. TGF-β1 is an autocrine negative growth regulator of human colon carcinoma FET cells *in vivo* as revealed by transfection of an antisense vector. J Cell Biol 1992; *116:*187–196.

147. Tsushima H, Kawata S, Tamura S, Ito N, Shirai Y, Kiso S, Imai Y, Shimomukai H, Nomura Y, Matsuda Y, Matsuzawa Y. High levels of transforming growth factor beta 1 in patients with colorectal cancer: association with disease progression. Gastroenterology 1996; *110:*375–382.

148. Robson H, Anderson E, James RD, Schofeld PF. Transforming growth factor β1 expression in human colorectal tumours: and independent prognostic marker in a subgroup of poor prognosis patients. Brit J Cancer 1995; *74:*753–758.

149. Picon A, Gold LI, Wang J-P, Klimstra D, Cohen A, Friedman E. Metastatic human colon cancers express elevated levels of TGF-β1, submitted for publication.

150. Hsu S, Huang F, Friedman E. Paracrine PDGF-B increases colon cancer growth in vivo. J Cell Physiol 1995; *165:*230–245.

151. Morson BC. The polyp-cancer sequence in the large bowel. Proc Royal Soc Med 1974; *67:*451–454.

152. Risio M, Lipkin M, Candelaresi G, Bertone A, Coverlizza S, Rossini PF. Correlations between rectal mucosal cell proliferation and the clinical and pathological features of nonfamilial neoplasia of the large intestine. Cancer Res. 1991; *51:*1917–1921.

153. Bedi A, Pasricha PJ, Akhtar AJ, Barber JP, Bedi GC, Giardiello FM, Zehnbauer BA, Hamilton SR, Jones RJ. Inhibition of apoptosis during development of colorectal cancer. Cancer Res 1995; *55:*1811–1816.

154. Loda M, Cukor B, Tam SW, Lavin P, Fiorentino M, Draetta GF, Jessup JM, Pagano M. Increased proteasome-dependent degradation of the cyclin-dependent kinase inhibitor p27 in aggressive colorectal carcinomas. Nature Med 1997; *3:*152–154.

155. Leach FS, Elledge SJ, Sherr CJ, Willson JKV, Markowitz S, Kinzler KW, Vogelstein B. Amplification of cyclin genes in colorectal cancer. Cancer Res 1993; *53:*1986–1989.

156. Eshelman JR, Markowitz SD. Microsatellite instability in inherited and sporadic neoplasms. Curr Opin Oncol 1995; *7:*83–89.

157. Ionov Y, Peinado AM, Malkhosyan S, Shibata D, Perucho M. Ubiquitous somatic mutations in simple repeated sequences reveal a new mechanism for colonic carcinogenesis. Nature 1993; *363:*558–561.

158. Marra G, Boland CR. Hereditary nonpolyposis colorectal cancer: the syndrome, the genes, and historical perspectives. J Natl Cancer Inst 1995; *87:*114–1125.

159. Risinger JI, Berchuk A, Koheler MF, Watson P, Lynch HT, Boyd J. Genetic instability of microsatellites in endometrial carcinoma. Cancer Res 1993; *53:*5100–5103.

160. Dos Santos NR, Seruca R, Constancia M, Sobrinho-Simoes M. Microsatellite instability at multiple loci in gastric carcinoma: clinicopathological implications and prognosis. Gastroenterology 1996; *110:*38–44.

161. Risio M, Reato G, Francia di Celle P, Fizzotti M, Rossini FP, Foa R. Microsatellite instability is associated with the histological features of the tumor in nonfamilial colorectal cancer. Cancer Res 1996; *56:*5470–5474.

162. Markowitz S, Wang J, Myeroff L, Parsons R, Sun L, Lutterbaugh J, Fan R, Zborowska E, Kinzler K, Vogelstein B, Brattain M, Willson K. Inactivation of the type II TGF-β receptor in colon cancer cells with microsatellite instability. Science 1995; *268:*1336–1338.

163. Myeroff LL, Parsons R, Kim S-J, Hedrick L, Cho KR, Orth K, Mathis M, Kinzler KW, Lutterbaugh J, Park K, Bang Y-J, Lee HY, Park J-G, Lynch HT, Roberts AB, Vogelstein B, Markowitz S. A transforming growth factor β receptor type II gene mutation common in colon and gastric but rare in endometrial cancers with microsatellite instability. Cancer Res 1995; *55:*5545–5547.

164. Lu S-L, Akiyama Y, Nagasaki H, Saitoh K, Yuasa Y. Mutations of the transforming growth factor-β type II receptor gene and genomic instability in hereditary nonpolyposis colorectal cancer. Biochem Biophys Res Commun 1995; *216:*452–457.

165. Parsons R, Myeroff LL, Liu B, Willson JKV, Markowitz SD, Kinzler KW, Vogelstein B. Microsatellite instability and mutations of the transforming growth factor β type II receptor gene in colorectal cancer. Cancer Res 1995; *55:*5548–5550.

166. Wright PA, Quirke P, Attanoos R, Williams GT. Molecular pathology of gastric carcinoma: progress and prospects. Human Pathol 1992; *23:*848–859.

167. Correa P. Human gastric carcinogenesis: a multistep and multifactorial process—First American Cancer Society Award lecture on cancer epidemiology and prevention. Cancer Res. 1992; *52:*6735–6740.

168. Fuchs CS, Mayer RJ. Gastric carcinoma. N Engl J Med 1995; *333:*32–41.

169. Hirayama D, Fujimori T, Satonaka K, Nakamura T, Kitazawa S, Horio M, Maeda S, Nagasako K. Immunohistochemical study of epidermal growth factor and transforming growth factor-β in the penetrating type of early gastric cancer. Human Pathol 1992; *23:*681–685.

170. Mizoi T, Ohtani H, Miyazono K, Miyazawa M, Matsuo S, Nagura H. Immunoelectron microscopic localization of transforming growth factor beta 1 and latent transforming growth factor beta 1 binding protein in human gastrointestinal carcinomas: qualitative differences between cancer stromal cells. Cancer Res 1993; *53:*183–190.

171. Wheater PR, Burkitt KG, Daniels VG. Wheater's Functional Histology. 3rd ed., Churchill Livingstone. Edinburgh, London, New York, Tokyo 1993.

172. Mahara K, Kato J, Terui T, Takimoto R, Horimoto M, Murakami T, Mogi Y, Watanabe N, Kohogo Y, Niitsu Y. Transforming growth beta 1 secreted from scirrhous gastric cancer cells is associated with excess collagen deposition in the tissue. Brit J Cancer 1994; *69:*777–783.

173. Ura H, Obara T, Yokota K, Shibata Y, Okamura K, Namik M. Effects of transforming growth factor beta released from gastric carcinoma cells on the contraction of collagen-matrix gels containing fibroblasts. Cancer Res 1991; *51:*3550–3554.

174. Yoshiura K, Ota S, Terano A, Takahashi M, Hata Y, Kawabe T, Mutoh H, Hiraishi H, Nakata R, Okano K. Growth regulation of rabbit gastric epithelial cells and proto-oncogene expression. Dig Dis Sci 1994; *39:*1454–1463.

175. Yamaoto M, Maehara Y, Sakagichi Y, Kusmoto T, Ichiyoshi Y, Sugimachi K. Transforming growth factor-beta1 induces apoptosis in gastric cancer cells through a p53-independent pathway. Cancer 1996; *77:*1628–1633.

176. Tahara E. Growth factors and oncogenes in human gastrointestinal carcinomas. J Cancer Res Clin Oncol 1990; *116:*121–131.

177. Akiyama Y, Nakasaki H, Nihei Z, Iwama T, Nomizu T, Utsunomiya J, Yuasa Y. Frequent microsatellite instabilities and analyses of the related genes in familial gastric cancers. Jap J Cancer Res 1996; *87:*595–601.

178. Morrow CP, Curtin JP, Townsend DE. Tumors of the endometrium. In: Synopsis of Gynecologic concology, fourth ed. Churchill Livingstone, New York, pp. 153–188.

179. Gurpide E. Endometrial cancer: biochemical and clinical correlates. J Natl Cancer Inst 1991; *83:*405–416.

180. Silverberg SG. Hyperplasia and carcinoma of the endometrium. Semin Diagn Pathol. 1988; *5:*135–153.

181. Creasman WT, Eddy GL. Recent advances in endometrial cancer. Semin Surg Oncol 1990; *6:*405–416.

182. Holinka C. Aspects of hormone replacement therapy. In: The Human Endometrium (Bulletti C, Gurpide E, Flamigni C, eds.) Ann NY Acad. Sci. 1994; *734:*271–284.

183. Jovanovic AS, Boynton KA, Mutter GL. Uteri of women with endometrial carcinoma contain a histopathological spectrum of monoclonal putative precancers, some with microsatellite instability. Cancer Res 1996; *56:*1917–1921.

184. Smith DC, Prentice RI, Bauermeister DE. Endometrial carcinoma: histopathology, survival, and exogenous estrogens. Gynecol Obstet Invest 1981; *12:*169–173.

185. Hulka BS. Links between hormone replacement therapy and neoplasia. Fertil Steril 1994; *62:*1688–1755.

186. Fisher B, Costantino JP, Redmond CK, Fisher ER, Wickerman DL, and Cronin WM. Endometrial cancer in Tamoxifen-treated and nontreated asymptomatic, post menopausal breast cancer patients. Gynecol Oncol 1994; *86:*527–537.

187. Lanza A, Alba E, Re A, Tessarolo M, Leo L, Bellino R, Lauricella A, Wierdis J. Endometrial carcinoma in breast cancer patients treated with Tamoxifen. Rev Eur J Gynecol Oncol 1994; *15:*455–459.

188. Yang NN, Venugopalan M, Hardikar S, Glasebrook A. Identification of an estrogen response element activated by metabolites of 17β-estradiol and Raloxifene. Science 1996; *273:*1222–1224.

189. Hayward SW, Cunha GR, Dahiya R. Normal development and carcinogenesis of the prostate: a unifying hypothesis. Basis for cancer management. Ann NY Acad Sci 1994; *784:*50–62.

190. Cunha GR, Foster BA, Sugimura Y, Hom YK. Keratinocyte growth factor as mediator of mesenchymal-epithelial interactions in the development of androgen target organs. Cell Devel Biol 1996; *7:*203–210.

191. Cunha GR, Young P, Brody JR. Role of uterine epithelium in the development of myometrial smooth muscle cells. Biol Reproduc 1989; *40:*861–871.

192. Cooke PS, Uchima FDA, Fujii DK, Bern HA. Restoration of normal morphology and estrogen responsiveness in cultured vaginal and uterine epithelia transplanted with stroma. Proc Natl Acad Sci USA 1986; *83:*2109–2113.

193. Bruner K, Rodger W, Gold L, Korc M, Hargrove J, Matrisian L, Osteen K. Transforming growth factor-β mediates the progesterone suppression of an epithelial metalloproteinase by adjacent stroma. Proc Natl Acad Sci USA 1995; *92:*7362–7366.

194. Boyd J, Kauffman D. Expression of transforming growth factor-β1 by human endometrial carcinoma cell lines: inverse correlation with effects on growth rate and morphology. Cancer Res 1990; *50:*3394–3399.

195. Sakata M, Kurachi H, Ikegam H, Jikihara H, Morishige K, Miyake A, Terakawa N, Tanizawa O. Autocrine growth mechanism by transforming growth factor-β (TGF-β1) and TGF-β1-receptor regulation by epidermal growth factor in a human endometrial cancer cell line IK-90. Int J Cancer 1993; *54:*862–867.

196. Presta M, Maier JAM, Rusnati M, Moscatelli D, Ragnotti G. Modulation of plasminogen activator activity in human endometrial adenocarcinoma cell lines by basic fibroblast growth factor and transforming growth factor-β. Cancer Res 1988; *48:*6384–6389.

197. Tan P, Cady B, Wanner M, Worland P, Cukor B, Magi-Galluzzi C, Lavin P, Draetta G, Pagano M, Loda M. The cell cycle inhibitor p27kip1 is an independent prognostic marker in small (T1a,b) invasive breast carcinomas.Cancer Res 1997; *57:*1259–1263.

198. Valverius EM, Walker-Jones D, Bates SE, Stampher MR, Clark R, McCormick F, Dickson RB, Lippman ME. Production and responsiveness to transforming growth factor β in normal and oncogene transformed human mammary epithelial cells. Cancer Res 1989; *49:*6269–6274.

199. Knabbe C, Lippman ME, Wakefield LM, Flanders KC, Kasid A, Derynck R, Dickson RB. Evidence that transforming growth factor-β is a hormonally regulated negative growth factor in human breast cancer cells. Cell 1987; *48:*417–428.

200. Arteaga CL, Coffey RJ, Dugger TC, McCutchen CM, Moses HL, Lyons RM. Growth stimulation of human breast cancer cells with anti-transforming growth factor β antibodies: evidence for negative autocrine regulation by transforming growth factor β. Cell Growth Different 1990; *1:*367–374.

201. Kalkhoven E, Roelen BA, de Winter JP, Mummery CL, van den Eijnden-van Raaij AJ. Resistance to transforming growth factor beta and activin due to reduced receptor expression in human breast tumor cell lines. Cell Growth Differen 1995; *6:*1151–1161.

202. Dickens T-A, Colletta A. The pharmacological manipulation of members of the transforming growth factor beta family in the chemoprevention of breast cancer. BioEssays 1993; *15:*71–74.

203. Perry RR, Kang Y, Greaves BR. Relationship between tamoxifen-induced transforming growth factor-β1 expression, cytostasis and apoptosis in human breast cancer cells. Brit J Cancer 1995; *72:*1441–1446.

204. Chen H, Tritton TR, Kenny N, Absher M, Chiu JF. Tamoxifen induces TGF-β 1 activity and apoptosis of human MCF-7 breast cancer cells. J Cell Biochem 1996; *61:*9–17.

205. Knabbe C, Kopp A, Hilgers W, Land D, Muller V, Zugmaier G, Jonat W. Regulation and role of TGF-beta production in breast cancer. Ann NY Acad Sci 1996; *784:*263–276.

206. MacCallum J, Keen JC, Barlett JM, Thompson AM, Dixon JM, Miller WR. Changes in expression of transforming growth factor beta mRNA isoforms in patients undergoing tamoxifen therapy. Brit J Cancer 1996; *74:*474–478.

207. Dickson RB, Bates SE, McManaway ME, Lippman ME. Characterization of estrogen-responsive transforming activity in human breast cancer cell lines. Cancer Res 1986; *46:*1701–1713.

208. Travers MT, Barrett-Lee PJ, Berger U, Luqmani YA, Gazet JC, Powles TJ, Coombes RC. Growth factor expression in normal, benign and malignant breast tissue. Brit J Cancer 1988; *296:*1621–1624.

209. Welch DR, Fabra A, Nakajima M. Transforming growth factor-β stimulates mammary adenocarcinoma cell invasion and metastatic potential. Proc Natl Acad Sci USA 1990; *87:*7678–7682.

210. Arteaga CL, Carty-Dugger T, Moses HL, Hurd SD, Pietenpol JA. Transforming growth factor (TGF)-β1 can induce estrogen-independent tumorigenicity of human breast cancer cells in athymic mice. Cell Growth Differen 1993; *4:*193–201.

211. Pierce DF, Johnson MD, Matsui Y, Robinson SD, Gold LI, Purchio AF, Daniel CW, Hogan BLM, Moses HL. Inhibition of mammary duct development but not alveolar outgrowth during pregnancy in transgenic mice expressing active TGF-β1. Genes Devel 1993; *7:*2308–2317.

212. Sun LZ, Wu G, Willson JKV, Zborowska E, Yang J, Rajkarunanayake I, Wang J, Gentry LE, Wang X-F, Brittain MG. Expression of transforming growth factor β type II receptor leads to reduced malignancy in human breast cancer MCF-7 cells. J Biol Chem 1994; *269:26*, 449–26, 455.

213. Sicinski P, Donaher JL, Parker SB, Li T, Fazeli A, Gardner G, Haslam S, Bronson T, Elledge SJ, and Weinberg RA. Cyclin D1 provides a link between development and oncogenesis in the retina and breast. Cell 1995; *82:*621–630.

214. Buckley MF, Sweeney KJE, Hamilton JA, Sini RL, Manning DL, Nicholson RI, DeFazio A, Watts CKW, Musgrove EA, Sutherland RL. Expression and amplification of cyclin genes in human breast cancer. Oncogene 1993; *8:*2127–2133.

215. Brenner AJ, Aldaz CM. Chromosome 9p allelic loss and p16/CDKN2 in breast cancer and evidence of p16 inactivation in immortal breast epithelial cells. Cancer Res 1995; *55:*2892–2895.

216. Burger PC. Malignant astrocytic neoplasms: classification, pathologic anatomy, and response to treatment. Semin Oncol 1986; *13:*16–26.

217. Torre-Amione G, Beauchamp RD, Koeppen H, Park BH, Schreiber H, Moses HL, Rowley DA. A highly immunogenic tumor transfected with a murine transforming growth factor β1 cDNA escapes immune surveillance. Proc Natl Acad Sci USA 1990; *87:*1486–1490.

218. Wrann M, Bodmer S, de Martin R, Siepl C, Hofer-Warbinek R. T cell supressor factor from human glioblastoma cells is a 12.5 kd protein closely related to transforming growth factor-β. EMBO J 1987; *6:*1633–1636.

219. Weller M, Fontana A. The failure of current immunotherapy for malignant glioma. Tumor-derived TGF-beta, T-cell apoptosis, and immune privilege of the brain. Brain Res 1995; *21:*128–151.

220. Wallick SC, Figari IS, Morris RE, Levinson AD, Palladino MA. Immunoregulatory role of transforming growth factor-β (TGF-β) in development of killer cells: comparison of active and latent TGF-β1. J Exp Med 1990; *172:*1777–1784.

221. Venter DJ, Bevan KL, Ludwig RL, Riley TEW, Jat PS, Thomas DGT, Noble MD. Retinoblastoma gene deletions in human glioblastoma. Oncogene 1991; *6:*445–448.

222. Hermanson M, Funa K, Hartman M, Cleasson-Wels L, Heldin C-H, Westermark B, Nister M. Platelet-derived growth factors and its receptors in human glioma tissue: expression of mRNA and protein suggests the presence of autocrine and paracrine loops. Cancer Res. 1992; *52:*3213–3219.

223. Kiefer R, Supler ML, Tpyka KV, Streit WJ. In situ detection of transforming growth factor-beta mRNA in experimental rat glioma and reactive glial cells. Neurosci Lett 1994; *166:*161–164.

224. Yamada N, Kato M, Yamashita H, Nister M, Miyazono K. Enhanced expression of transforming growth factor-β and its type I and type II receptors in human glioblastoma. Int J Cancer 1995; *62:*386–392.

225. Helseth E, Unsgaard G, Dalen A. The effects of type beta transforming growth factor on proliferation and epidermal growth factor expression in a human glioblastoma cell line. J Neuro-Oncol 1989; *6:*269–276.

226. Sasaki A, Naganuma H, Satoh E, Nagasaka M, Isoe S, Nakano S, Nukui H. Secretion of transforming growth factor-beta 1 and -beta 2 by malignant glioma cells. Neurologia Medico-Chirurgica 1995; *35:*423–430.

227. Toru-Delbauffe D, Baghdassarian-Chalaye D, Gavaret JM. Effects of TGF-β1 on astroglial cells in culture. J Neurochem 1990; *54:*1056–1061.

228. Jennings MT, Maciunas RJ, Carver R, Bascom CC, Juneau P, Misulis K, Moses HL. TGF-β1 and TGF-β2 are potential growth regulators for low-grade and malignant gliomas *in vitro*: evidence in support of an autocrine hypothesis. Int J Cancer 1991; *49:*129–139.

229. Jachimczak P, Hessdorfer B, Fabel-Schulte K, Wismeth C, Brysch W, Schlingensiepen

KH, Bauer A, Blesch A, Bogdahn U. Transforming growth-factor-beta-mediated autocrine growth regulation of gliomas as detected with phosphorothioate antisense oligonucleotides. Int J Cancer 1996; *65:*332–337.

230. Riffini PA, Rivoltini L, Silvani A, Boiardi A, Parmiani G. Factors, including transforming growth factor beta, released in the glioblastoma residual cavity, impair cavity of adherent lymphokine-activated killer cells. Cancer Immunol Immunother 1993; *36:*409–416.

231. Jachimczak P, Bogdahn U, Schneider J, Behl C, Meixensberger J, Rainer A, Dorries R, Schlingensiepen KH, Brysch W. The effect of transforming growth factor-β2-specific phosphorothioate-anti-sense oligodeoxynucleotides in reversing cellular immunosuppression in malignant glioma. J Neurosurg 1993; *78:*944–951.

232. Fakhrai H, Dorigo O, Shawler DL, Lin H, Mercola D, Black KL, Royston I, Sobol RE. Eradication of established intracranial rat gliomas by transforming growth factor beta antisense gene therapy. Proc Natl Acad Sci USA 1996; *93:*2902–2914.

233. Adams Pearson C, Pearson D, Shibahara S, Hofsteenge J, Ciquet-Erishmann R. Tenascin: cDNA cloning and induction by TGF-β. EMBO J 1988; *10:*2677–2981.

234. Zagzag D. Angiogenic growth factors in neural embryogenesis and neoplasia. Am J Pathol 1995; *146:*293–309.

235. Merzak A, McCrea S, Koocheckpour S, Pilkington GJ. Control of human glioma cell growth, migration, and invasion in vitro by transforming growth factor beta 1. Brit J Cancer 1994; *70:*199–203.

236. Grundmann E, Rossner A, Ueda Y et al. Current aspects of the pathology of osteosarcomas. Anitcancer Res 1995; *15:*1023–1033.

237. Robey PG, Young MF, Flanders KC et al. Osteoblasts synthesize and respond to transforming growth factor-type β (TGF-β) in vitro. J Cell Biol 1987; *105:*457–463.

238. Joyce ME, Roberts AB, Sporn MB, and Bolander ME. Transforming growth factor-β and the initiation of chrondrogenesis and osteogenesis in the rat femur. J Cell Biol 1990; *110:*2195–2207.

239. Beck LS, Amenot EP, Deguzman L, et al. TGF-β1 induces bone closure of skull defects temporal dynamics of bone formation in defects exposed to rh-TGF-β1. J Bone Min Res 1993; *8:*753–761.

240. Centrella M, Horowitz MC, Wozney JM et al. Transforming growth factor-β gene family members in bone. Endocrinol Rev 1994; *15:*27–39.

241. Kloen P, Jennings CL, Gebhardt MC et al. Expression of transforming growth factor-beta (TGF-β) receptors, TGF-β1 and TGF-β2 production and autocrine growth control. Int J Cancer 1994; *58:*440–445.

242. Erlebacher A, Dernyck R. Increased expression of TGF-β2 in osteoblasts results in an osteoporosis-like phenotype. J Cell Biol 1996; *132:*195–210.

243. McCune BK, Patterson K, Chandra RS et al. Expression of transforming growth factor-β isoforms in small round cell tumors of childhood. Am J Pathol 1993; *142:*1098–1100.

244. Teot LA, O'Keefe RJ, Rosier RN, O'Connell JX, Fox EJ, Hicks DG. Extraosseous primary and recurrent giant cell tumors: transforming growth factor-β1 and -β2 expression may explain metaplastic bone formation. Hum Pathol 1996; *27:*625–632.

245. Barton R, Neff L, Louvard CA et al. Cell-mediated extracellular acidification and bone resorption: evidence for a low pH in resorbing lacunae and localization of a 100 kDa lysosomal membrane protein at the osteoclast ruffled border. J Cell Biol 1985; *101:*2210–2222.

246. Yoshikawa H, Rettig WJ, Takaoka K et al. Expression of bone morphogenetic proteins in human osteosarcomas. Cancer 1994; *73:*85–91.

247. Fuegas O, Guriec N, Babin-Boilletot A et al. Loss of heterozygosity of the RB gene is a poor prognostic factor in patients with osteosarcoma. J Clin Oncol. 1996; *14:*467–472.

248. Friend SH, Horowitz JM, Gerber MR, et al. Deletions of DNA sequence in both retinoblastomas and mesenchymal tumors: organization of the sequence and its encoded protein. Proc Natl Acad Sci 1987; *24:*9059–9063.

249. Shew J-Y, Chen P-L, Bookstein R, Lee Y-HP, Lee W-H. Antibodies detecting abnormalities of the retinoblastoma susceptibility gene product (pp110[RB]) in osteosarcomas and synovial sarcomas. Oncogene Res 1989; *1:*205–214.

250. Kim J, Johnson K, Chen HJ, Carroll S, Laughton A. Drosophila Mad binds to DNA and directly mediates activation of vestigial by Decapentaplegic. Nature 1997; *388:*304–308.

251. Hayashi H, Abdollah S, Qiu Y, Cai J, Yong-Yao X, Grinnell BW, Richardson MA, Topper JN, Gimbrone MA, Wrana JL, Falb D. The MAD-related protein Smad7 associates with the TGFβ receptor and functions as an antagonist of TGFβ signaling. Cell 1997; *89:*1165–1173.

252. Takanami I, Tanaka F, Hashizume T, Kodaira S. Roles of the transforming growth factor beta 1 and its type I and II receptors in the development of a pulmonary adenocarcinoma: results of an immunohistochemical study. J Surg Oncol 1997; *64:*262–267.

253. Tu H, Jacobs SC, Borkowski A, Kyprianou N. Incidence of apoptosis and cell proliferation in prostate cancer: relationship with TGF-β1 and bcl-2 expression. Int J Cancer 1996; *69:*357–363.

254. Eastham JA, Truong LD, Rogers E, Kattan M, Flanders KC, Scardio PT, Thompson TC. Transforming growth factor-beta1: comparative immunohistochemical localization in human primary and metastatic prostate cancer. Lab Invest 1995; *73:*628–635.

255. Troung LD, Kadmon D, McCune BK, Flanders KC, Scardino PT, Thompson TC. Association of transforming growth factor-β1 with prostate cancer: an immunohistochemical study. Hum Pathol 1993; *24:*4–9.

256. Chen X, Rubock MJ, Whitman M. A transcriptional partner for MAD proteins in TGF-β signalling. Nature 1996; *383:*691–696.

257. Kretzchmar M, Lui F, Hata A, Doody J, Massague J. The TGF-β family mediator Smad1 is phosphorylated directly and activated functionally by the BMP receptor kinase. Genes Dev 1997; *11:*984–995.

258. Lui F, Hata A, Baker JC, Doody J, Carcamo J, Harland RM, Massague J. A human Mad protein as a BMP-regulated transcriptional activator. Nature 1996; *381:*620–623.

259. Hoodless PA, Haerry T, Abdollah S, Stapleton M, O'Connor MB, Attisano L, Wrana JL. MADR1, a MAD-related protein that functions in BMP2 signaling pathways. Cell 1996; *85:*489–500.

260. Sekelsky JJ, Newfield SJ, Raftery LA, Chartoff EH, Gelbart WM. Genetic characterization and cloning of Mothers against dpp, a gene required for decapentaplegic function in Drosophila melanogaster. Genetics 1995; *139:*1347–1358.

261. Parekh TV, Del Priore G, Schatz F, Demopoulos R, Korc M, Gold LI. Decreased growth inhibitory responses of primary cultures of endometrial carcinoma cells to TGF-β1 is accompanied by altered response to gonadal steroids. Proc Am Assoc Cancer Res *38:*3025.

262. Parekh TV, Schatz F, Del Priore G, Demopoulos R, Gold LI. Altered expression of TGF-β isoforms and TGF-β receptors in stromal cells derived from endometrial cancer patients in response to gonadal steroids. Gynecol Oncol 1997; *64:*310.

263. Yamaguchi T, Toguchida J, Yamamuro T, Kotoura Y, Takada, N, Kauaguchi N, Kaneko Y, Nakamura T, Sasaki MS, Ishizaki K. Allotype analysis in osteosarcomas: frequent allele loss on 3q, 13q, 17p, and 18q. Cancer Res 1992; *52:*2419–2423.

II
Diagnosis and Staging

Screening for Pancreatic Cancer Using Techniques to Detect Altered Gene Products

Robb E. Wilentz, Robbert J. C. Slebos, and Ralph H. Hruban

INTRODUCTION

Although cancer of the pancreas accounts for only 2% of new cancer cases in the United States, it is the fifth leading cause of cancer death *(1)*. This is true because many patients with pancreatic cancer are not diagnosed until late in the course of the disease, when the carcinoma has already metastasized or spread locally, and is no longer curable. Although 5-yr survival for all patients with cancer of the pancreas is 3% *(2)*, 5-yr survival after successful pancreaticoduodenectomy (Whipple procedure) approaches 20% overall, and may be as high as 40% in patients with small tumors, negative lymph nodes, and negative surgical margins *(3–4)*. Therefore, methods that can detect pancreatic cancers earlier, when they are still surgically resectable, will improve patient outcome.

The fundamental premise on which screening tests for the early detection of cancer are based is that *clinically early tumors are biologically late*. The smallest clinically detectable tumor weighs about 1 g and contains at least 10^9 cells. At this point the original tumor clone has already undergone approx 30 doublings. After only 10 more doublings, the tumor will weigh 1 kg, a mass no longer compatible with life. Therefore, by the time the average tumor is clinically detected, it has exhausted three-fourths of its lifespan *(5–7)*. This presents an enormous window of opportunity. If techniques can be developed to detect cancers based on properties other than their size, then smaller and therefore more curable tumors will be found.

Clinically early tumors are also genetically late. By this we mean that, at the time of clinical detection, most cancers already have accumulated a large number of molecular changes *(5)*. For example, in colorectal neoplasia, cells successively accumulate mutations that enable them to progress from hyperplasia to adenoma to invasive carcinoma. Mutations in the adenomatous polyposis coli (APC) gene occur early in this neoplastic progression, and usually are followed by mutations in K-*ras* and inactivation of the DCC (deleted in colorectal carcinoma) and *p53* genes *(8–9)*. There is evidence that cancers of other organs move through similar genetic paradigms, although these have not been elucidated as completely as they have been for tumors in the colorectum. For example, human papilloma virus (HPV) inactivates the products of the *p53* and *RB* (retinoblastoma) tumor-suppressor genes in the initial steps in cervical cancer progression *(10)*. Similarly, activating point mutations in K-*ras* are present very early in the development of adenocarcinoma of the lung, in microscopic lesions called atypical alveolar hyperplasias *(11)*. Thus, most neoplasms accumulate multiple genetic alterations long before they are large enough to be detected by current techniques. This suggests that molecular-based tests to identify genetic mutations can be used to detect early, and therefore curable, neoplasms.

THE DEVELOPMENT OF PANCREATIC CANCER

Pancreatic cancer is no exception to the general rules of neoplasia. Clinically early pancreatic cancers are indeed biologically late lesions. Histologic examination of pancreata resected for pancreatic cancer has revealed striking changes in the pancreatic ducts and ductules adjacent to the infiltrating cancers *(3)*. These changes have been called "hyperplasias" and "pancreatic intraepithelial neoplasias," and they include the replacement of the normal cuboidal epithelial lining of the ducts and ductules by a proliferative epithelium with varying degrees of cytologic and architectural atypia *(3,12)*. These lesions can be flat, papillary without atypia, papillary with atypia, or may even meet histopathologic criteria for carcinoma *in situ (13)*. For example, Cubilla and Fitzgerald *(13)* compared the duct changes in 227 pancreata with pancreatic cancer with the duct changes in 100 age- and sex-matched controls without pancreatic cancer. They found that papillary duct lesions were three times more common in the pancreata obtained from patients with pancreatic cancer than they were in pancreata obtained from patients without pancreatic cancer, and that the atypical papillary duct lesions were seen only in pancreata with pancreatic cancer *(13)*. Similar findings have been obtained by Kozuka et al. and Pour et al. *(14–15)*. More recently, Furukawa et al. *(16)*, using three-dimensional mapping techniques, have demonstrated a stepwise progression from mild dysplasia to severe dysplasia in these pancreatic duct lesions. These results suggest that, just as there is progression from adenoma to infiltrating adenocarcinoma in colonic neoplasia, so too is there progression in the pancreas from flat duct lesions to papillary duct lesions without atypia, to papillary duct lesions with atypia, and finally to infiltrating adenocarcinoma *(3,12)*.

Clinically detectable pancreatic cancers are also genetically late lesions. Most pancreatic cancers have accumulated numerous genetic alterations by the time they come to clinical presentation. For example, 85% or more of pancreatic adenocarcinomas contain activating point mutations in codon 12 of the K-*ras* oncogene *(17–24)*. In addition, three tumor-suppressor genes are inactivated frequently in pancreatic carcinomas: *p53* in up to 70% *(22–26)*, *p16* (multiple tumor suppressor 1 [*MTS1*]) in early 80% *(27–28)*, and deleted in pancreatic carcinoma 4 (*DPC4*) in 50% *(29)*. *RB* inactivation has been demonstrated in a small minority of pancreatic cancers, and germ line *BRCA2* (breast cancer 2) mutations have also been reported in 5 to 10% of patients with pancreatic cancer *(30–31)*. Indeed, Rozenblum et al. *(32)* recently determined the status of the K-*ras*, *p53*, *p16* (*MTS1*), *DPC4*, and *BRCA2* genes in a series of 42 pancreatic carcinomas. All 42 carcinomas harbored a mutation in codon 12 of K-*ras*, and inactivation of the *p53*, *p16* (*MTS1*), and *DPC4* genes occurred together in 37% of the cancers. Remarkably, one carcinoma had a germline mutation in *BRCA2* and eight additional selected genetic events *(32)*. Thus, multiple genetic alterations have already occurred by the time most pancreatic cancers are detected.

Even the biologically early duct lesions in the pancreas have genetic changes. Clonal activating point mutations in codon 12 of K-*ras* have been demonstrated in papillary and atypical papillary duct lesions. In contrast, K-*ras* mutations have not been found in morphologically normal pancreatic ducts *(33–41)*. Thus, duct lesions in the pancreas are the earliest microscopically recognizable lesions in the development of adenocarcinoma of the pancreas, and even these lesions harbor genetic changes.

The early duct lesions in the pancreas not only provide an opportunity to study the early genetic events in the development of adenocarcinoma of the pancreas, but they also suggest that molecular tests can be used to detect early neoplastic lesions in the pancreas before they have spread beyond the gland. These molecular tests center on detecting genetic changes resulting from mutations in three general types of genes: oncogenes, tumor-suppressor genes, and mutator genes (*see* Chapter 1 of this book). This chapter will examine techniques that can be used to detect mutations in an oncogene (K-*ras*), in a tumor-suppressor gene (*p53*), and in mutator genes (by way of microsatellite instabilities), and it will discuss how each of these techniques, in turn, could be used to develop novel tests to detect early pancreatic cancers.

MOLECULAR DETECTION OF K-RAS MUTATIONS

Of all the genes involved in pancreatic neoplasia, K-*ras* is currently the most attractive target for a molecular-based test to detect early pancreatic cancers. As described in detail in Chapter 1, K-*ras* is an oncogene that produces a G protein involved in signal transduction *(42)*, and it is an attractive target for four reasons. First, mutations in the K-*ras* gene are extremely common in pancreatic neoplasia. Between 80 and 100% of pancreatic carcinomas harbor activating point mutations in K-*ras (17–24)*. This suggests that K-*ras* will be a sensitive marker for the presence of a pancreatic cancer. Second, most of these mutations are single amino-acid changes restricted to codon 12 of the K-*ras* gene *(17–24)*. This greatly reduces the number of probes that need to be employed to detect these changes, thus markedly simplifying the assays. Third, K-*ras* mutations occur very early in the development of pancreatic cancer, so that tests for K-*ras* mutations could detect early neoplasms and allow for curative treatment *(33–41,43–53)*. Fourth, with modern molecular techniques, mutations in K-*ras* are detectable, even when cells harboring the mutations are admixed with much larger numbers of normal cells. In some studies, mutant cells have been detected in samples in which the cancer cells comprise as few as 1 in 10,000 of the cells in the sample *(36,38,43–53)*.

Techniques for Detecting Mutant K-ras

In Surgically Resected Tissue

In 1988, Almoguera et al. *(17)* were the first to describe mutations in the K-*ras* gene in resected adenocarcinomas of the pancreas. They already knew that K-*ras* played a significant role in the pathogenesis of a variety of cancers. In fact, their own group and another had previously shown that activating K-*ras* mutations were present in approx 40% of colorectal tumors *(54–55)*. In addition, the techniques they needed to detect K-*ras* mutations in pancreatic cancer already had been developed. These included tumor microdissection from slides cut from paraffin-embedded tissue, a technique in which areas of tumor with as little nonneoplastic tissue as possible are scraped from unstained microscope slides *(56–57)*; extraction and purification of DNA from the microdissected tissue *(56–57)*; amplification of the DNA by polymerase chain reaction (PCR) *(58–59)*; and mutation detection by RNase cleavage at sites of mismatch between DNA–RNA hybrids *(60)*. In this fourth procedure, amplified DNA is hybridized to artificially made wild-type K-*ras* RNA and then cleaved with RNase. Cleavage by RNase identifies a mutation, because the mutant DNA–RNA hybrids are cleaved by the RNase, but wild-type DNA–RNA hybrids are protected from the RNase cleavage. With this foundation, they analyzed 22 pancreatic carcinomas and found K-*ras* codon 12 mutations in 21. This study provided the first evidence that the vast majority of pancreatic cancers harbor activating-point mutations in K-*ras*.

DNA purification and PCR have not changed much since 1988. However, the techniques to detect mutations in clinical material eventually were improved by three developments: analysis of artificially created restriction fragment-length polymorphisms generated by PCR amplification (PCR-RFLP); hybridization with allele-specific oligodeoxynucleotides (ASOH); and enrichment of PCR products with mutant sequences at the expense of wild-type ones (mutant-enriched PCR). Each of these techniques may be important in the development of molecular screening tests for pancreatic cancer, and the following discussion gives examples of the uses of each technique and briefly describes the general methodologies of each.

An example of a study using PCR-RFLP analysis comes from Rall et al. *(24)*, who found codon 12 K-*ras* mutations in 14 of 20 (70%) surgically resected primary or metastatic pancreatic cancers. Briefly, this technique consists of amplifying with PCR DNA obtained from tumors. The PCR products then are digested with *Bst*NI, a restriction enzyme whose cleavage site is "built in" by PCR primers, so that *Bst*NI cleaves only wild-type codon 12 K-*ras* sequences. Mutant K-*ras* sequences are not cut with this enzyme. This procedure is possible because the first part of *Bst*NI's recognition site lies within the PCR primer; the remainder of the recognition site depends on the sequence present at codon 12 of K-*ras*. The PCR mixtures are then run on a gel. Because only the wild-type sequences are cut, wild-type and mutant samples produce different gel patterns. If the wild-type product has been completely digested, its gel contains only small fragments representing digested products. In contrast, carcinomas with mutant K-*ras* will contain a band representing the undigested product. In practice, tumors with mutations usually also contain digested products, because tumor samples almost always contain some admixed normal cells with wild-type DNA. Therefore, PCR-RFLP analysis identifies the presence of mutations. This technique, however, does not characterize the type of mutation, and nonmutant K-*ras* could mimic mutant K-*ras*, if the PCR products are incompletely digested by the restriction enzyme *(49)*. In such cases, laborious DNA sequence analysis is needed to correctly characterize the K-*ras* status of the sample *(49)*.

As a quicker alternative to this DNA sequencing, ASOH was developed to characterize and confirm the mutations *(18,54,61)*. In this technique, PCR products are denatured and spotted onto nylon membranes. The nylon membranes are then hybridized to radioactively labeled, sequence-specific oligodeoxynucleotide probes and washed under highly stringent conditions. As a result, the oligodeoxynucleotide probes will bind only to spots on the nylon membranes that harbor their exact corresponding sequences. The normal K-*ras* codon 12 DNA sequence is GGT, which encodes for glycine. There are six possible mutations at this site; GGT can be mutated to TGT (cysteine), AGT (serine), CGT (arginine), GTT (valine), GAT (aspartic acid), or GCT (alanine). Probes have been developed for wild-type K-*ras* and for each of these possible K-*ras* mutations. ASOH therefore can be used to identify the specific type of mutation present in a sample. With this method, Motojima et al. *(21)* detected K-*ras* codon 12 mutations in 46 of 53 (87%) pancreatic carcinomas. Importantly, they also were able to characterize the types of mutations and showed that the wild-type GGT was converted to GAT in 30 cases, to GTT in 12, to CGT in 5, and to TGT in 1. Forty-eight mutations were found in 46 cases because two patients had cancers with two different mutations, in both cases GAT and GTT *(21)*. ASOH therefore allows one not only to identify mutations, but also to characterize the exact type of mutation present.

Finally, mutant-enriched PCR was developed to detect mutations with greater sensitivity. With a combination of mutant-enriched PCR, PCR-RFLP, and ASOH, Hruban et al. *(19)* found K-*ras* mutations in 68 of 82 (83%) formalin-fixed, paraffin-embedded, surgically resected pancreatic adenocarcinomas. Their study essentially combined aspects of both PCR-RFLP and ASOH. Also, as the term "mutant enriched" suggests, they detected rare mutant sequences admixed with much larger numbers of wild-type sequences. This ability to detect rare mutant sequences will form an essential part of any molecular-based test to find cancers, because most samples that will be analyzed (e.g., blood and stool) will contain large numbers of normal cells harboring wild-type DNA. The following section will therefore describe this technique in detail.

First, as summarized in Fig. 1A, DNA prepared from a cancer is amplified by PCR. This PCR is performed with primers that generate a *Bst*NI restriction site in wild-type alleles of K-*ras*, but not in mutant alleles. The PCR products are then split into two equal portions. Next, only one of the two portions is digested with *Bst*NI. This digestion with *Bst*NI will cleave only wild-type K-*ras*. The specimen treated with *Bst*NI therefore will be enriched for mutant K-*ras*, but the portion of the specimen which was not treated with *Bst*NI will not be enriched. The difference between the two can be used to demonstrate the effectiveness of the enrichment. Both the unenriched and enriched sets are amplified again, and the products of this second amplification are then examined using PCR-RFLP, to detect mutations, and ASOH, to confirm and characterize them. Because mutant-enriched PCR increases the proportion of mutant sequences at the expense of wild-type ones, the PCR-RFLP of the enriched sample will identify mutations in samples in which the tumor cells make up only a small minority of the cells in the sample. These mutations may not have been detected without the enrichment procedure. A summary of these procedures is provided in Fig. 1B.

Similarly, the ASOH analyses of the enriched samples can be used to characterize mutations in samples in which the tumor cells make up only a small fraction of the cells in the sample. The effect of this enrichment and the power of this technique can be appreciated best by comparing unenriched and enriched samples on ASOH membranes (Fig. 1C). Each membrane is hybridized to one specific oligodeoxynucleotide probe, either wild-type or mutant. The first column on each membrane is the unenriched product, and the second, the enriched. A mutant sample should create a weak signal in the unenriched column and a strong signal in the enriched, when probed for the appropri-

A

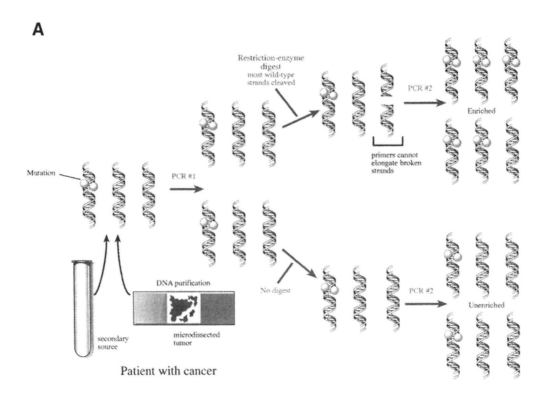

Fig. 1. (A) DNA purification and mutant-enriched polymerase chain reaction (PCR). DNA purified from either primary cancers or from secondary sources is amplified by PCR, possibly digested with the restriction enzyme *Bst*NI, and then amplified again. The specimen treated with *Bst*NI will be enriched for mutant K-*ras*, but the specimen which was not treated with *Bst*NI will not be enriched. **(B)** Artificially created restriction fragment-length polymorphisms generated by PCR amplification (PCR-RFLP). The restriction enzyme does not cleave mutant K-*ras*. Tumors with mutations, which contain both mutant and wild-type K-*ras*, will produce three bands. In contrast, pure wild-type samples show solely cleaved products (two bands) in both the unenriched and enriched lanes. Because mutant-enriched PCR (A) increases the proportion of mutant sequences at the expense of wild-type ones, the PCR-RFLP of the enriched sample will identify mutations in samples in which the tumor cells make up only a small fraction of the cells. Without the enrichment procedure, mutant genes appear as only very faint uncleaved bands. **(C)** Allele-specific oligodeoxynucleotide hybridization (ASOH). A mutant sample will create a weak signal in the unenriched column and a strong signal in the enriched, when probed for the appropriate mutation, since enrichment increases the proportion of mutant DNA. All samples with wild-type DNA, including tumor samples, will create a strong signal in the unenriched column and a weak signal in the enriched when probed for wild-type K-*ras*, since enrichment decreases the proportion of wild-type DNA. Pure wild-type samples show no signal when probed for mutant K-*ras*.

ate mutation, since enrichment increases the proportion of mutant DNA. All samples with wild-type DNA should create a strong signal in the unenriched column and a weak signal in the enriched when probed for wild-type K-*ras*, since enrichment decreases the proportion of wild-type DNA. Actual ASOH hybridization membranes are illustrated in Fig. 2. Figure 2 is complicated, but basically it shows four distinct membranes onto

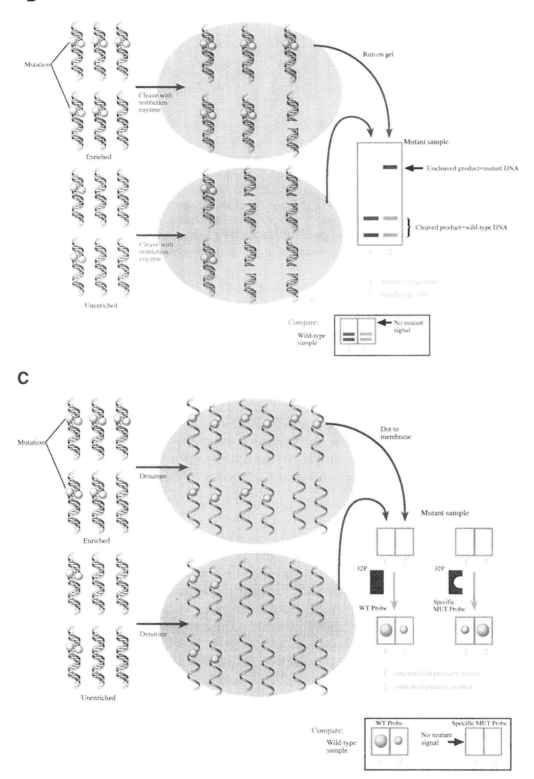

Fig. 1. (*continued*)

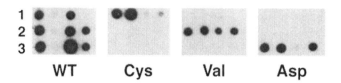

Fig. 2. Representative allele-specific oligodeoxynucleotide hybridization (ASOH). The first membrane has been probed for wild-type K-*ras*, and the second, third, and fourth for mutant K-*ras* (cys, val, asp). The first two columns on each membrane contain DNA prepared from a primary pancreatic cancer, and the third and fourth columns contain duodenal fluid-derived DNA from the same patient. The first and third columns are unenriched; the second and fourth columns are enriched for mutant K-*ras*. Patient 1 has a cysteine mutation; patient 2, a valine mutation; and patient 3, an aspartic acid mutation. Note how the enrichment procedure decreases wild-type signals and increases mutant signals. This ASOH also demonstrates that this technique can be used to detect mutant K-*ras* in duodenal fluid samples obtained from patients with pancreas cancer.

which PCR products have been spotted in identical positions. Each membrane, which consists of four columns, is hybridized to one specific oligodeoxynucleotide probe. The first two columns on each membrane contain DNA prepared from a primary pancreatic cancer, and the third and fourth columns contain duodenal fluid-derived DNA from the same patient. The first and third columns are unenriched; the second and fourth columns are enriched for mutant K-*ras*. Figure 2 demonstrates that the enrichment procedure decreases the wild-type signals and increases the mutant signals.

One can see quickly that the techniques described above provide the means both to enrich for mutant DNA and to identify definitively the type of mutation present in a sample. These advances will prove vital in developing molecular screening tests for early cancers.

K-ras in Secondary Sources

Now that the techniques to screen for rare mutations have been developed, the next natural question is, "What specimens should be screened?" Using mutant-enriched PCR, PCR-RFLP, and ASOH, several groups have probed for K-*ras* mutations in pure pancreatic juice, in fine needle aspirations (FNAs) of the pancreas, in endoscopic retrograde cholangiopancreatography (ERCP) brushings, in archived cytology smears, in blood, in stool, and in duodenal fluid. These specimen sources can be divided into two basic groups: those in which the detection of mutant K-*ras* could be used to confirm or belie the presence of cancer in a specimen obtained from a patient with abnormal radiology or cytology, and those in which the identification of K-*ras* mutations may lead to the development of population-based screening tests for pancreatic cancer.

For example, pure pancreatic juice, FNAs, and ERCP brushings are obtained by invasive procedures and therefore cannot be used in screening tests *(43–53)*. However, the identification of mutations in these sources can improve the sensitivity of cytology in establishing the diagnosis of a periampullary cancer. Indeed, two groups have found that the combination of cytology and K-*ras* mutation analysis raises the sensitivity of cancer identification over cytology alone, in one study from 76 to 83%, and in the other from 89 to 96% *(43,50)*. Cytology can be equivocal in as many as 50% of the cases be-cause chronic pancreatitis and well-differentiated adenocarcinoma may be histologi-cally indistinguishable *(62)*, and because there may be too few neoplastic cells in a cy-tology specimen for recognition by light microscopy *(2,43,50,63–68)*. The finding of mutant K-*ras* in an equivocal cytology specimen could be used to favor the diagnosis of cancer.

In contrast, samples of stool, blood, and perhaps even duodenal fluid could be used on a broader scale to screen for pancreatic cancers. For example, Tada et al. *(46)* found K-*ras* codon 12 mutations in the blood of two of six patients with adenocarcinoma of the pancreas, but the blood of two patients with insulinomas did not harbor mutant K-*ras* (sensitivity = 33%, specificity = 100%). Similarly, K-*ras* mutations have been iden-tified in the stools of patients with either pancreatic adenocarcinoma or cholangiocar-cinoma, but the sensitivity of this test proved to be only 57% and the specificity only 67% *(36)*. Finally, using mutant-enriched PCR and ASOH, K-*ras* mutations were iden-tified in only 13 of 51 samples (25%) of duodenal fluid (Fig. 2) obtained from patients undergoing pancreaticoduodenectomy for cancer *(38)*. Although these sensitivities and specificities are relatively disappointing, these studies do demonstrate that mutant DNA shed from the pancreas can be detected in duodenal juice, in stool, and even in the blood. Indeed, Berthélemy et al. have recently used a test for K-*ras* to diagnose two pancreas cancers 18 and 40 mo before they were clinically apparent (68*a*).

If these sources are, however, ever used in future screening tests, there are a few caveats that should be noted. First, stool and blood specimens do not sample lesions just from the pancreas. DNA in the stool can come from anywhere in the digestive tract, and DNA in the blood can come from anywhere in the body. Thus, mutant K-*ras* in the stool could originate from an adenoma in the colon, and mutant K-*ras* in the blood could originate from a lung tumor. Simply stated, K-*ras* mutations are not organ specific. Sec-ond, because even very early duct lesions may contain genetic alterations such as K-*ras* mutations, a positive test is not specific for an infiltrating cancer. Indeed, Caldas et al. *(36)* demonstrated that the K-*ras* mutations in stool specimens obtained from four patients in their series were derived from noninvasive pancreatic duct lesions. These duct lesions also appear to be the source of some of the mutations found in duodenal fluid and pancreatic juice *(38,46)*. Early duct lesions, however, do not necessarily progress to cancer. One would hate to perform radical surgery because of a mutation found in a screening test, only to learn that the only lesion present was an early duct lesion that may never have caused the patient any harm.

K-ras Conclusions

K-*ras* mutations can be detected in primary tumors and secondary sources, with sen-sitivities and specificities that depend on both the source and method used. K-*ras* mu-tations can be detected in pure pancreatic juice, in FNAs, and in ERCP brushings, with higher sensitivities than in blood, stool, and duodenal fluid. K-*ras* detection in the for-mer sources can be used to clarify diagnoses when histology is equivocal. More research is needed, however, to devise tests that are more sensitive and specific for cancer in the latter sources before K-*ras* mutational analyses are applied to screening the general pop-ulation. These tests must be quick, easy, and cost-effective, certainly a difficult task to achieve.

In conclusion, mutations at codon 12 of K-*ras* are the most common molecular genetic alterations in pancreatic cancer. The detection of K-*ras* mutations in secondary sources may form the basis for the development of new approaches to detect pancreatic cancer earlier and less invasively, and to differentiate it from benign conditions of the pancreas.

MOLECULAR DETECTION OF P53 MUTATIONS

Another gene associated with the development of pancreas cancer is the *p53* tumor-suppressor gene (*see* Chapter 1). Although the genetic changes in *p53* are not as easy to detect as are mutations in K-*ras*, the identification of *p53* mutations and deletions eventually may help identify patients with pancreatic cancer. *p53* is an attractive target for two reasons. First, *p53* is frequently inactivated in pancreas cancer; it is mutated and/or deleted in 50–70% of pancreatic adenocarcinomas *(22–26,69–78)*. Second, mutations in the *p53* gene can be detected at a variety of levels: the *p53* gene, the *p53* protein, or the cell cycle control pathway.

Unfortunately, screening for cancer using techniques to detect mutations that inactivate *p53* has two major problems. First, the *p53* gene is large, and mutations can occur throughout the gene; therefore, one must search a large stretch of DNA to identify the majority of genetic changes *(69–74)*. This means that, with the current technology, screening tests for mutant *p53* DNA will be very time-consuming. In addition, although alternative tests for *p53* inactivation based upon the detection of the *p53* protein are less time-consuming, they will not detect mutant *p53* in all cases *(24,75,77–78)*. Second, K-*ras* mutations appear to occur early in the development of pancreatic cancer, but the timing of most *p53* mutations in the progression of pancreatic cancer is not well established *(78–79)*. Although some *p53* mutations have been identified in pancreatic carcinoma *in situ*, in other organ systems *p53* is primarily a marker for invasive cancer *(69–73)*. *p53* mutations may therefore best be used to clarify diagnoses of cancer, rather than to screen patients for early cancers.

Despite these problems, several investigators have explored the detection of *p53* genetic changes in pancreatic cancer, primarily because genetic alterations of *p53* are so common, and because *p53* has proven a useful target in other organs, especially the colon.

Techniques for Detecting p53

In Surgically Resected Tissue

Mutations in the *p53* gene have been detected using a variety of techniques, including PCR and single-strand conformation polymorphism (SSCP) analysis. SSCP is a technique that can be used to screen larger genes for mutations, and it has been used to detect single base-pair changes, with sensitivities of up to 95% in human leukocytes and tumor cell lines *(80)*. The procedure consists of tagging DNA with a radioactive label during PCR, separating the amplification products on a nondenaturing polyacrylamide gel, and then autoradiographing the gels. This method identifies mutations, because, under conditions that allow for the formation of secondary structures, a single base-pair alteration can cause conformational, and hence gel mobility, changes in DNA *(24,80)*. For example, after amplifying all the coding exons in the *p53* gene and analyzing these PCR products by SSCP, Rall et al. *(24)* identified *p53* mutations in three of 14 (21%) primary periampullary carcinomas and three of six (50%) metastases. Direct sequencing confirmed that all six cases harbored *p53* mutations. The sensitivity of the SSCP technique, however, can vary greatly from laboratory to laboratory.

Immunohistochemical staining for the *p53* gene product can serve as a surrogate screen for *p53* mutations, because wild-type *p53* protein has a half-life of only 20–30 min, and usually does not reach immunohistochemically detectable levels; mutant p53 frequently has a longer half-life, and therefore reaches immunohistochemically detectable levels *(75,77–78,81–85)*. Although it is only an indirect marker for the presence of mutations, immunohistochemical staining for the p53 protein is a sensitive and specific marker for mutant *p53* in colorectal tumors *(86–90)*. In the pancreas, 25–70% of primary adenocarcinomas have been reported to stain for p53. In addition, *in situ* carcinomas adjacent to pancreatic adenocarcinoma have been reported to stain for the *p53* gene product; staining in the nonneoplastic pancreas has not been reported *(3,24,75,77–78)*.

Rall et al. *(24)* compared the results they obtained from both SSCP and immunohistochemical staining in a series of pancreatic carcinomas. Immunochemical staining was positive in 9 of 14 (64%) primary carcinomas, but SSCP analysis detected mutations in only three (21%) of the cancers. In this same study, three of six (50%) metastatic carcinomas stained for the *p53* protein, and all three also produced gene mobility changes on an SSCP gel. SSCP analysis or immunohistochemistry did not identify *p53* mutations in any of the control samples (from patients with normal pancreatic tissue or with chronic pancreatitis). Thus, in only one-third of the immunohistochemically positive primary cancers could a mutation be confirmed by SSCP.

Some of the discrepancies between immunohistochemical staining and sequence analysis can be explained by considering the types of mutations that can occur in the *p53* gene. *p53* can be inactivated by mutation or deletion. Although missense mutations cause the production of mutant proteins, which could be detected immunohistochemically, nonsense mutations or deletions result in truncated gene products, which may not be detectable immunohistochemically. Indeed, in Rall et al.'s study described above *(24)*, one cancer that did not stain for *p53* protein actually contained a mutation by SSCP analysis. The *p53* gene was sequenced, and a nonsense mutation was found. Similarly, when Slebos et al. *(90)* studied the inactivation of *p53* by DNA sequence analysis and immunohistochemistry in colorectal carcinomas, they found five cases that harbored mutations that would result in truncated proteins, and none of these samples were positive for p53 protein by immunohistochemistry. Thus, immunohistochemical staining for p53 is an imperfect marker for the presence of mutations in the *p53* gene.

Because of these limitations in staining for p53, others have looked at different proteins that reflect p53 function. This approach is possible because wild-type, and not mutant, p53 acts indirectly to suppress tumor growth by inducing the synthesis of a cascade of factors. The absence of these cascade constituents therefore may indicate a mutation in *p53 (90–99)*. For example, wild-type *p53* protein activates transcription of the *WAF1* gene. The gene product of *WAF1*, p21, in turn inactivates complexes necessary for cell growth. In the absence of wild-type p53 protein, p21 is not produced, complexes are not inhibited, and cell growth occurs unchecked. Because wild-type p53 protein results in the production of p21, the presence of p21 theoretically could signal a wild-type p53 gene *(90–99)*. Unfortunately, theory does not play out in practice. DiGiuseppe et al. *(100)* recently demonstrated that *WAF1* expression does not correlate with *p53* mutational status in pancreatic cancer. These findings are consistent with the recent discovery of other pathways, independent of p53, by which *WAF1* is activated *(90,100–102)*. To summarize, the *p53* tumor-suppressor gene is frequently inactivated in pancreatic cancers, but this inactivation can be difficult to detect, even in the primary cancers.

p53 in Secondary Sources

p53 mutations have also been detected in secondary sources from patients with pancreatic cancer. van Es et al. *(43)* immunohistochemically stained a series of pancreatic cancers and compared the staining patterns in the primary cancers with those seen in cytology specimens from the same patients. In their series, immunocytochemical staining for the *p53* gene product demonstrated the accumulation of p53 protein in six of seventeen (35%) cytology samples. The patients' tumors were resected, and 11 of the 17 (66%) primary tumors stained positively. All five discrepancies between the cytologies and the primary cancers were from cytology specimens that originally had been processed with Giemsa stain. Significantly, staining for p53 confirmed the diagnosis of malignancy in one cytology sample originally read as atypical cells suspicious for malignancy. From these results, van Es and colleagues *(43)* concluded that immunohistochemical staining for the p53 protein, combined with cytological analysis, may be useful in identifying cancers with a greater sensitivity than cytological analysis alone. Thus, the immunohistochemical detection of *p53* protein in cytology samples can be used in much the same way as the detection of K-*ras* mutations, i.e., to clarify equivocal diagnoses.

Mutations in *p53* also have been detected in more accessible secondary sources, although not yet from patients with pancreatic cancer. For example, *p53* mutations have been identified in the urine of patients with bladder cancer *(103)*, and recently *p53* genetic changes were detected in the stool of patients with colon cancer *(104)*. The genetic alterations in the stool were identified by amplifying exons 5–8 of the *p53* gene by PCR and then using SSCP. When this was done, SSCP changes were noted in 11 of 25 (44%) primary adenocarcinomas of the colon and in 7 of 25 (28%) stool samples from these same patients. All seven of the stool-positive patients had *p53* mutations in their primary carcinomas. More significantly, the same patients were also screened for colon cancer using fecal occult blood detection. Three of five patients (60%) who had a negative fecal occult blood screen produced stool with detectable *p53* mutations. Thus, molecular genetic testing of stool for *p53* mutations may be more sensitive for cancer than fecal occult blood detection. Clearly, there are enormous technical hurdles to overcome before *p53*-based detection tests can be used to screen for pancreatic cancer. Nonetheless, screening for mutant *p53* may provide the specificity not provided by screening for mutant K-*ras*.

p53 Conclusions

Although genetic changes in *p53* are almost as common in pancreatic cancer as are K-*ras* mutations, the methods used to detect *p53* mutations will be difficult to apply on a large scale for three reasons. First, a quick and easy test to probe the gene has not yet been developed, because mutations occur throughout the *p53* gene. Second, immuno-histochemical stains for p53 can never detect all of the genetic changes in *p53*, because immunohistochemistry stains only stable mutant products of *p53*. Nonsense mutations and deletions do not produce immunohistochemically stable products. Third, as is true for mutations in K-*ras*, mutations in *p53* are seen in other organs besides the pancreas. Nevertheless, even if detection of *p53* mutations is tedious and costly, tests to identify these mutations may be cost-effective if their use eliminates unnecessary surgical procedures, or if they can be used to save lives by identifying early cancers.

MOLECULAR DETECTION OF MICROSATELLITE INSTABILITIES

An exciting advance in the molecular detection of cancers has been the identification of microsatellite instabilities. Microsatellite instability results from mutations in DNA repair genes (the "mutator phenotype"), or possibly from saturation of a normal DNA repair system *(105–112)*. Because their DNA repair process goes awry, tumors with the mutator phenotype possess multiple di-, tri-, or quadranucleotide repeat expansions or deletions throughout their genome. Such changes have been described in tumors with colorectal and bladder cancers, and they may serve as markers for cancer in these cases *(109–112)*. In fact, Mao et al. *(112)* have used the detection of microsatellite instabilities as an adjunct to urine cytology to diagnose and screen for bladder cancer. Using PCR with radioactively labeled primers targeted to areas prone to microsatellite instability, they were able to identify either microsatellite instabilities (by the presence of shifted bands) and/or losses of alleles (by the loss of bands) in 19 of 20 patients (95%) with bladder cancer. In contrast, urine cytology identified only 9 of the 18 patients (50%) with bladder cancer in this series. Of note, however, instabilities and/or allelic losses were also discovered in 2 of 5 patients (40%) with an inflammatory condition of the bladder, although cytology identified atypical cells in these two patients as well *(112)*. Thus, just as molecular tests have shown the potential to be more sensitive than fecal blood tests, so too may molecular tests be more sensitive than urine cytology.

Unfortunately, the detection of microsatellite instabilities probably will not be applicable in the widespread diagnosis of, and screening for, pancreatic cancer. First, although these changes have been described in patients with pancreatic cancer *(107–108,108a)*, the frequency with which they occur is probably very low *(25,108)*. Goggins et al. found microsatellite instabilities in 3 (4%) of 82 pancreatic cancers *(108a)*. Second, although it has not been confirmed, microsatellite instabilities may occur in pancreata with benign conditions, such as pancreatitis. Brentnall et al. *(107)* found microsatellite instabilities at one or more loci in pancreatic juice-derived DNA from 5 of 5 patients (100%) with pancreatitis, and in primary tissue-derived DNA from 8 of 9 patients (89%) with pancreatitis *(107)*. Therefore, the detection of microsatellite instabilities may not distinguish pancreatic cancer from benign conditions. Third, the detection of microsatellite instabilities requires the analysis of numerous areas of the genome, and so, at present, the technique is costly and time-consuming.

Thus, although the detection of microsatellite instabilities is proving useful in other organ systems, it seems unlikely that microsatellite instabilities can be applied to the diagnosis of, and screening for, pancreatic cancer.

SCREENING POPULATIONS AND FAMILIAL PANCREATIC CANCER

Genetic changes no doubt will be used to clarify equivocal diagnoses. However, the identification of genetic changes as a method of screening the general population for cancer has one major disadvantage. Pancreas cancer is a relatively rare disease, and as a consequence, screening large numbers of people may generate too many false-positive results. A much more logical approach would be to screen a population known to be at increased risk for the development of pancreas cancer. Narrowing the application of molecular tests to screening only persons at risk would decrease false positives and could make the test worth the costs of its clinical application. Familial pancreatic cancer cases may account for up to 5–10% of all cases of pancreatic cancer *(113–130)*, and patients with a family history of pancreatic cancer may represent a population worth screening.

Patients with familial pancreatic cancer can be divided into three general groups. First, some patients have well-characterized syndromes that predispose them to the development of pancreatic cancer. These syndromes include hereditary pancreatitis, ataxia-telangiectasia, hereditary nonpolyposis colorectal carcinoma syndrome (HNPCC, or Lynch syndrome), familial atypical multiple-mole melanoma (FAMMM) syndrome, and Peutz-Jeghers syndrome *(3,113,115,117,120–122)*. Second, some patients have a family history of pancreatic cancer but do not have a clinically definable syndrome. For example, the authors have collected over 114 families *(130a)* and Lynch has reported over 30 families, in which two or more family members had pancreas cancer. In some of these families, the pancreas cancer appeared to be inherited in an autosomal dominant pattern *(113–115,118)*. Third, some patients with pancreatic cancer have a family history of extrapancreatic cancer, and others with extrapancreatic cancer have a family history of pancreatic cancer *(115)*. For example, Tulinius et al. *(123)* have found an increased risk of pancreas cancer in male first-degree relatives of women with breast cancer, and Kerber et al. *(124)* have demonstrated an increased risk of ovarian cancer in patients with a family history of pancreatic cancer. In addition, some patients with familial forms of melanoma and breast cancer are at increased risk for developing pancreatic cancer *(125–130)*. Because they are at increased risk for developing pancreatic cancer, family members in all three of these groups would be attractive candidates for molecular-based screening tests.

Furthermore, these families could be screened for germline mutations in known cancer-causing genes. For a long time, the specific genetic alterations that cause the hereditary forms of pancreatic cancer were not known, but, recently, germline mutations in the *BRCA2* gene (often also present in familial forms of breast cancer) and in the *p16 (MTS1)* gene have been shown to be responsible for some familial pancreatic cancers *(31,127–131)*. For example, Moskaluk et al. *(131)* screened 21 families with a familial aggregation of pancreatic cancer, and they identified one family with germline *p16 (MTS1)* mutations in two members. Both family members with germline *p16 (MTS1)* mutations developed pancreatic cancer. Similarly, Goggins et al. *(31)* found germline mutations in the *BRCA2* gene in 3 of 41 patients (7%) with pancreatic adenocarcinomas. Thus, molecular biology-based tests may serve two functions in families with an aggregation of pancreatic cancer. Family members could be tested for germline mutations in known cancer-causing genes, such as *BRCA2* and *p16 (MTS1)*, and family members also could be screened for early cancers using molecular-based screening tests.

In order to study the pathogenesis of familial pancreatic cancer and the possibility of screening this population, The National Familial Pancreas Tumor Registry (NFPTR) has been established at The Johns Hopkins Hospital. This database now includes over 114 families in which at least two first-degree relatives have had pancreatic cancer. The address of the registry is The National Familial Pancreatic Tumor Registry, The Johns Hopkins Hospital, Department of Pathology, Meyer 7-181, 600 N. Wolfe Street, Baltimore, MD 21287-6971. The telephone and facsimile numbers are (410) 955-9132 and (410) 955-0115. The NFPTR also can be accessed on the World Wide Web at http://www.path.jhu.edu/pancreas.

FUTURE PERSPECTIVES: SERIAL ANALYSIS OF GENE EXPRESSION (SAGE)

The detection of genetic changes thus far has focused on the identification of mutations in one gene, but technology is now available to characterize the expression of multiple genes simultaneously. One such method, called serial analysis of gene expression (SAGE), can be used to identify the transcriptional activity of thousands of genes at once *(132)*. This technique holds enormous promise; it will be described briefly, as a preview of what the future might hold for the molecular detection of pancreatic cancer (132a, 132b).

The SAGE technique is illustrated in Fig. 3. Briefly, complementary DNA (cDNA), coupled to biotin, is produced from a cell's mRNA. Because it is made from mRNA, this cDNA represents only transcribed gene sequences. The cDNA then is cleaved into fragments of varying lengths with a particular restriction enzyme ("anchoring enzyme"). Binding the biotin-labeled 3' ends of these cDNA fragments to streptavidin beads leaves only 5' ends of the cleaved cDNA exposed. The cDNA fragments are then split into two portions, and to each portion a synthetic DNA linker, containing a type IIS restriction enzyme ("tagging enzyme") recognition site, is added. The linkers are then coupled to the exposed 5' ends of the cDNA fragments. Because Type IIS restriction enzymes cleave at a fixed distance downstream from their recognition sites, treatment of each of the portions of cDNA with the tagging enzyme results in free-floating fragments that contain a linker at one end and a short stretch of cDNA, recently cleaved by the tagging enzyme, at the other end. The two portions of cDNA fragments attached to the linkers now are mixed together, and ligation allows any two random cDNA fragments to join together back-to-back at the sites where the tagging enzyme had cleaved them. These difragments then are amplified by PCR with primers specific for each linker. The resulting mixture contains fragments in roughly the same concentrations as in the initial mixture, with the more actively transcribed genes producing more fragments. The amplified products then are cleaved with the anchoring enzyme. Because the linkers had been attached originally at these sites, they fall off. The result is a difragment of two pieces of DNA oriented back-to-back and surrounded by anchoring enzyme sites. Then, because these restriction enzyme sites are easily coupled by ligation, many difragments can be linked together, and a large number of short DNA fragments now can be cloned and sequenced in one long stretch of DNA.

The technical advantages of SAGE are twofold. First, fragments of DNA are oriented and tagged by restriction enzyme site sequences, enabling their easy identification during sequencing. Second, by placing two cDNA fragments together in one difragment

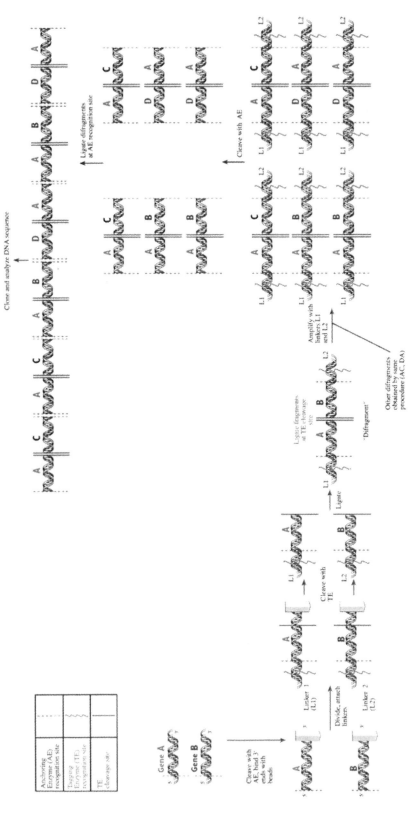

Fig. 3. Serial analysis of gene expression (SAGE). SAGE results in a difragment of two pieces of cDNA oriented back-to-back and surrounded by anchoring enzyme sites. Because these restriction enzyme sites are easily coupled by ligation, many difragments can be linked together, and a large number of short cDNA fragments can then be cloned and sequenced in one long stretch of DNA. SAGE can be used to characterize all of the genes expressed in a cancer, and it may help identify new markers of pancreatic cancer.

before the application of PCR, any bias in the amplification procedure, with a particular difragment predominating, is obvious. Without difragments, one cannot determine if a prevalent fragment represents PCR bias or the true transcriptional activity of a gene.

One of the first tissues to be examined using the SAGE technique was the pancreas. Eight hundred forty SAGE sequences were generated from normal pancreas. Three hundred fifty-one of these occurred once, and 77 occurred multiple times. The 10 most commonly occurring SAGE sequences, and thus the 10 most commonly expressed genes in the pancreas, matched database sequences for genes of known pancreatic function. For example, the three most common sequences were from the procarboxypeptidase A1, pancreatic trypsinogen 2, and chymotrypsinogen genes *(132)*.

The power of SAGE and other techniques that analyze multiple mRNAs simultaneously is clear. First, by comparing the transcriptional activity of different genes in benign and cancerous tissue, these techniques can be used to characterize the genes involved in neoplastic transformation *(132a)*. Second, when applied to cancers, they can be used to identify new genes expressed in cancer cells, and these new genes may lead to new assays to detect cancers *(132b)*. For example, SAGE can be used to discover an abundantly expressed sequence that could serve as a serum marker specific for pancreas cancer *(132b)*. Just as there is a PSA marker for prostate cancer, so too could SAGE be used to discover a pancreas-specific antigen. Finally, SAGE eventually could be used as a diagnostic or screening test to determine a specimen's malignant potential. The invention of SAGE is a first step in the development of clinically applicable tests that can analyze numerous transcription fragments at once. These tests will provide a molecular fingerprint that may identify cells with malignant potential.

CONCLUSIONS

The identification of molecular genetic changes in human tissues may serve four purposes. First, it may be used to clarify ambiguous morphology. In this regard, the detection of molecular genetic changes will prove a useful adjunct to cytology. Second, molecular genetic changes can be used to detect the presence of a neoplasm, even when the neoplasm is too small to be detected clinically, using current technology. Third, molecular genetics can be used to identify patients with germline mutations in cancer-causing genes who would be at increased risk for the development of cancer. Finally, molecular genetics can be used to identify the recurrence of disease by detecting the return of cancer-specific genetic changes in clinical samples.

Tests serving each of these purposes are in various stages of development for a variety of extrapancreatic organs. For example, in cases in which the histopathology is equivocal, microsatellite instabilities and allelic losses have been used to verify the presence of cancer in urine cytology specimens *(112)*. In addition, *p53* mutations have been used to screen the urine of patients with preinvasive bladder cancer *(103,133)*. In families with an aggregation of breast cancer, noninvasive tests have been used to characterize the *BRCA1* and *BRCA2* breast cancer genes in at-risk family members. Germline mutations in *BRCA1* or *BRCA2* indicate an increased risk for the development of breast cancer *(134)*. Finally, in squamous carcinoma of the head and neck, the detection of *p53* mutations may be used to identify residual cancer after treatment, with greater sensitivity than does histological analysis alone *(135–136)*.

Molecular biology is also applicable to pancreas cancer on all four of these fronts. Molecular-based tests one day may be used to confirm the presence of pancreatic cancer in cytology specimens, to detect genetic changes consistent with pancreatic cancer in screening sources, to identify germline mutations in patients at risk for pancreatic cancer, and to predict recurrences of pancreatic cancer. Each of these applications may, in turn, improve survival in patients with pancreatic cancer.

We are on our way to applying molecular-based tests to pancreatic cancer. However, before these tests can be applied to a large number of patients, more development is needed to generate quick, easy, cost-efficient, sensitive, specific, and noninvasive tests. Although we know what genes to probe, we cannot do it yet with the speed, ease, efficiency, and accuracy that are required for clinical application. Much more effort is needed. It will be worth the effort, however, because the application of molecular biology to clinical practice will impact greatly the prevention and effective treatment of pancreatic cancer.

REFERENCES

1. Parker SL, Tong T, Bolden S, et al. Cancer statistics. Ca Cancer J Clin 1996; *46:*5–27.
2. Warshaw AL and Castillo CF. Pancreatic carcinoma. N Engl J Med 1992; *326:*455–465.
3. DiGiuseppe JA, Yeo CJ, and Hruban RH. Molecular biology and the diagnosis and treatment of adenocarcinoma of the pancreas. Adv Anat Path 1996; *3:*139–155.
4. Yeo CJ, Cameron JL, Lillemoe KD, et al. Pancreaticoduodenectomy for cancer of the head of the pancreas: 201 patients. Ann Surg 1995; *221:*721–733.
5. Cotran RS, Kumar V, and Robbins SL, eds. Robbins pathologic basis of disease, 5th ed., WB Saunders, Philadelphia, 1994; p. 272.
6. Tannock IF. Biology of tumor growth. Hosp Pract 1983; *18:*81–93.
7. Tannock IF. Cell proliferation. In: Tannock IF, and Hill RP (eds), Basic science of oncology, 2nd ed., McGraw-Hill, New York, 1992; p. 154.
8. Vogelstein B and Kinzler KW. The multistep nature of cancer. Trends Genet 1993; *9:*138–141.
9. Fearon ER and Vogelstein B. A genetic model for colorectal tumorigenesis. Cell 1990; *61:*759–767.
10. zur Hausen H. Viruses in human cancers. Science 1991; *254:*1167–1173.
11. Westra WH, Baas IO, Hruban RH, et al. K-*ras* oncogene activation in atypical alveolar hyperplasias of the human lung. Cancer Res 1996; *56:*2224–2228.
12. Hruban RH, DiGiuseppe JA, and Offerhaus GJA. K-*ras* mutations in pancreatic ductal proliferative lesions: author's reply. Am J Pathol 1994; *145:*1548–1550.
13. Cubilla A and Fitzgerald PJ. Morphological lesions associated with human primary invasive nonendocrine pancreas cancer. Cancer Res 1976; *36:*2690–2698.
14. Kozuka S, Sassa R, Taki T, et al. Relation of pancreatic duct hyperplasia to carcinoma. Cancer 1979; *43:*1418–1428.
15. Pour PM, Sayed S, and Sayed G. Hyperplastic, preneoplastic, and neoplastic lesions found in 83 human pancreases. Am J Clin Pathol 1982; *77:*13–52.
16. Furukawa T, Chiba R, Kobari M, et al. Varying grades of epithelial atypia in the pancreatic ducts of humans. Arch Pathol Lab Med 1994; *118:*227–234.
17. Almoguera C, Shibata D, Forrester K, et al. Most human carcinomas of the exocrine pancreas contain mutant c-K-*ras* genes. Cell 1988; *53:*549–554.
18. Smit VT, Boot AJ, Smits AM, et al. K-*ras* codon 12 mutations occur very frequently in pancreatic adenocarcinomas. Nuclei Acid Res 1988; *16:*7773–7782.
19. Hruban RH, van Mansfield ADM, Offerhaus GJA, et al. K-*ras* oncogene activation in adenocarcinoma of the human pancreas: a study of 82 carcinomas using a combination of mu-

tant-enriched polymerase chain reaction analysis and allele-specific oligonucleotide hybridization. Am J Pathol 1993; *143:*545–554.

20. Grünewald K, Lyons J, Frohlich A, et al. High frequency of Ki-*ras* codon 12 mutations in pancreatic adenocarcinomas. Int J Cancer 1989; *43:*1037–1041.

21. Motojima K, Urano T, Nagata Y, et al. Detection of point mutations in the Kirsten-*ras* oncogene provides evidence for the multicentricity of pancreatic carcinoma. Ann Surg 1993; *217:*138–143.

22. Kalthoff H, Schmiegel W, Roeder C, et al. *p53* and K-*ras* alterations in pancreatic epithelial cell lesions. Oncogene 1993; *8:*289–298.

23. Pellegata NS, Sessa F, Renault B, et al. K-*ras* and *p53* gene mutations in pancreatic cancer: ductal and non-ductal tumors progress through different genetic lesions. Cancer Res 1994; *54:*1556–1560.

24. Rall CJN, Yan Y, Graeme-Cook F, et al. Ki-*ras* and *p53* mutations in pancreatic ductal adenocarcinoma. Pancreas 1996; *12:*10–17.

25. Seymour AB, Hruban RH, Redston MS, et al. Allelotype of pancreatic adenocarcinoma. Cancer Res 1994; *54:*2761–2764.

26. Redston MS, Caldas C, Seymour AB, et al. *p53* mutations in pancreatic carcinoma and evidence of common involvement of homocopolymer tracts in DNA microdeletions. Cancer Res 1994; *54:*3025–3033.

27. Caldas C, Hahn SA, da Costa LT, et al. Frequent somatic mutations and homozygous deletions of the *p16 (MTS1)* gene in pancreatic adenocarcinoma. Nature Genet 1994; *8:*27–32.

28. Huang L, Goodrow TL, Zhang S, et al. Deletion and mutation analyses of the *p16/MTS-1* tumor-suppressor gene in human ductal pancreatic cancer reveal a higher frequency of abnormalities in tumor-derived cell lines than in primary ductal adenocarcinomas. Cancer Res 1996; *56:*1137–1141.

29. Hahn SA, Schutte M, Shamsul Hoque ATM, et al. *DPC4*, a candidate tumor-suppressor gene at human chromosome 18q21.1. Science 1996; *271:*350–353.

30. Huang L, Lang D, Geradts J, et al. Molecular and immunochemical analyses of RB1 and cyclin D1 in human ductal pancreatic carcinomas and cell lines. Mol Carcinog 1996; *15:*85–95.

31. Goggins M, Schutte M, Lu J, et al. Germline *BRCA2* gene mutations in patients with apparently sporadic pancreatic carcinomas. Cancer Res 1996; *56:*5360–5364.

32. Rozenblum E, Schutte M, Goggins M, et al. Co-existent inactivations infer distinct tumor-suppressive pathways in pancreatic cancer. Cancer Res 1997; *57:*1731–1734.

33. Cerny WL, Mangold KA, and Scarpelli DG. K-*ras* mutations is an early event in pancreatic duct carcinogenesis in the Syrian golden hamster. Cancer Res 1992; *52:*4507–4513.

34. DiGiuseppe JA, Hruban RH, Offerhaus GJA, et al. Detection of K-*ras* mutations in mucinous pancreatic duct hyperplasia from a patient with a family history of pancreatic carcinoma. Am J Pathol 1994; *144:*889–895.

35. Yanagisawa A, Ohtake K, Ohashi K, et al. Frequent c-Ki-*ras* oncogene activation in mucous cell hyperplasias of pancreas suffering from chronic inflammation. Cancer Res 1993; *53:*953–956.

36. Caldas C, Hahn SA, Hruban RH, et al. Detection of K-*ras* mutations in the stool of patients with pancreatic adenocarcinoma and pancreatic ductal hyperplasia. Cancer Res 1994; *54:*3568–3573.

37. Lemoine NR, Jain S, Hughes CM, et al. Ki-*ras* oncogene activation in preinvasive pancreatic cancer. Gastroenterology 1992; *102:*230–236.

38. Wilentz RE, Chung CH, Musler A, et al. Detection of K-*ras* mutations in duodenal fluid-derived DNA from patients with periampullary cancer. 1998; *82:*96–103.

39. Smith RC, Kneale K, and Goulston K. *In situ* carcinoma of the pancreas. Aust NZ J Surg 1986; *56:*369–373.

40. Tabata T, Fujimori T, Maeda S, et al. The role of *ras* mutation in pancreatic cancer, precancerous lesions, and chronic pancreatitis. Int J Pancreatol 1993; *14:*237–244.

41. Tada M, Ohashi M, and Shiratori Y. Analysis of K-*ras* gene mutations in hyperplastic duct cells of the pancreas without pancreas disease. Gastroenterology 1996; *110:*227–231.

42. Barbacid M. *Ras* genes. Annu Rev Biochem 1987; *56:* 779–827.

43. van Es JM, Polak MM, van den Berg FM, et al. Molecular markers for diagnostic cytology of neoplasms in the head region of the pancreas: mutation of K-*ras* and overexpression of the p53 protein product. J Clin Pathol 1995; *48:*218–222.

44. Berthélemy P, Bouisson M, Escourrou J, et al. Identification of K-*ras* mutations in pancreatic juice in the early diagnosis of pancreatic cancer. Ann Intern Med 1995; *123:*188–191.

45. Watanabe H, Sawabu N, Songür Y, et al. Detection of K-*ras* point mutations at codon 12 in pure pancreatic juice for the diagnosis of pancreatic cancer by PCR-RFLP analysis. Pancreas 1996; *12:*18–24.

46. Tada M, Omata M, Kawai S, et al. Detection of ras gene mutations in pancreatic juice and peripheral blood of patients with pancreatic adenocarcinoma. Cancer Res 1993; *53:*2472–2474.

47. Watanabe H, Sawabu N, Ohta H, et al. Identification of K-*ras* oncogene mutations in the pure pancreatic juice of patients with pancreatic adenocarcinoma and pancreatic cancers. Jpn J Cancer Res 1993; *84:*961–965.

48. Shibata D, Almoguera C, Forrester K, et al. Detection of c-Ki-*ras* gene codon 12 mutations in fine needle aspirates from human pancreatic adenocarcinomas. Cancer Res 1990; *50:*1279–1283.

49. van Laethem J-L, Vertongen P, Deviere J, et al. Detection of c-Ki-*ras* gene codon 12 mutations from pancreatic duct brushings in the diagnosis of pancreatic tumors. Gut 1995; *36:*781–787.

50. Apple SK, Hecht JR, Novak JM, et al. Polymerase chain reaction-based K-*ras* mutation detection of pancreatic adenocarcinoma in routine cytology smears. Am J Clin Pathol 1996; *105:*321–326.

51. Miki H, Matsumoto S, Harada H, et al. Detection of c-Ki-*ras* point mutations from pancreatic juice. Int J Pancreatol 1993; *14:*145–148.

52. Kondo H, Sugano K, Fukayama N, et al. Detection of point mutations in the K-*ras* oncogene at codon 12 in pure pancreatic juice for diagnosis of pancreatic carcinoma. Cancer 1994; *73:*1589–1594.

53. Liu T, Wang Z, and Cui Q. Significance of the detection of Ki-*ras* codon 12 mutation in the diagnosis and differential diagnosis of pancreatic carcinoma. Int J Surg Pathol 1995; *3:*93.

54. Bos JL, Fearon ER, Hamilton SR, et al. Prevalence of *ras* gene mutations in human colorectal cancers. Nature 1987; *327:*293–297.

55. Forrester K, Almoguera C, Han K, et al. Detection of high incidence of K-*ras* oncogenes during human colon tumorigenesis. Nature 1988; *327:*298–303.

56. Vogelstein B, Fearon ER, Hamilton SR, et al. Genetic alterations during colorectal-tumor development. New Eng J Med 1988; *319:*525–532.

57. Fearon ER, Hamilton SR, and Vogelstein B. Clonal analysis of human colorectal tumors. Science 1987; *238:*193–197.

58. Mullis KB and Faloona FA. Specific synthesis of DNA *in vitro* via a polymerase catalyzed chain reaction. Methods Enzymol 1987; *155:*335–350.

59. Winter E, Yamamoto F, Almoguera C, et al. A method to detect and characterize point mutations in transcribed genes: amplification and overexpression of the mutant c-K-*ras* allele in human tumor cells. Proc Natl Acad Sci USA 1985; *82:*7575–7579.

60. Meyers RM, Lann Z, and Maniatis T. Detection of single base substitutions by ribonuclease cleavage at mismatches in RNA:DNA duplexes. Science 1985; *230:*1242–1246.

61. Verlaan-de Vries M, Bogaard M, van den Elst H, et al. A dot-blot screening procedure for mutated ras oncogenes using synthetic oligodeoxynucleotides. Gene 1986; *50:*313–320.

62. Tao LC. Liver and pancreas. In: Bibbo M. (ed), Comprehensive cytopathology, Saunders, Philadelphia, 1991; p. 844.

63. Venu RP, Geenen JE, Kini M, et al. Endoscopic retrograde brush cytology: a new technique. Gastroenterology 1990; *99:*1475–1479.

64. Goodale RL, Gajl-Peczalaka K, Dressel T, et al. Cytologic studies for the diagnosis of pancreatic cancer. Cancer 1981; *47:*1652–1655.

65. Nakaizumi A, Tatsuta M, Vehara H, et al. Cytologic examination of pure pancreatic juice in the diagnosis of pancreatic carcinoma. Cancer 1992; *70:*2610–2614.

66. Edoute Y, Lemberg S, and Malberger E. Preoperative and intraoperative fine-needle aspiration cytology of pancreatic lesions. Am J Gastroenterol 1991; *86:*1015–1019.

67. Hyoty MK, Mattila JJ, and Salo K. Intraoperative fine-needle aspiration cytology examination of pancreatic lesions. Surg Gynecol Obstet 1991; *173:*193–197.

68. Schadt ME, Kline TS, Neal HS, et al. Intraoperative pancreatic fine-needle aspiration biopsy: results in 166 patients. Am Surg 1991; *57:*73–75.

68a. Berthélemy P, Bouisson M, Escorerrou J, et al. Identification of K-*ras* mutations in pancreatic juice in the early diagnosis of pancreatic cancer. Ann Intern Med 1995; *123:*188–191.

69. Levine AJ. The *p53* tumor-suppressor gene. N Engl J Med 1992; *326:*1350,1351.

70. Weinberg RA. Tumor-suppressor genes. Science 1991; *254:*1138–1146.

71. Bartek J, Bartkova J, Vojtesek B, et al. Aberrant expression of the p53 oncoprotein is a common feature of a wide spectrum of human malignancies. Oncogene 1991; *6:*1699–1703.

72. Hollstein M, Sidransky D, Vogelstein B, et al. *p53* mutations in human cancers. Science 1991; *253:*49–53.

73. Nigro JM, Baker SJ, Preisinger AC, et al. Mutations in the *p53* gene occur in diverse human tumour types. Nature 1989; *342:*705–708.

74. Scarpa A, Capelli P, Mukai K, et al. Pancreatic adenocarcinomas frequently show *p53* gene mutations. Am J Surg Pathol 1993; *142:*1534–1543.

75. DiGiuseppe JA, Hruban RH, Goodman SN, et al. Overexpression of p53 protein in adenocarcinoma of the pancreas. Amer J Clin Pathol 1994; *101:*684–688.

76. Barton CM, Stoddon SL, and Hughes CM. Abnormalities of the *p53* tumor-suppressor gene in human pancreatic cancer. Br J Cancer 1991; *64:*1076–1082.

77. Zhang SY, Ruggeri B, Agarwal P, et al. Immunohistochemical analysis of p53 expression in human pancreatic carcinomas. Arch Pathol Lab Med 1994; *118:*150–154.

78. Boschman CR, Stryker S, Reddy JK, et al. Expression of p53 protein in precursor lesions and adenocarcinoma of human pancreas. Am J Pathol 1994; *145:*1291–1295.

79. Baker SJ, Preisinger AC, Jessup JM, et al. *p53* gene mutations occur in combination with 17p allelic deletion as late events in colorectal tumorigenesis. Cancer Res 1990; *50:*7717–7722.

80. Orita M, Iwahana H, Kanazawa H, et al. Detection of polymorphisms of human DNA by gel electrophoresis as single-strand conformation polymorphisms. Proc Natl Acad Sci USA 1989; *86:*2766–2770.

81. Reich NC, Oren M, and Levine AJ. Two distinct mechanisms regulate the levels of a cellular tumor antigen, p53. Mol Cell Biol 1983; *3:*2143–2150.

82. Hall PA and Lane DP. p53 in tumour pathology: can we trust immunohistochemistry?... Revisited! J Pathol 1994; *172:*1–4.

83. Wynford-Thomas D. p53 in tumor pathology: can we trust immunocytochemistry? J Pathol 1992; *166:*329,330.

84. van den Berg FM, Baas IP, Polak M, et al. Detection of *p53* overexpression in routinely paraffin-embedded tissue of human carcinomas using a novel target unmasking fluid (TUF). Am J Pathol 1993; *142*:381–385.

85. Midgley CA, Fisher CJ, Bartek J, et al. Analysis of *p53* expression in human tumors: an antibody raised against human p53 expressed in *Escherichia coli*. J Cell Sci 1992; *101 (Part 1)*:183–189.

86. Rodrigues NR, Rowan A, Smith ME, et al. *p53* mutations in colorectal cancer. Proc Natl Acad Sci USA 1990; *87*:7555–7559.

87. Baas IO, Mulder JWR, Offerhaus GJA, et al. Immunohistochemistry of altered p53 suppressor gene product in colorectal neoplasms. Lab Invest 1993; *68*:43A (abstract).

88. Baas IO, Mulder JWR, Offerhaus GJA, et al. An evaluation of six antibodies for immunohistochemistry of mutant *p53* gene product in archival colorectal neoplasms. J Pathol 1994; *172*:5–12.

89. van den Berg FM, Tigges AJ, Schipper MEI, et al. Expression of the nuclear oncogene *p53* in colon tumours. J Pathol 1989; *157*:193–199.

90. Slebos RJC, Baas IO, Clement M, et al. Clinical and pathological associations with *p53* tumour-suppressor gene mutations and expression of p21[WAF1/Cip1] in colorectal carcinoma. Br J Cancer 1996; *74*:165–171.

91. El-Deiry WS, Tokino T, Velculescu VE, et al. WAF1, a potential mediator of p53 tumor suppression. Cell 1993; *75*:817–825.

92. Peters G. Stifled by inhibitors. Nature 1994; *371*:204,205.

93. White E. p53, guardian of Rb. Nature 1994; *371*:21,22.

94. El-Deiry WS, Kern SE, Pietenpol JA, et al. Definition of a consensus binding site for p53. Nature Genet 1992; *1*:45–49.

95. Kern SE, Kinzler KW, Bruskin A, et al. Identification of p53 as a sequence-specific DNA-binding protein. Science 1991; *252*:1708–1711.

96. O'Rourke RW, Miller CW, Kato GJ, et al. A potential transcriptional activation element in the p53 protein. Oncogene 1990; *5*:1829–1832.

97. Harper JW, Adami GR, Wei N, et al. The p21 cdk-interacting protein Cip1 is a potent inhibitor of G1 cyclin-dependent kinases. Cell 1993; *75*:805–816.

98. Xiong Y, Hannon GJ, Zhang H, et al. p21 is a universal inhibitor of cyclin kinases. Nature 1993; *366*:701–704.

99. Kern SE. *p53*: tumor suppression through control of the cell cycle. Gastroenterology 1994; *106*:1708–1711.

100. DiGiuseppe JA, Redston MS, Yeo CJ, et al. *p53*-independent expression of the cyclin-dependent kinase inhibitor p21 in pancreatic carcinoma. Amer J Pathol 1995; *147*:884–888.

101. Halevy O, Novitch BG, Spicer DB, et al. Correlation of terminal cell cycle arrest of skeletal muscle with induction of p21 by MyoD. Science 1995; *267*:1018–1024.

102. Michieli P, Chedid M, Lin D, et al. Induction of WAF1/CIP1 by a *p53*-independent pathway. Cancer Res 1994; *54*:3391–3395.

103. Sidransky D, Eschenbach DV, Tsai YC, et al. Identification of *p53* gene mutations in bladder cancers and urine samples. Science 1991; *252*:706–709.

104. Eguchi S, Kohara N, Komuta K, et al. Mutations of the *p53* gene in the stool of patients with resectable colon cancer. Cancer 1996; *77(8 Suppl)*:1707–1710.

105. Schaaper RM, and Radman M. The extreme mutator effect of *Escherichia* mutD5 results from saturation of mismatch repair by excessive DNA replication errors. EMBO J 1989; *8*:3511–3516.

106. Mao L, Lee DJ, Tockman MS, et al. Microsatellite alterations as clonal markers for the detection of human cancer. Proc Natl Acad Sci USA 1994; *91*:9871–9875.

107. Brentnall TA, Chen R, Lee JG, et al. Microsatellite instability and K-*ras* mutations associated with pancreatic adenocarcinoma and pancreatitis. Can Res 1995; *55*:4264–4267.

108. Han H-J, Yanagisawa A, Kato Y, et al. Genetic instability in pancreatic cancer and poorly differentiated type of gastric cancer. Cancer Res 1993; *53:*5087–5089.

108a.Goggins M, Offerhaus GJA, Hilgers W, et al. Adenocarcinomas of the pancreas with DNA replication errors (RER+) are associated with a characteristic histopathology. Am J Pathol 1998; in press.

109. Aaltonen LA, Peltomaki P, Leach FS, et al. Clues to the pathogenesis of familial colorectal cancer. Science 1993; *260:*812–816.

110. Ionov Y, Peinado M, Malkhosyan S, et al. Ubiquitous somatic mutations in simple repeated sequences reveal a new mechanism for colonic carcinogenesis. Nature 1993; *363:*558–561.

111. Thibodeau SN, Bren G, and Schaid D. Microsatellite instability in cancer of the proximal colon. Science 1993; *260:*816–819.

112. Mao L, Schoenberg MP, Scicchitano M, et al. Molecular detection of primary bladder cancer by microsatellite analysis. Science 1996; *271:*659–662.

113. Lynch HT. Genetics and pancreatic cancer. Arch Surg 1994; *129:*266–268.

114. Lynch HT, Fusaro L, and Lynch JF. Familial pancreatic cancer: a family study. Pancreas 1992; *7:*511–515.

115. Lynch HT, Smyrk TC, and Kern SE. Familial pancreatic cancer: a review. Semin Oncol 1996; *23:*251–275.

116. Fernandez E, La Vecchia C, D'Avanzo B, et al. Family history and the risk of liver, gallbladder, and pancreas cancer. Cancer Epidemiol Biomarkers Prev 1994; *3:*209–212.

117. Lumadue JA, Griffin CA, Osman M, et al. Familial pancreatic cancer and the genetics of pancreatic cancer. Surg Clin N Am 1995; *75:*845–855.

118. Lynch HT, Fusaro L, Smyrk TC, et al. Medical genetic study of eight pancreatic cancer-prone families. Cancer Invest 1995; *13:*141–149.

119. Ghadirian P, Boyle P, Simard A, et al. Reported family aggregation of pancreatic cancer within a population-based case-control study in the Francophone community in Montreal, Canada. Int J Pancreatol 1991; *10:*183–196.

120. Lynch HT, and Fusaro RM. Pancreatic cancer and the familial atypical multiple-mole melanoma (FAMMM) syndrome. Pancreas 1991; *6:*127–131.

121. Bergman W, Watson P, de Jong J, et al. Systemic cancer and the FAMMM syndrome. Br J Cancer 1990; *61:*932–936.

122. Lynch HT, Smyrk TC, Watson P, et al. Genetics, natural history, tumor spectrum, and pathology of hereditary non-polyposis colorectal cancer: an updated review. Gastroenterol 1993; *104:*1535–1549.

123. Tulinius H, Olafsdottir GH, Sigvaldeson H, et al. Neoplastic diseases in families of breast cancer patients. J Med Genet 1994; *31:*618–621.

124. Kerber RA and Slattery ML. The impact of family history on ovarian cancer risk. Arch Int Med 1995; *155:*905–912.

125. Whelan AJ, Bartsch D, and Goodfellow PI. Brief report: a familial syndrome of pancreatic cancer and melanoma with a mutation in the *CDKN2* tumor-suppressor gene. N Eng J Med 1995; *333:*975–977.

126. Goldstein AM, Fraser MC, Struewing JP, et al. Increased risk of pancreatic cancer in melanoma-prone kindreds with *p16^{INK4}* mutation. N Engl J Med 1995; *333:*970–974.

127. Thorlacius S, Olafsdottir G, Gryggvadottir L, et al. A single *BRCA2* mutation in male and female breast carcinoma families from Iceland with varied cancer phenotypes. Nat Genet 1996; *13:*117–119.

128. Phelan CM, Lancaster JM, Tonin P, et al. Mutation analysis of the *BRCA2* gene in 49 site-specific breast cancer families. Nat Genet 1996; *13:*120–122.

129. Couch FJ, Farid LM, DeShano ML, et al. *BRCA2* germline mutations in male breast cancer cases and breast cancer families. Nat Genet 1996; *13:*123–125.

130. Berman DB, Costalas J, Schultz DC, et al. A common mutation in *BRCA2* that predisposes to a variety of cancers is found in both Jewish Ashkenazi and non-Jewish individuals. Cancer Res 1996; *56:*3409–3414.

130a. Hruban RH, Petersen GM, Hoo PK, et al. Genetics of pancreatic cancer: from genes to families. Surg Oncol Clin North Am 1998; 7: in press.

131. Moskaluk CA, Hruban RH, Lietman A, et al. Low prevalence of *p16^{INK4a}* and *CDK4* mutations in familial pancreatic carcinoma. Hum Mutat 1998; in press.

132. Velculescu VE, Zhang L, Vogelstein B, et al. Serial analysis of gene expression. Science 1995; *270:*484–487.

132a. Zhang L, Zhou W, Velculescu VE, et al. Gene expression profiles in normal and cancer cells. Science 1997; *276:*1268–1272.

132b. Zhou W, Sokoll LJ, Bruzek DS, et al. Identifying markers for pancreatic cancer by gene expression analysis. Cancer Epidemiol Biomarkers Prev 1998; 7: in press.

133. Hruban RH, van der Riet P, Erozan YS, et al. Brief report: molecular biology and the early detection of carcinoma of the bladder–the case of Hubert H. Humphrey. N Eng J Med 1994; *330:*1276–1278.

134. Sidransky D. Advances in cancer detection. Sci Am 1996; *275:*104–109.

135. Brennan JA, Mao L, Hruban RH, et al. Molecular assessment of histopathological staging in squamous-cell carcinoma of the head and neck. N Eng J Med 1995; *332:*429–435.

136. Koch WM, Boyle JO, Mao L, et al. *p53* gene mutations as markers of tumor spread in synchronous oral cancers. Arch Otolaryngol Head Neck Surg 1994; *120:*943–947.

Tumor Antigens in Pancreatic Cancer

Carlos Rollhauser and William Steinberg

INTRODUCTION

A wide array of tumor markers, including enzymes, oncofetal antigens, tumor-associated antigens, and other markers, has been used in the diagnosis and management of pancreatic cancer. The advent of hybridoma technology, with the development of monoclonal probes for tumor markers, has represented an important step in this regard, with significant contributions to both the diagnosis and management of patients with pancreatic carcinoma.

Table 1 lists most of the tumor markers evaluated at one time or currently employed for pancreatic carcinoma. This chapter will focus on tumor-associated antigens (TAAs) and will only cover those that have clinical or experimental application, and that appear promising for future clinical use. These include CA 19-9, CA 50, Span-1, Dupan-2, CA 242, CA 494, tissue polypeptide antigen (TPA), insulin amyloid polypeptide (IAPP), and the testosterone:dihydrotestosterone ratio (T:DHT). TAAs that have low sensitivity or that have not stood the test of time, such as Tag72 (1,2), CEA (3), tumor-associated trypsin inhibitor (4,5), CA 125 (6), elastase (7–10), galactosyl transferase II, ribonuclease, and leukocyte adherence inhibition assay, will not be covered. Likewise, those limited to experimental use, such as CA 195, the pancreatic oncofetal antigen, and fetoacinar antigen, and those that may turn out to be useful markers, such as cathepsin E (11) and CAM 17.1/WGA (12,13), but on whom only preliminary information is available, will not be covered in this review.

Table 2 presents the biochemical structure of the serological carbohydrate markers. Oncogenic transformation of mucin-producing cells is associated with the release into circulation of complex carbohydrates whose structures resemble that of the Lewis Blood Group antigen. These substances are 80% carbohydrate by weight and have a ceramide or protein residue linked to oligosaccharide chains, which constitute the target of the different monoclonal antibodies.

CA 19-9

This is the TAA most frequently used in clinical practice for the diagnosis and management of patients with pancreatic carcinoma. The monoclonal antibody that detected

Table 1
Tumor Markers in Pancreatic Carcinoma

Oncoproteins
    K-*ras* mutations
Tumor-associated antigens
    CA 19-9
    Span-1
    Dupan-2
    CA 50
    CA 242
    CA 494
    TPA (tissue polypeptide antigen)
    CA 12-5
    CA 195
    TAG72
Enzymes
    Elastase 1
    Galactosyl transferase III
    Ribonuclease
    Tumor-associated trypsin inhibitor (TATI)
Oncofetal antigens
    Carcinoembryonic antigen (CEA)
    Pancreatic oncofetal antigen
    Fetoacinar antigen
Other tumor markers
    Testosterone/dihydrotestosterone ratio (T/DHT)
    IAPP (insulin amyloid polypeptide)
    Leukocyte adherence inhibition assay

this antigen was first isolated by Koprowski et al. in 1979, using an immunogen derived from a colon carcinoma cell line *(14)*. This monoclonal antibody-defined antigen is a ganglioside containing sialyl-lacto-*N*-fucopentaose, the same oligosaccharide chain that defines Lewis[a] blood group antigen *(15)* (Table 2). About 7–10% of the population are genotypically Lewis[(a,b)] negative and cannot synthesize CA 19-9 antigen *(16,17)*. Although this would limit the maximum achievable sensitivity of the assay to 90–95% *(18)*, reports of detectable CA 19-9 levels in patients with Lewis[(a,b)] negative phenotype and pancreatic cancer have been published *(19–21)*. It has been hypothesized that malignant transformation may be associated with activation of fucosyl transferase (Lewis enzyme), leading to synthesis and secretion of Lewis A type of oligosaccharide in those cases *(21)*.

    The CA 19-9 antigen is produced by a variety of normal epithelial tissues, including liver, bile, and pancreatic duct cells, as well as gastric, colonic, and esophageal epithelia *(22,23)*. Small amounts of CA 19-9 antigen can be detected in the serum of patients with benign disorders of these organs, and, occasionally, in normal individuals *(24,25)*.

Table 2
Biochemical Structure of Lewis and Tumor-Associated Antigens

Antigen	Epitope(s)	Structure
Lewis[a] (blood group Ag.)	Lacto-*N*-fucopentaose	Gal-GlcNAc-Gal-R | Fuc
Dupan-2 (sialyl Lewis[c])	Sialyl-lacto-*N*-tetraose	Gal-GlcNAc-Gal-R | NANA
CA 19-9 (sialyl-Lewis[a])	Sialyl-lacto-*N*-fucopentaose	Gal-GlcNAc-Gal-R | | NANA Fuc
CA 50	Sialyl-lacto-*N*-fucopentaose + sialyl-lacto-*N*-tetraose	Gal-GlcNAc-Gal-R | | NANA Fuc + Gal-GlcNAc-Gal-R | NANA
SPan-1	Sialyl-lacto-*N*-fucopentaose + ?	Gal-GlcNAc-Gal-R | | NANA Fuc + ?
CA 242	Not completely defined. Sialylated carbohydrate located on the same macromolecule as CA 50, but with different antigenic epitope(s)	
CA 494	Unknown. Carbohydrate structure not related to sialyl Lewis[a]	
TPA	Glycoprotein, single polypeptide chain with both keratin-like and Lewis antigen-like determinants	
TPS	Antigen corresponding to a specific epitope (M3) of the TPA molecule	

Gal, galactose; GlcNAc, *N*-acetyl-glucoseamine; Glc, glucose; R, ceramide or protein; NANA, *N*-acetyl-neuraminic acid (sialic acid); Fuc, fucose; TPA, tissue polypeptide antigen; TPS, tissue polypeptide specific antigen.

Malignancies of these same organs are associated with increased serum quantities of this tumor marker in the following decreasing order of frequency, excluding pancreatic cancer: bile duct, 67%; hepatocellular carcinoma, 49%; stomach, 41%; colon, 34%; esophagus, 22%; and nongastrointestinal cancers, 14% (*3*).

Concerning pancreatic cancer, Steinberg pooled data from more than 20 studies that evaluated the sensitivity and specificity of the CA 19-9 antigen at various cutoff levels in more than 4000 subjects (*3*). Using the recommended cutoff value of 37 U/mL, he found that the sensitivity ranged from 68 to 93%, with a specificity of 76–99%. Increasing the cutoff value predictably affects the operating characteristics of the test, skewing the ratio in favor of specificity at the expense of sensitivity. Thus, the specificity of the assay at a level greater than 1000 U/mL is close to 100%, but the sensitivity falls to 40% (*3*).

The specificity of CA 19-9 decreases in the presence of jaundice of both hepatocellular and extrahepatic origin. Craxi et al. *(26)* found a 62% rate of CA 19-9 elevation in cirrhosis. Albert et al. *(27)* reported marked elevation of CA 19-9 antigen in acute cholangitis, but not in common duct obstruction without cholangitis, with a rapid decrease of its concentration after decompression of the bile duct. This elevation is probably caused by injury of the biliary epithelium, rather than by interference of bile acids or bilirubin with the antigen assay, since the addition of bile salts and bilirubin to sera with known concentration of CA 19-9 produced no change in the measurable quantity of CA 19-9 in one experiment *(28)*.

False-positive rates of 5–20% have been reported in chronic pancreatitis, which frequently presents a difficult differential diagnosis with pancreatic cancer. The determination of CA 19-9 in pure pancreatic juice (PPJ) has been evaluated for this purpose, with different results *(29–32)*. Tatsuta *(29)* did not find that the level of CA 19-9 in PPJ discriminated between pancreatic cancer and chronic pancreatitis. However, Malesci et al. *(31)* described an almost perfect separation between pancreatic cancer vs chronic pancreatitis and controls by dividing the CA 19-9 concentration in PPJ by the total amount of pancreatic secretory protein. More recently, another study reported that the combined determination of serum CA 19-9 and the so-called 90K protein in PPJ, a marker of immune and inflammatory activity, correctly identified 84.2% of the patients with pancreatic cancer and 90% of those with chronic pancreatitis *(33)*.

The most important characteristic of a test is its predictive value, which in turn depends on its sensitivity and specificity and the prevalence of the target disease in the population tested. The prevalence of pancreatic cancer in the population older than 50 yr in the United States has been estimated around 0.05%, or 50 cases per 100,000 individuals *(34)*. Table 3 shows the predictive value calculated for this prevalence, according to the different cutoff levels and their respective sensitivity and specificity values obtained from Steinberg's study *(3)*. The positive predictive value of a CA 19-9 level, even at a value >1000 U/mL, is only 2%. Thus, the limitations of this assay as a screening test for pancreatic cancer become obvious. At a cutoff of 37 U/mL, its cost-effectiveness ratio would be very poor, yielding only 40 accurate diagnoses per 100,000 individuals, and producing almost 10,000 false-positive results. The cost of investigating these patients would be enormous and the risk for the patients subjected to invasive procedures, such as ERCP, or endoscopic ultrasound, prohibitive.

On practical grounds, there is no role for screening of asymptomatic individuals. Only four cases were detected among 10,152 subjects older than 40 yr of age in a screening program carried out in Japan, using a combination of elastase 1, CA 19-9 antigen, and ultrasound, and only one patient underwent curative resection *(35)*. Similarly, the prospective evaluation of 866 patients with benign disorders found 135 patients with an elevated CA 19-9 level, of which only one had pancreatic cancer *(36)*.

As expected, the predictive value of CA 19-9 improves significantly when it is used in a population with a higher prevalence of disease, such as in patients presenting with weight loss, jaundice, or an abdominal mass found on radiological studies. Thus, at a 20% prevalence, for example, a CA 19-9 level >1000 U/mL would have a negative predictive value (NPV) of 87% and a positive predictive value (PPV) of 100%, using sensitivity and specificity figures from Table 3.

Table 3
Positive Predictive Value of CA 19-9 Level at 0.05%
Prevalence of Pancreatic Carcinoma[a]

Cutoff values (U/mL)	Sensitivity (%)	Specificity (%)	PPV (%)
>37	81	90	0.04
>100	68	98	0.35
>300	54	99	0.5
>1000	41	99.8	2

[a] Sensitivity and specificity values obtained with permission from ref. *3*.

Table 4
Correlation of CA 19-9 Sensitivity According to Size of Tumor[a]

Author	Ref. no.	≤2 cm		<3 cm		>3 cm	
		N	%	N	%	N	%
Satake	7	24	62.5				
Furukawa	9	31	58.1				
Tatsuta	29			7	57	7	86
Kobayashi	55	5	40			63	87
Satake	107	2	0	3	33	6	67
Sakahara	108			8	12	47	91
Iishi	109			14	78		
Total		62	40	32	45	123	83

[a] Modified with permission from ref. *3*.

N, number of patients with tumor of specified size; %, percentage of those patients with abnormally elevated CA 19-9 levels.

The sensitivity of CA 19-9, according to size of pancreatic tumor, is shown in Table 4. The sensitivity of this assay for tumors <3 cm in size is approx 50%. The stage of pancreatic cancer also has an influence on the detectable amount of CA 19-9, with increasing sensitivity of the assay as the disease progresses to more advanced stages. Satake et al. *(8)* reported sensitivities of 62.5 and 77.7% for T1 and T2 lesions, respectively. Similarly, Chang and Takeuchi *(37)* found a sensitivity of 37.5 vs 88.9% in relationship with T1 and T2 lesions, respectively. In Pleskow's series *(38)*, CA 19-9 antigen was elevated in only 50% of the patients with local or regional disease, but in 71% of those with distant metastases. Despite some unusually optimistic results from isolated series *(39)*, the available data clearly reveal less than optimal sensitivity of CA 19-9 as a marker of early disease. In a recent report, 58% of patients with tumors ≤2 cm in diameter had a CA 19-9 elevation above 37 U/mL, but when subjected to surgical exploration, over two-thirds had lymphatic involvement, roughly 50% had vascular invasion, and 45% had retroperitoneal invasion *(9)*.

Table 5
CA 19-9 Level and Resectability[a]

Author	Ref. no.	Number of resectable patients with level >1000 U/mL	Number of unresectable patients with level >1000 U/mL[b]
Schmiegel	*30*	2/3	16/37
Malesci	*31*	0/3	22/45
Forsmark	*41*	0/5	21/40
Satake	*107*	0/2	2/7
Steinberg	*110*	1/14	9/23
Safi	*111*	0/3	8/45
Del Favero	*112*	0/3	8/45
Wang	*113*	0/3	14/21
Total		3/49 (6%)	93/245 (38%)

[a] Modified with permission from ref. *3*.

[b] Of 245 cases of unresectable disease, 93 (38%) had levels >1000 U/mL and 62% had levels <1000 U/mL.

Recent studies have evaluated the potential use of CA 19-9 in the determination of significant clinical end points, including prognosis and resectability, in addition to postsurgical recurrence and survival based on pre- and postoperative levels of this tumor marker. The answer to some of these important questions can be gleaned from the literature.

CA 19-9 and Resectability of the Tumor

Table 5 compares a single level of CA 19-9 with tumor resectability. Only 3 of 49 (6%) of resectable patients had a level higher than 1000 U/mL, but 93 of 245 (38%) unresectable patients had a level this high. In other words, 93 of 96 patients (97%) with a serum CA 19-9 concentration higher than 1000 U/mL were found to be unresectable.

The prognostic value of lower levels of CA 19-9 is not well defined from the available literature. Bosch et al., using a much lower cutoff of 37 U/mL, found this marker to lack discriminatory power for resectability in 36 patients with pancreatic carcinoma who underwent laparotomy to evaluate the extent of tumor spread *(40)*. Other studies suggest that a level of more than 300 U/mL may also correlate with unresectability, but to a lesser extent than levels higher than 1000 U/mL. Forsmark et al. *(41)* retrospectively compared the value of CA 19-9 with imaging studies (ultrasound, abdominal CT, and MRI) in their ability to predict resection. Almost three-quarters of patients (29/40) who were found unresectable by either radiological studies or surgical exploration had a level greater than 300 U/mL. Likewise, 18/25 or 72% of patients predicted resectable by imaging studies, but found to be unresectable at the time of surgical exploration, also had a level higher than 300 U/mL. In a recent study, 18% of 126 patients with resectable tumors had a level greater than 400 U/mL *(42)*. Thus, resection may still be possible in a tangible proportion of 20–30% of patients with a CA 19-9 level of more than 300 U/mL. On the other hand, a cutoff of 1000 U/mL closely correlates with unresectability, and hence would convey the same implication as any other imaging criteria used to predict resectability. In this regard, studies that prospectively compare the

CA 19-9 assay to other diagnostic modalities, such as abdominal helical CT and endoscopic ultrasound, would be helpful to clarify the usefulness of this marker to predict resectability or unresectability.

CA 19-9 Level and Prognosis

Lundin et al. reported on the prognostic value of preoperative CA 19-9 determination in a group of patients with histologically proven adenocarcinoma of the pancreas *(43)*. There was a statistically significant difference in survival according to the CA 19-9 level for all analyzed patients, with a mean survival of 12.8 mo for the patients who had a level <370 U/mL vs 6.7 mo in the patients who had a level above that value. The determination of CA 19-9 was particularly helpful in prognosticating survival in patients with stages II and III, most of which underwent palliative procedures, and in whom the distinction between localized and advanced disease was difficult to establish even at surgery. In another study, Sperti et al. *(44)* found the CA 19-9 level to be an independent prognosticator of survival, regardless of tumor size or histological grade; it also correlated with spread of disease (lymph node involvement), and could be interpreted to portend the same prognosis as cancer staging *(44)*. A significant difference in postoperative survival time (17.3 vs 7.1 mo), according to preoperative CA 19-9 levels, was also found in another study *(42)*.

A recent study evaluated the prognostic role of CA 19-9 in survival of 24 patients with unresectable stage III pancreatic cancer, treated with combined radiotherapy and chemotherapy. The authors found that pretreatment levels discriminated between two groups of patients in terms of outcome, with a threefold 1-yr survival difference, 60 vs 20%, according to levels below and above 2000 U/mL, respectively *(45)*. In the same study, the combined use of CA 19-9 and CA 125 provided additional prognostic information, with a median survival of 7.4 mo in patients with elevation of both markers, in comparison to 12.8 mo in those patients with low levels of one or both markers. CA 19-9 level was also found to be an important parameter of response in 42 patients subjected to neoadjuvant chemoradiation, followed by abdominal CT or laparotomy restaging, with a statistically significant association of CA 19-9 increase and decrease to disease progression or stabilization, respectively *(46)*.

The results of four studies that evaluated the prognostic value of postoperative CA 19-9 determinations are shown in Table 6. In these studies, normalization of CA 19-9 levels within 15 d after surgery correlated with a statistically significant longer 1-yr survival *(44,47–49)*. On the other hand, persistently elevated levels were associated with mortality within a year following surgical treatment. Survival was also significantly longer in 14 of 84 resected patients who had normalization of CA 19-9 levels a median of 4 wk after surgery *(42)*.

CA 19-9 is an early marker of recurrent disease. The lead time of CA 19-9 re-elevation before clinical or radiological recurrence of pancreatic cancer was evident ranged from 1 to 20 mo in five studies (Table 7).

Although debatable, the available data suggest a role for preoperative and postoperative determination of the CA 19-9 assay in most patients undergoing surgical resection. Serum CA 19-9 concentration correlates with tumor burden, so that any effective therapy, surgical or medical (radiation and chemotherapy), should lead to a fall in the level after an appropriate length of time. Failure to show this adequate response

Table 6
Early (<15 d) Postoperative Normalization of CA 19-9 as a Prognosticator
of Survival

Author[a]	Ref. no.	N^b	Survival with normalized levels[c]	N	Survival with persistent elevation[c]	P value
Sperti	44	14	22	16	7	<0.001
Glenn	47	7/8	>18	6	<12	<0.005
Beretta	48	7	17.3 ± 9.05	7	4.8 ± 1.57	<0.005
Tian	49	7	21.9	4	8.7	<0.05

[a] Cutoff for CA 19-9 >37 U/mL, except for Beretta: >40 U/mL.
[b] N, number of patients.
[c] Survival measured in months.

Table 7
Lead Time of CA 19-9 Re-Elevation Before Clinical Evidence
of Pancreatic Cancer Recurrence[a]

Author	Ref. no.	Lead time in months[a] (range)
Safi	42	5–20
Sperti	44	1–10
Glenn	47	1–7
Beretta	48	2–6
Tian	49	2–9

[a] "Lead time" refers to the time elapsed since CA 19-9 levels became abnormal after therapy (surgery, chemotherapy, or radiation therapy), until the first sign of pancreatic cancer recurrence was clinically apparent.

might indicate persistence of disease and should prompt consideration of additional therapy. After a reduction in the CA 19-9 concentration following surgical resection, a secondary rise should be regarded as an early indicator of cancer recurrence.

CA 50 ANTIGEN

The murine monoclonal antibody CA 50, described originally by Lindholm et al. in 1983 (50), is directed to an epitope present in two glycolipids: sialyl-lacto-fucopentaose (sialyl Lewis[a], similar to CA 19-9) and sialyl-lactotetraose, which is also found in Lewis[(a,b)]-negative individuals (51; Table 2).

Table 8 compares this marker with CA 19-9. Its overall sensitivity ranges from 65 to 88%, with a specificity between 73 and 93% (6,7,28,52–56), depending on the cutoff chosen. Positive rates of CA 50 in T1, T2, and T3 pancreatic cancer lesions were 20, 80, and 89%, respectively, in one series (55). Its contribution to early diagnosis is negligible. In general, no advantage of using CA 50 over CA 19-9 or other TAA in pancreatic cancer has been found. This antigen is not routinely used in clinical practice.

Table 8
Comparison of CA 19-9 vs CA 50

Author	Ref. no.	N^a	Sensitivity CA 19-9 (%)	CA 50 (%)	n^b	Specificity CA 19-9 (%)	CA 50 (%)
Saito	6	35	82.6	80	32	87.5	81.3
Satake	7	572	79.4	65[c]	1394	72.5	73.2[d]
Paganuzzi	28	26	84.6	80.7	80	88.8	73
Haglund	52	95	77	69	81	77	80
Pasquali	53	50	80	82	121	91.6	88.7
Molina	54	20	94	88	58	95	97.5
Kobayashi	55	200	81	84	652	79	85
Benini	56	25	92	88	168	85	86.5
Total		1023	84	80	2586	85	83

[a] N, patients with pancreatic carcinoma.

[b] n, includes healthy controls and patients with benign pancreatic and biliary disorders and other gastrointestinal malignancies.

[c] $N = 94$ patients.

[d] $n = 97$ patients.

Cutoff values: CA 19-9: Molina and Saito, 100 U/mL, other studies 37 U/mL; CA 50: Paganuzzi, 17 U/mL; Haglund, 20 U/mL; Satake and Pasquali, 40 U/mL; Molina, 170 U/mL; Kobayashi and Saito, 35 U/mL; Benini 28 U/mL.

SPAN-1

Originally described by Chung et al. Span-1 monoclonal antibody was produced by immunization of Balb/c mice with the mucin-producing human pancreatic cancer cell line, SW 1990 *(57)*. In addition to sialyl Lewis A, this antibody also reacts with tissue samples from patients with Lewis[(a,b)]-negative phenotype *(57)*, which could explain the slightly higher sensitivity than CA 19-9. The exact antigenic determinant corresponding to this epitope is not known, although one study suggested a structure related to sialyl-lactotetraose *(58;* Table 2). Table 9 presents six studies that compared this marker to CA 19-9 *(7,8,10,55,57,59)*. The sensitivity and specificity of both markers are equivalent, although the specificity of Span-1 is particularly low in the setting of liver cirrhosis, in which a false-positive rate as high as 50% has been described *(55)*.

One study evaluating both markers found a similar positive rate of 40% in T1 lesions *(55)*; another study reported a sensitivity of 50 and 0% for Span-1 and CA 19-9 antigens, respectively *(57)*. Analogous to most TAAs, no substantial superiority over CA 19-9 has been demonstrated. The use of this marker remains limited to experimental research.

DUPAN-2

This monoclonal antibody recognizes as its epitope sialyl-lacto-tetraose, which is converted to sialyl-lacto-fucopentaose or sialyl-Lewis[a] by the action of the enzyme fucosyl-transferase *(58)*. Thus, Dupan-2 is thought to be the precursor of CA 19-9, and is apparently the reason that this marker accumulates in the sera of patients with pan-

Table 9
Comparison of Span-1 vs CA 19-9

Author	Ref. no.	N^a	Sensitivity Span-1 (%)	Sensitivity CA 19-9 (%)	n^a	Specificity Span-1 (%)	Specificity CA 19-9 (%)
Satake	7	641	81.4	79.4	$1,231^b$	67.5	72.5
Satake	8	74	73	73		n/a	n/a
Kuno	10	47	89.4	87.2	356	84	82
Kobayashi	55	200	82	81	662	85	79
Chung	57	57	94	85	30	93	90
Kiriyama	59	64	81.3	73.4	344^b	75.6	80.1
Total		1083	83.5	80	2623	81	81

[a] N, number of patients with pancreatic cancer; n, number of patients with other conditions.
[b] CA 19-9 specificity was determined in 1394 patients and 337 patients, respectively.
Cutoff values: >37 U/mL for all studies; Span-1: Chung >400 U/mL, others >30 U/mL.
n/a, not available.

Table 10
Sensitivity and Specificity of Dupan-2 Compared with CA 19-9

Author	Ref. no.	N^a	Cutoff (U/mL)	Sensitivity Dupan-2 (%)	Sensitivity CA 19-9[b] (%)	n^c	Specificity Dupan-2 (%)	Specificity CA 19-9 (%)
Saito	6	35	>150	80	88.6	32	75	62.5
Satake	7	239	>400	47.7	79.4	564	85.3	72.5
Satake	8	39	n/a	47	79^e			
Takasaki	18	22	>300	67	73			
Kawa	60	200	>150	64	81			
Ferrara	61	23	>300	57	83	44	59	43
Ohshio	62	87^d	>150	63	70	60	62	80
Cooper	63	49	>100	76	73			
Total		694		63	78	700	70	64.5

[a] N, number of patients with pancreatic cancer.
[b] CA 19-9 cutoff value in all studies was 37 U/mL.
[c] n, number of patients with nonmalignant biliary, hepatic, and pancreatic diseases.
[d] Includes 29 patients with biliary tract carcinoma.
[e] Sensitivity calculated in 74 patients with pancreatic cancer.
n/a, not available.

creatic cancer and Lewis[a]-negative phenotype *(58,60)*. Table 10 shows the general characteristics of Dupan-2 in relation to the CA 19-9 antigen. In multiple studies using a wide range of cutoff values, the average sensitivity of Dupan-2 was 63 vs 78% for CA 19-9. No significant differences were found in the specificity rates *(6–8,18,60–63)*, including a high false-positive rate in the presence of jaundice and liver dysfunction *(64)*. The sensitivity of Dupan-2 in early, resectable disease is approx 30–40% *(61,63)*; its ability as a postoperative prognosticator is not defined. This marker has not been widely employed in clinical practice.

Table 11
Sensitivity and Specificity of CA 19-9 vs CA 242

Author	Ref. no.	Number of patients		Sensitivity		Specificity	
		PC[a]	Other[b]	CA 19-9[c] (%)	CA 242[d] (%)	CA 19-9 (%)	CA 242 (%)
Rothlin	66	68	262	70	66	n/a	n/a
Plebani	67	27	232	69	63	89	85
Kuusela	68	42	262	70.6	66	74	95
Haglund	71	179	112	83	74	81	91
Kawa	72	151	447	82	79	85	93
Banfi	73	41	60	79	57	80	88.5
Total		508	1375	76	67.5	82	90.5

[a] PC, pancreatic cancer.

[b] Other includes healthy controls, blood donors, and patients with benign biliary and pancreatic disorders, including cholestasis and cholangitis, chronic hepatitis, cirrhosis, and other gastrointestinal malignancies.

[c] CA 19-9 cutoffs: >37 U/mL in all studies.

[d] CA 242 cutoffs: Haglund and Rothlin, >20 U/mL; Kawa, Kuusela, and Plebani, >30 U/mL; Banfi >34 U/mL.

n/a, not available.

CA 242 ANTIGEN

Ca 242 is a relatively new tumor marker that was first isolated by Lindholm et al. in 1985 (65). It was obtained by immunization of mice with the human adenocarcinoma cell line COLO 205, and fusion with the SP 2/0 mouse myeloma cell line. The epitope recognized by the CA 242 antibody is a sialylated carbohydrate coexpressed with sialylated Lewis[a] antigen (CA 19-9) and CA 50 on the same macromolecular complex. Although CA 242 was thought to be completely different from those cancer antigens (66), a recent report has put this issue into question by showing high crossreactivity between the CA 242 antigen and the CA 19-9 antibody (67).

The comparison with CA 19-9 is shown in Table 11. Several studies have compared CA 242 against other tumor markers, and, although the sensitivity of this test is inferior to that of CA 19-9 and CA 50 (68–70), its specificity seems to be superior (66–68,70–75). In chronic pancreatitis, higher false-positive rates for CA 19-9 have been reported by several authors, on the order of 24% for CA 19-9 and 14% for CA 242 (66,67,76,77). Tissue expression of CA 242 has been found to be very similar to that of CA 19-9 in histologic sections of normal pancreatic tissue (71). In chronic calcific pancreatitis, CA 242 expression was found to be less prominent than CA 19-9 in centroacinar and ductal cells, possibly explaining lower release of CA 242 antigen into the circulation in that setting (78). The sensitivity for stage I and for resectable disease is approx 50% (66,72). Positive correlation with tumor size and lymph node status has been reported (66,72). Serum levels of CA 242 did not correlate with tumor grading in one trial (66).

The usefulness of this marker as an adjunct in evaluating resectability and selecting patients for surgical treatment, and as a prognostic indicator before and after surgery, remains to be established.

CA 494

CA 494 monoclonal antibody was initially obtained after immunization of Balb/C mice with tissue-culture cells from the De-Ta colon carcinoma cell line, and subsequent fusion of spleen cells with the Sp2/o-Ag mouse myeloma cell line *(79)*. The epitope recognized by this monoclonal antibody, chiefly expressed on well-differentiated adenocarcinoma of the pancreas, has been described as a high-mol-wt glycoprotein, but the structure of CA 494 is not exactly known.

CA 494 monoclonal antibody was first evaluated as passive immunotherapy in patients with pancreatic cancer, based on its ability to bind to more than 90% of human pancreatic cancers, and to mediate antibody-dependent cellular cytotoxicity against radiolabeled malignant pancreatic cells *(80,81)*. Unfortunately, in a randomized controlled trial evaluating patients with resectable disease, there was no difference in survival between treatment and placebo groups *(80)*.

Only one study has compared the use of CA 494 as a diagnostic tool for pancreatic carcinoma *(82)*. The sensitivity of CA 494 was the same as that of CA 19-9 (90%), with a higher specificity of 96%. There was no statistical difference in CA 494 among the individual stages of pancreatic cancer. No details are provided regarding the clinical course of these patients, to estimate the role of CA 494 in terms of its power to predict resectability, survival, or disease recurrences. More studies are needed to establish the role of this marker in pancreatic cancer.

TISSUE POLYPEPTIDE ANTIGEN (TPA)

TPA, a marker of cellular proliferation released from the membranes of human cancer cells, was originally described by Bjorklund in 1957 *(83)*. It consists of a single polypeptide chain with more than 100 amino acids, variable mol wt, and both keratin-like and Lewis antigen-like determinants *(84)*. The results of nine studies evaluating its role, and that of the tissue polypeptide specific antigen (TPS) in the setting of adenocarcinoma of the pancreas, are shown in Table 12 *(6,56,73,85–90)*. TPS is directed to an epitope (M_3) of the TPA molecule. Data summarized from these studies show a low sensitivity and specificity for both TPA and TPS, although interpretation of these results is hampered by the wide range of cutoff values selected in the different studies. Comparisons with other tumor markers have shown better profiles for CA 19-9, CA 50, CA 242, and even CEA, in relation to TPA *(88,89)*.

The false-positive rate for chronic pancreatitis has ranged from 0 to 24%, and, for benign liver diseases, from 30 to 42% *(87,89,91)*. No definite correlation could be found between TPA levels and stage of pancreatic cancer in one series *(87)*; another study found a positive rate of TPA in approx 40% of 13 patients with stages I and II *(89)*. Information is lacking regarding the use of TPA in monitoring for recurrences or as a prognosticator after surgery; TPS was shown to provide useful prognostic information in a small number of patients after palliative chemotherapy *(90)*. Collectively, these data suggest that TPA and TPS are not as useful as CA 19-9 in the diagnosis and management of pancreatic adenocarcinoma.

THE TESTOSTERONE:DIHYDROTESTOSTERONE RATIO (T:DHT)

The relationship between the pancreas and sex hormones was initially suggested by the discovery of estrogen receptors in malignant pancreatic tissue in 1981 by Green-

Table 12
**Tissue Polypeptide Antigen (TPA) and Tissue Polypeptide Specific Antigen (TPS)
in Pancreatic Cancer**

Author	Ref no.	Tumor marker	Cutoff level	N^a	Sensitivity (%)	n^b	Specificity (%)
Saito	6	TPA	110 U/L	35	74.3	32	75
Benini	56	TPA	150 U/mL	25	48	168	80.2
Meduri	85	TPA	150 U/L	30	97	82	37
Andriulli	86	TPA	200 U/L	83	37	143	92
Panucci	87	TPA	105.5 U/L	28	96.4	53	67.3
Pasanen	88	TPA	320 U/L	25	52	132	85
Total				226	67.5	610	73
Banfi	73	TPS	40 Au/L	41	98	19	22
Pasanen	88	TPS	630 U/L	26	50	149	69.6
Plebani	89	TPS	340 U/L	42	74	100^c	61
Kornek	90	TPS	80 U/L	20	95	n/a	n/a
Total				129	79	268	51

[a] N, number of patients with pancreatic cancer.
[b] n, number of controls and patients with benign biliary, hepatic, and pancreatic diseases.
[c] Included 29 patients with other gastrointestinal malignancies.

way et al. *(92)*, setting the stage for a potential role of antihormonal therapy in pancreatic cancer. In 1983, two separate reports by the same investigators described low testosterone levels in patients with pancreatic cancer, and the presence of enzymes involved in androgen metabolism in operative specimens of human pancreatic cancer *(93,94)*.

Decreased serum testosterone levels have been reported in pancreatic cancer patients, when compared to controls *(95,96)*. Although this finding has been correlated to nutritional status *(97,98)*, other evidence points to an active role of the pancreatic gland in androgen metabolism, including the conversion of testosterone to both dihydrotestosterone and androstenedione *(99,100)*.

Fernandez Del Castillo et al. *(100)* first evaluated the application of the T:DHT ratio in 1987. A T:DHT ratio < 5 correctly identified 20 of 22 (91%) male patients with pancreatic cancer, with a specificity of 99% for controls. These results stimulated the comparison of the T:DHT ratio with the CA 19-9 antigen in a group of 83 male patients with pancreatic, ampullary, biliary tract, and other gastrointestinal cancers, with benign pancreatobiliary disorders *(101)*. The sensitivity of T:DHT was 66.7% and the specificity 98.4%, against CA 19-9 figures of 90.5 and 61.3%, respectively.

The detection rate for stage I pancreatic cancer was a surprising 100%. This exceptionally high result, however, should be considered preliminary, because of the small number of patients included in this group. A major hindrance to the potential application of this marker is that it is only relevant to male patients.

ISLET AMYLOID POLYPTIDE (IAPP)

IAPP is a 37-amino-acid polypeptide produced in the beta cells of the islets, which has been invoked in the pathogenesis of noninsulin dependent diabetes mellitus

(NIDDM) *(102,103)*. The deposition of this peptide in the form of islet amyloidosis is the most common lesion found in the endocrine pancreas of the majority of the patients with NIDDM *(102,103)*. In rats, a significant reduction in food intake has been observed after infusion of IAPP *(104)*. The production of this hormonal factor and *its* presence in increased amounts in the serum of some patients with pancreatic cancer has been suggested, to explain, at least in part, the anorexia seen in patients with this disorder. Increased circulating levels of IAPP have also been reported to occur in patients with neuroendocrine tumors, including both the sporadic type of pancreatic endocrine tumors and those related to multiple endocrine neoplasia syndrome *(105)*. These findings prompted the evaluation of IAPP as a diagnostic marker for pancreatic cancer. Permert et al. measured IAPP by radioimmunoassay in 30 patients with pancreatic cancer, 46 patients with other cancers, 23 patients with diabetes, and 25 normal individuals *(106)*. The sensitivity was 57% and the specificity 99%, with a cutoff of 18 pmol/L. This study did not include patients with chronic pancreatitis. More data are needed before the role of IAPP as a tumor marker can be judged.

CONCLUSIONS

Despite its limitations, CA 19-9 antigen remains the gold standard tumor-associated antigen, against which any new tumor marker should be compared. It appears to be superior to other TAAs such as CEA, elastase-1, TPA, and TPS. No significant differences can be found when compared to CA 50, DUPAN-2, and Span-1, and its preferred use over these tumor antigens probably reflects a larger clinical experience with CA 19-9. On the basis of preliminary information, the T:TDHT ratio may be promising in diagnosing early pancreatic cancer in males only. The appropriate use of CA 494 and IAPP in diagnosis of pancreatic malignancy remains to be defined by further studies. CA 242 appears promising by virtue of a somewhat greater specificity than CA 19-9, but it has lower sensitivity.

Further studies should emphasize the application of CA 19-9 antigen in predicting unresectability and recurrence after surgery for pancreatic cancer. The use of this TAA, in general, should evolve from a supporting role in diagnosis to an important role in prognosis and other important clinical end points in patients with this malignancy.

REFERENCES

1. Pasquali C, Sperti C, D'Andrea AA, et al. Clinical value of serum tag 72 as a tumour marker for pancreatic carcinoma. Comparison with CA 19-9. Int J Pancreatol 1994; *15:*171–177.
2. Sperti C, Pasquali C, Guolo P, Polverosi R, Liessi G, and Pedrazzoli S. Serum tumour markers and cyst fluid analysis are useful for the diagnosis of pancreatic cystic tumors. Cancer 1996; *78:*237–243.
3. Steinberg W: Clinical utility of the CA 19-9 tumor associated antigen. Am J Gastroenterol 1990; *85:*350–355.
4. Taccone W, Mazzon W, and Belli M. Evaluation of TATI and other markers in solid tumors. Scand J Clin Lab Invest 1991; *51:*25–32.
5. Aroasio E and Piantino P. Tumor-associated inhibitor in pancreatic diseases. Scand J Clin Lab Invest 1991; *51:*71–73.
6. Saito S, Taguchi K, Nishimura N, et al. Clinical usefulness of computer-assisted diagnosis using combination assay of tumor markers for pancreatic carcinoma. Cancer 1993; *72:*381–388.

7. Satake K and Takeuchi T. Comparison of CA 19-9 with other tumor markers in the diagnosis of cancer of the pancreas. Pancreas 1994; *9:*720–724.

8. Satake K, Chung YS, Umeyama K, et al. The possibility of diagnosing small pancreatic cancer (less than 4.0 cm) by measuring various tumor markers. Cancer 1991; *68:*149–152.

9. Furukawa H, Okada S, Ariyama J, et al. Clinicopathologic features of small pancreatic adenocarcinoma. Cancer 1996; *78:*986–990.

10. Kuno N, Kurimoto K, Fukushima M, Hayakawa T, Shibata T, Suzuki T, et al. Effectiveness of multivariate analysis of tumor markers in diagnosis of pancreatic carcinoma: a prospective study in multiinstitutions. Pancreas 1994; *9:*725–730.

11. Azuma T, Hira M, Ito S, et al. Expression of cathepsin E in pancreas: a possible tumor marker for pancreas, a preliminary report. Int J Cancer 1996; *67:*492–497.

12. Parker N, Makin CA, Ching CK, et al. A new enzyme-linked lectin/mucin antibody sandwich assay (CAM17.2/WGA) assessed in combination with CA 19-9 and peanut lectin binding assay for the diagnosis of pancreatic cancer. Cancer 1992; *70:*1062–1068.

13. Yiannakow JY, Newland P, Calder F, et al. Prospective study of CAM 17.1/WGA mucin assay for serological diagnosis of pancreatic cancer. Lancet 1997; *349:*389–392.

14. Kropowski H, Stepleweski Z, Mitchell K, et al. Colorectal carcinoma antigens detected by hybridoma antibodies. Somat Cell Genet 1979; *5:*957–972.

15. Magnani J, Nilsson B, Brockhaus M, et al. A monoclonal antibody-defined antigen associated with gastrointestinal cancer is a ganglioside containing sialylated lacto-N-fucopentaose II. J Biol Chem 1982; *257:*14365–14369.

16. Itkowitz SH and Kim YS. New carbohydrate tumor markers. Gastroenterology 1986; *90:*491–494.

17. Tempero MA, Uchida E, Tkasaki H, et al. Relationship of carbohydrate antigen CA 19-9 and Lewis antigen in pancreatic cancer. Cancer Res 1987; *47:*5501–5503.

18. Takasaki H, Uchida E, Tempero M, et al. Correlative study on expression of CA 19-9 and DUPAN-2 in tumor tissue and in serum of pancreatic cancer patients. Cancer Res 1988; *48:*1435–1438.

19. Von Rosen A, Linder S, Harmenberg U, and Pegert S. Serum levels of CA 19-9 and CA 50 in relation to Lewis blood cell status in patients with malignant and benign pancreatic disease. Pancreas 1993; *8:*160–165.

20. Yazawa S, Asao T, Izawa H, et al. The presence of CA 19-9 in serum and saliva from Lewis negative cancer patients. Japn J Cancer Res 1987; *79:*538.

21. Masson P, Pålsson B, and Andrén-Sandberg Å: Cancer associated tumor markers CA 19-9 and CA 50 in patients with pancreatic cancer with special reference to the Lewis blood cell status. Br J Cancer 1990; *62:*118–121.

22. Arends JW. Distribution of monoclonal antibody-defined monosialoganglioside in normal and cancerous human tissues: an immunoperoxidase study. Hybridoma 1983; *2:*219–229.

23. Atkinson BF, Ernst CS, Herlyn M, et al. Gastrointestinal immunoperoxidase assay. Cancer Res 1982; *42:*4820–4823.

24. Ritts RE, Del Villano BC, Go VLW, et al. Initial clinical evaluation of an immunoradiometric assay for CA 19-9 using NCI serum bank. Int J Cancer 1984; *33:*339–345.

25. Del Villano BC, Brennan S, Brock P, et al. Radioimmunometric assay for a monoclonal antibody-defined tumor marker, CA 19-9. Clin Chem 1983; *29:*549–552.

26. Craxi A, Patti C, and Aragona E. Serum CA 19-9 levels in patients with hepatocellular carcinoma or cirrhosis. Ital J Gastroenterol 1985; *17:*288–289.

27. Albert MB, Steinberg W, and Henry JP. Elevated serum levels of tumor marker CA 19-9 in acute cholangitis. Dig Dis Sci 1988; *33:*1223–1225.

28. Paganuzzi M, Onetto M, Marroni P, et al. CA 19-9 and CA 50 in benign and malignant pancreatic and biliary disease. Cancer 1988; *61:*2100–2108.

29. Tatsuta M, Yamamura H, Iishi H, et al. Values of CA 19-9 in the serum, pure pancreatic juice and aspirated pancreatic material in the diagnosis of malignant pancreatic tumor. Cancer 1985; 2669–2673.

30. Schmiegel WH, Kreiker W, Eberl W, et al. Monoclonal antibody defines CA 19-9 in pancreatic juices and sera. Gut 1985; 26:456–460.

31. Malesci A, Tommasini MA, Bonato C, et al. Determination of CA 19-9 antigen in serum and pancreatic juice for differential diagnosis of pancreatic adenocarcinoma from chronic pancreatitis. Gastroenterology 1987; 92:60–67.

32. Chen YF, Mai CR, Tie ZJ, et al. The diagnostic significance of carbohydrate antigen CA 19-9 in serum and pancreatic juice in pancreatic carcinoma. Chinese Med J 1989; 102:333–337.

33. Gentiloni N, Caradonna MD, Costamagna G, et al. Pancreatic juice 90K and serum CA 19-9 combined determination can discriminate between pancreatic cancer and chronic pancreatitis. Am J Gastroenterol 1995; 90:1069–1072.

34. Podolsky DK: Serologic markers in the diagnosis and management of pancreatic carcinoma. World J Surg 1984; 8:822.

35. Satake K, Takeuchi T, Homma T, and Ozaki H. CA 19-9 as a screening and diagnostic tool in symptomatic patients: the Japanese experience. Pancreas 1994; 9:703–706.

36. Frebourg T, Bercoff E, Manchon N, et al. The evaluation of CA 19-9 antigen level in the early detection of pancreatic cancer: a prospective study of 866 patients. Cancer 1988; 62:2287–2290.

37. Chang JH and Takeuchi T. Clinical significance of measurement of Span-1 antigen in the diagnosis of pancreatic cancer. J Japn Pancreas Soc 1990; 5:80–88.

38. Pleskow DK, Berger H, Gyves J, et al. Evaluation of a serologic marker, CA 19-9, in the diagnosis of pancreatic cancer. Ann Intern Med 1989; 110:704–709.

39. Ji-yao W, Fu-Zhen C, and Yong-Zhang Y. Evaluation of non-invasive diagnostic tests in detecting cancer of the pancreas. Chinese Med J 1990; 103:817–820.

40. Van den Bosch RP, van Eijck CHJ, Mulder PGH, Jeekel J: Serum CA 19-9 determination in the management of pancreatic cancer. Hepatogastroenterology 1996; 43:710–713.

41. Forsmark CE, Lambiase L, and Vogel S. Diagnosis of pancreatic cancer and prediction of unresectability using the tumor-associated antigen CA 19-9. Pancreas 1994; 9:731–734.

42. Safi F, Schlosser W, Falkenreck S, and Beger H. CA 19-9 serum course and prognosis of pancreatic cancer. Int J Pancreatol 1996; 20:155–161.

43. Lundin J, Roberts P, and Haglund C. The prognostic value of preoperative serum levels of CA 19-9 and CEA in patients with pancreatic cancer. Br J Cancer 1994; 69:515–519.

44. Sperti C, Pasquali C, Catalini S, et al. CA 19-9 as a prognostic index after resection for pancreatic cancer. Oncology 1993; 52:137–141.

45. Gattani AM, Mandeli J, and Bruckener HW. Tumor markers in patients with pancreatic carcinoma. Cancer 1996; 78:57–62.

46. Willet C, Daly W, and Warshaw A. CA 19-9 is an index of response to neoadjuvant chemoradiation therapy in pancreatic cancer. Am J Surg 1996; 172:350–352.

47. Glenn J, Steinberg W, Kurtzman S, et al. Evaluation of the utility of a radioimmunoassay for serum CA 19-9 levels in patients before and after treatment of carcinoma of the pancreas. J Clin Oncol 1988; 6:462–468.

48. Beretta E, Malesci A, Zerbi A, et al. Serum CA 19-9 in the postsurgical follow-up of patients with pancreatic cancer. Cancer 1987; 60:2428–2431.

49. Tian F, Appert H, Myles J, and Howard J. Prognostic value of serum CA 19-9 levels in pancreatic adenocarcinoma. Ann Surg 1992; 215:350–355.

50. Lindholm L, Holmgren J, Svennerholm L, et al. Monoclonal antibodies against gastrointestinal tumour-associated antigens isolated as monosialogangliosides. Int Arch Allergy Appl Immunol 1983; *71:*178–181.

51. Mansson JE, Fredman P, Nilsson O, et al. Chemical structure of carcinoma ganglioside antigens defined by monoclonal antibody C-50 and some allied gangliosides of human pancreatic adenocarcinoma. Biochim Biophys Acta 1985; *834:*110–117.

52. Haglund C, Roberts PJ, Jalanko H, and Kuusela P. Tumor markers CA 19-9 and CA 50 in digestive tract malignancies. Scand J Gastroenterol 1992; *27:*169–174.

53. Pasquali C, Sperti C, D'Andrea AA, et al. CA 50 compared with CA 19-9 as serum tumour marker for pancreatic carcinoma. Ital J Gastroenterol 1994; *26:*169–173.

54. Molina LM, Diez M, Cava MT, et al. Tumor markers in pancreatic cancer: a comparative clinical study between CEA, CA 19-9 and CA 50. Int J Biol Markers 1990; *5:*127–132.

55. Kobayashi T, Kawa S, Tokoo M, et al. Comparative study of CA 50 (time-resolved fluoroimmunoassay), Span-1, and CA 19-9 in the diagnosis of pancreatic cancer. Scand J Gastroenterol 1991; *26:*787–797.

56. Benini L, Cavallini G, Zordan D, Rizzotti P, Rigo L, Brocco G, et al. A clinical evaluation of monoclonal (CA 19-9, CA 50, CA 12-5) and polyclonal (CEA, TPA) antibody-defined antigens for the diagnosis of pancreatic cancer. Pancreas 1988; *3:*61–66.

57. Chung YS, Ho JJ, Kim YS, et al. The detection of human pancreatic cancer-associated antigen in the serum of cancer patients. Cancer 1987; *60:*1636–1643.

58. Kawa S, Tokoo M, Oguchi H, et al. Epitope analysis of SPan-1 and DUPAN-2 using synthesized glyconconjugates sialyllact-N-fucopentaose II and sialyllact-N-tetraose. Pancreas 1994; *9:*692–697.

59. Kiriyama S, Hayakawa T, Kondo T, et al. Usefulness of a new tumor marker, Span-1, for the diagnosis of pancreatic cancer. Cancer 1990; *65:*1557–1561.

60. Kawa S, Oguchi H, Kobayashi T, et al. Elevated serum levels of Dupan-2 in pancreatic cancer patients negative for Lewis blood group phenotype. Br J Cancer 1991; *64:*899–902.

61. Ferrara C, Basso D, Fabris C, et al. Comparison of two newly identified tumor markers (CAR-3 and DU-PAN-2) with CA 19-9 in patients with pancreatic cancer. Tumori 1991; *77:*56–60.

62. Ohshio G, Manabe T, Watanabe Y, et al. Comparative studies of DU-PAN-2, carcinoembryonic antigen, and CA 19-9 in the serum and bile of patients with pancreatic and biliary tract diseases: evaluation of the influence of obstructive jaundice. Am J Gastroenterol 1990; *85:*1370–1376.

63. Cooper EH, Forbes MA, and Taylor M. An evaluation of DUPAN-2 in pancreatic cancer and gastrointestinal disease. Brit J Cancer 1990; *62:*1004–1005.

64. Fabris C, Malesci A, Basso D, et al. Serum DU-PAN-2 in the differential diagnosis of pancreatic cancer: influence of jaundice and liver dysfunction. Br J Cancer 1991; *63:*451–453.

65. Lindholm L, Johansson C, Jansson EL, et al. An immuno-radiometric assay (IRMA) for the CA 50 antigen. In: Holmgren J (ed), Tumor marker antigen, Studentlitteratur, Lund, Sweden, 1985; pp. 123–133.

66. Rothlin M, Joller H, and Largiadèr F. CA 242 is a new tumor maker for pancreatic cancer. Cancer 1993; *71:*701–707.

67. Plebani M, Basso D, Navaglia F, et al. Is CA 242 really a new tumor marker for pancreatic adenocarcinoma? Oncology 1995; *52:*19–23.

68. Kuusela P, Haglund C, and Roberts PJ. Comparison of a new tumour marker CA 242 with CA 19-9, CA 50 and carcinoembryonic antigen (CEA) in digestive tract diseases. Br J Cancer 1991; *63:*636–640.

69. Pasanen PA, Eskelinen M, Partanen K, et al. A prospective study of serum tumour markers carcinoembryonic antigen, carbohydrate antigens 50 and 242, tissue polypeptide antigen and tissue polypeptide specific antigen in the diagnosis of pancreatic cancer with special reference to multivariate diagnostic score. Br J Cancer 1994; *69:*562–565.

70. Pasanen PA, Eskelinen M, Partanen K, Pikkarainen P, Penttilä I, and Alhava E. Clinical value of serum tumour markers CEA, CA 50 and CA 242 in the distinction between malignant *versus* benign diseases causing jaundice and cholestasis; results from a prospective study. Anticancer Res 1992; *12:*1689–1694.

71. Haglund C, Lindgren J, Roberts PJ, and Nordling S. Tissue expression of the tumor associated antigen CA 242 in benign and malignant pancreatic lesions. Br J Cancer 1989; *60:*845.

72. Kawa S, Tokoo M, Hasebe O, et al. Comparative study of CA242 and CA19-9 for the diagnosis of pancreatic cancer. Br J Cancer 1994; *70:*481–486.

73. Banfi G, Zerbi A, Pastori S, et al. Behavior of tumor markers CA19.9, CA195, CAM43, CA242, and TPS in the diagnosis and follow-up of pancreatic cancer. Clin Chem 1993; *39:*420–423.

74. Pålsson B, Masson P, and Andrén-Sandberg Å. The influence of cholestasis on CA 50 and CA 242 in pancreatic cancer and benign biliopancreatic diseases. Scand J Gastroenterol 1993; *28:*981–987.

75. Pasanen PA, Eskelinen M, Partanen K, et al. A prospective study of the value of imaging, serum markers and their combination in the diagnosis of pancreatic carcinoma in symptomatic patients. Anticancer Res 1992; *12:*2309–2314.

76. Nilsson O, Johansson C, Glimelius B, et al. Sensitivity and specificity of CA 242 in gastrointestinal cancer. A comparison with CEA, CA 50 and CA 19-9. Br J Cancer 1988; *65:*215–221.

77. Pasanen PA, Eskelinen M, Pikkarainen P, et al. Clinical evaluation of a new serum tumor marker CA 242 in pancreatic carcinoma. Br J Cancer 1989; *60:*845.

78. Furuya N, Kawa S, Hasebe O, et al. Comparative study of CA 242 and CA 19-9 in chronic pancreatic. Br J Cancer 1996; *73:*372–376.

79. Bosslet K, Kern HF, Kanzy EJ, et al. A monoclonal antibody with binding and inhibiting activity towards human pancreatic carcinoma cells. Cancer Immunol Immunother 1986; *23:*185–191.

80. Büchler M, Friess H, Schultheiss K, et al. A randomized controlled trial of adjuvant immunotherapy (murine monoclonal antibody 494/32) in resectable pancreatic cancer. Cancer 1991; *68:*1507–1512.

81. Büchler M, Friess H, Malfertheiner P, et al. Studies of pancreatic cancer utilizing monoclonal antibodies. Int J Pancreatol 1990; *7:*151–157.

82. Friess H, Buchler M, Auerbach B, et al. CA 494—a new tumor marker for the diagnosis of pancreatic cancer. Int J Cancer 1993; *53:*759–763.

83. Bjöklund N and Björklund V. Antigenecity of pooled human malignant and normal tissues by cyto-immunological technique: presence of an insoluble, heatlabile tumor antigen. Int Arch Allergy 1957; *10:*153–184.

84. Ochi Y, Ura Y, Hamazu H, et al. Immunological study of tissue polypeptide antigen (TPA)—demonstration of keratin-like sites and blood group antigen-like sites on TPA molecules. Clin Chem Acta 1985; *151:*157–167.

85. Meduri F, Doni MG, Merenda R, et al. The role of the leukocyte adherence inhibition (LAI), CA 19-9, and the tissue polypeptide antigen (TPA) tests in the diagnosis of pancreatic cancer. Cancer 1989; *64:*1103–1106.

86. Andriulli A, Gindro T, Piantino P, et al. Efficacy of CA 19-9, TPA and CEA assays in pancreatic cancer. Digestion 1983; *28:*9–10.

87. Panucci A, Fabris C, Del Favero G, et al. Tissue polypeptide antigen (TPA) in pancreatic cancer diagnosis. Br J Cancer 1985; *52:*801–803.

88. Pasanen P, Eskelinen M, Partanen K, et al. Clinical evaluation of tissue polypeptide antigen (TPA) in the diagnosis of pancreatic carcinoma. Anticancer Res 1993; *13:*1883–1888.

89. Plebani M, Basso D, Del Favero G, et al. Clinical utility of TPS, TPA and CA 19-9 measurement in pancreatic cancer. Oncology 1993; *50:*436–440.

90. Kornek G, Schenk T, Djavarnmad M, and Scheithauer W. Tissue polypeptide-specific antigen (TPS) in monitoring palliative treatment response of patients with gastrointestinal tumors. Br J Cancer 1995; *71:*182–185.

91. Basso D, Fabris C, Piccoli A, et al. Serum tissue polypeptide antigen in pancreatic cancer and other gastrointestinal diseases. J Clin Pathol 1989; *42:*555–557.

92. Greenway B, Iqbal MJ, Johnson PJ, and Williams R. Oestrogen receptor protein in malignant and foetal pancreas. Brit Med J 1981; *283:*751–753.

93. Greenway B, Iqbal MJ, Johnson PJ, and Williams R. Low serum testosterone levels in patients with carcinoma of the pancreas. Br Med J 1983; *286:*93–95.

94. Iqbal MJ, Greenway B, Wilkinson ML, et al. Sex steroid enzymes aromatase and reductase in the pancreas: a comparison of normal adult, foetal and malignant tissue. Clin Sci 1983; *65:*71–75.

95. Fernandez del Castillo C, Díaz-Sanchez V, and Robles-Díaz G. Pancreatic cancer and androgen metabolism: high androstenedione and low testosterone serum levels. Pancreas 1990; *5:*515–518.

96. Shearer NG, Taggart D, and Gray C. Useful differentiation between pancreatic carcinoma and chronic pancreatitis by testosterone assay. Digestion 1984; *30:*106–107.

97. Todd BD. Pancreatic carcinoma and low serum testosterone: a correlation secondary to cancer cachexia? Eur J Surg Oncol 1988; *14:*199–202.

98. Sperti C, Bonadimani B, Militello C, et al. Testosterone and androgen metabolism in pancreatic cancer. J Clin Gastroenterol 1992; *15:*161–162.

99. Fernandez del Castillo C, Diaz-Sanchez V, Varela-Fascinetto V, et al. Testosterone biotransformation by the isolated perfused canine pancreas. Pancreas 1991; *6:*104–111.

100. Robles-Díaz G, Díaz-Sanchez V, Mendez JP, et al. Low serum testosterone/dihydrotestosterone ratio in pancreatic carcinoma. Pancreas 1987; *2:*684–687.

101. Robles-Díaz G, Díaz-Sanchez V, Fernandez-del Castillo C, et al. Serum testosterone/dihydrotestosterone ratio and CA 19-9 in the diagnosis of pancreatic cancer. Am J Gastroenterol 1991; *86:*591–594.

102. Clark A, de Koning EJ, Hattersley AT, et al. Pancreatic pathology in non-insulin dependent diabetes. Diabetes Res Clin Pract 1995; *28(Suppl):*S39–47.

103. Oosterwijk C, Hoppener JW, van Hulst KL, and Lips CJ. Pancreatic islet amyloid formation in patients with noninsulin-dependent diabetes mellitus. Implication for a therapeutic strategy. Int J Pancreatol 1995; *18:*7–14.

104. Arnelo U, Larsson J, Permert J, et al. Could islet amyloid polypeptide contribute to the cachexia of pancreatic cancer? Gastroenterology 1993; *104(Suppl):*A294.

105. Stridsberg M, Eriksson B, Skogseid B, et al. Islet amyloid polypeptide (IAPP) in patients with neuroendocrine tumors. Regul Peptides 1995; *55:*119–131.

106. Permert J, Larsson J, Westermark G, et al. Islet amyloid polypeptide in patients with pancreatic cancer and diabetes. N Engl J Med 1994; *330:*313–318.

107. Satake K, Kanazawa G, Kho I, et al. Evaluation of serum pancreatic enzymes, carbohydrate antigen 19-9 and carcinoembryonic antigen in various pancreatic diseases. Am J Gastroenterol 1985; *80:*630–636.

108. Sakahara H, Endo K, Nakajima K, et al. Serum CA 19-9 Concentrations and computed tomography findings in patients with pancreatic carcinoma. Cancer 1986; *57:*1324–1326.

109. Iishi H, Yamamura H, and Tatsuta M. Value of ultrasonic examination combined with measurement of serum tumor marker in the diagnosis of pancreatic cancer of less than 3 cm in diameter. Cancer 1986; *57:*1947–1951.

110. Steinberg WM, Gelfand R, Anderson KK, et al. Comparison of the sensitivity and specificity of the CA 19-9 and carcinoembryonic antigen assays in detecting cancer of the pancreas. Gastroenterology 1986; *90:*343–349.

111. Safi F, Beger H, Bittner R, et al. CA 19-9 and pancreatic adenocarcinoma. Cancer 1986; *57:*779–783.

112. Del Favero G, Fabris C, Plebani M, et al. CA 19-9 and carcinoembryonic antigen in pancreatic cancer. Cancer 1986; *57:*1576–1579.

113. Wang TH, Lin JW, Chen DS, et al. Noninvasive diagnosis of advanced pancreatic cancer by real-time ultrasonography, carcinoembryonic antigen and carbohydrate antigen 19-9. Pancreas 1986; *1:*219–223.

8

Radiologic Techniques for Diagnosis and Staging of Pancreatic Carcinoma

Mark E. Baker

INTRODUCTION

The purpose of imaging patients with pancreatic carcinoma is to detect the primary tumor, to determine whether the tumor is potentially resectable or unresectable, and, lastly, to guide a confirmatory percutaneous biopsy.

The purpose of this chapter will be to review the common and emerging radiologic technologies used for the diagnosis and staging of this tumor. This includes computed tomography, including the developing use of CT angiography derived from spiral-CT data sets, angiography, magnetic resonance imaging, including MR angiography, ultrasound (excluding endoscopic ultrasound), and, lastly, nuclear medicine. The chapter also discusses the role of image guided percutaneous biopsies in the diagnosis and management of these patients. The overall focus of the chapter will be on radiographic staging of this tumor.

BASIC PRINCIPLES OF PANCREATIC IMAGING

Before ordering a specific radiographic study, it is important for the internist or surgeon to understand the strengths and weaknesses of the study requested. Transabdominal ultrasound is considered by many the study of first choice in patients with jaundice. Using a decision analysis approach, however, if there is a high pretest probability that jaundice is caused by a pancreatic carcinoma, the study of first choice should probably be a CT, because more information than just the presence of the tumor will be gleaned than with an ultrasound (1,2).

The relatively poor performance of ultrasound, when compared to CT, in the detection of pancreatic carcinoma is in part because ultrasound is the study first performed in obstructive jaundice. In these cases, the patient is often scanned at night by an inexperienced operator when the patient has not been optimally prepared. Transabdominal or standard ultrasound is limited by large body habitus (a more significant problem in the United States) and upper abdominal bowel gas. Further, sonographers do not consistently visualize the entire pancreas, especially portions of the head–uncinate process and tail. Much of this is secondary to inexperience and lack of resolve on the part of the sonographer. In the United States, where CT is ubiquitous and easy to obtain, this lack of resolve is a particular problem. When the pancreas is not well seen on a cursory ultrasound, it is easy to defer to CT to evaluate the pancreas.

Endoscopic ultrasound requires a skilled endoscopist and sonographer. The field of view of the ultrasound probe is generally limited to the head and distal (downstream) body of the pancreas. Its use also requires sedation, with monitoring and postsedation recovery, all of which adds to the cost of care.

Computed tomography is considered by many to be the imaging procedure of choice for suspected pancreatic carcinoma. Because of the reasons previously stated, this is more true in the United States than in Europe, Asia, and other parts of the world.

In order for CT to detect most pancreatic carcinomas, iodinated contrast media enhancement is essential. Further, the contrast media must be injected rapidly into a centrally located arm vein in a patient with reasonable or good cardiac output. An excellent arterial bolus of contrast media to the pancreas and liver is essential to achieve a high sensitivity for primary tumor detection, vascular involvement by tumor, and the presence of liver metastases. Not all patients have adequate venous access or cardiac output to achieve these goals.

Over the past 5 yr, a new form of CT has developed: spiral or helical CT *(3)*. These CT machines continuously scan while the patient is moved through the X-ray beam. As a result, the machine produces images from a volume data set; information then can be sliced and diced in multiple ways. The most exciting spin-offs from this technology are convenient multiplanar reconstructions (coronal, sagittal, or oblique planes), CT-angiograms, and three-dimensional images. The state of these postprocessing options from spiral CT is rapidly evolving. Key to the process is a real-time, powerful postprocessing computer capable of parallel processing for real-time visualization and texture mapping. This requires multiple CPUs and extensive video RAM. Therefore, their cost is currently too high for routine clinical use; there are only a few manufacturers producing these postprocessing units. Further, software capable of rapid, real-time manipulation of image data is only in the development stage *(4)*.

Production software is now available for simple multiplanar reconstruction, as well as surface-rendered CT angiograms. However, for the angiograms, significant and time-consuming editing is necessary to produce interpretable images. In the next 5 yr, we hope to see relatively inexpensive (<$50,000), user-friendly, real-time visualization engines capable of rapidly rendering volume information helpful to both the radiologist, surgeon, and oncologist *(4)*. This technology will be much more helpful for the surgeon, both for operative planning and in the operating room, rather than for the diagnostic radiologist.

Magnetic resonance imaging has not been used extensively in the evaluation of patients with suspected pancreatic cancer for several reasons. Up until recently, motion artifact from nonbreath-held techniques obscured detail in the pancreas and peripancreatic regions. Further, high-quality images could not be obtained from breath-held techniques. Patient scanning took a minimum of 1 h or more, and the study was expensive. High-quality MR exams of the upper abdomen now take <45 min, and often 30 min. The spatial resolution of these images approaches CT quality and the sensitivity of MR to enhancement (using gadolinium based substances, rather than iodine) is extremely high. There are also some advantages of MR over CT that I will discuss. However, availability of MR time is limited and remains expensive.

Scintigraphy has the potential of high specificity, especially with tumor-specific agents, but lacks sufficient spatial resolution to guide surgery. The most exciting area in nuclear medicine involves the use of a glucose analog labeled with a fluorine isotope (so-called 2-[fluorine-18]-fluoro-2-deoxy-D-glucose-positron emission tomography or FDG-PET). At present, these techniques are investigational and show promise in patients with pancreatic carcinoma. However, they are expensive and have not yet been shown to be cost-effective.

PANCREATIC CARCINOMA: TUMOR DETECTION AND STAGING

Most radiologic literature states that cross-sectional imaging, especially CT, is 90–95% sensitive in the detection of pancreatic carcinoma *(5–8)*. However, there are several issues that must be considered. First, cross-sectional imaging often cannot detect pancreatic carcinomas <1 cm in size. Therefore, in most of the series published, patients with these small tumors could have easily been excluded, because they were not detected with CT. Second, most if not all of these series are based on surgical cases and/or discharge diagnoses. As a result, we do not know the true prevalence of disease in the population studied by imaging. We only know the sensitivity of CT in the patients with a confirmed diagnosis. Early diagnosis in patients with this aggressive tumor is key, yet we continue to have difficulty in detecting disease early. At least in some cases, this is because our imaging studies are inadequate.

COMPUTED TOMOGRAPHY

In the United States, CT is the imaging procedure of choice in the diagnosis and staging of patients with pancreatic carcinoma. In the best of hands, using the latest technology, CT should detect 90–95% of all pancreatic ductal adenocarcinoma *(5,6)*. In general, any mass >1–2 cm in size will be detected. In the absence of a visualized mass (<5%), there are almost always ancillary findings, such as biliary and/or pancreatic ductal dilatation and evidence for local invasion, especially when the tumor is in the head of the gland *(5)*.

There are, however, several caveats to CT detection and staging of pancreatic carcinoma. Some of these have been previously mentioned, but bear emphasis *(9)*. Modern CT equipment, capable of rapid scanning over 20–25 cm of the body within 60–120 s and using thin slices (3–5 mm), must be available. Spiral scanning is preferred, especially when CT angiography is contemplated; however, a spiral scanner is not necessary to detect the tumor. Further, the rapid injection of iodinated intravenous contrast material is essential, because tumor detection in the absence of enhancement is impaired. Therefore, good venous access is important to achieve adequate bolus enhancement. Lastly, if CT arteriography is contemplated, especially as a replacement for conventional angiography, a postprocessing workstation is mandatory.

Before discussing imaging staging of this tumor, we must understand the terms used. One must determine whether a tumor is resectable or unresectable on imaging findings. A pancreatic tumor that is resectable on the basis of imaging findings is <2–3 cm in size, shows no vascular involvement, no nodal, hepatic, or mesenteric/peritoneal disease, and has no soft-tissue infiltration into the peripancreatic fat adjacent to vessels. It has been the author's experience that surgeons use these terms differently.

According to the American Joint Committee on Cancer (AJCC) staging classification of this tumor, stage I tumors are T1 or T2 tumors without nodal or distant metastatic involvement. T1a tumors are 2 cm or less in greatest dimension and T1b tumors are 2 cm or greater in greatest dimension. T2 tumors extend directly to duodenum, bile duct, or peripancreatic tissues (10). Therefore, only certain T1 tumors are resectable. Stage II tumors are T3 tumors without nodal or distant metastatic involvement (T3 tumors extend directly to involve the stomach, spleen, colon, or adjacent large vessels); stage III tumors are T1–3 with nodal disease. Stage IV tumors are T1–3, N1, M1 lesions (10). Very few stage II or III tumors are resectable. Based on the experience at the Johns Hopkins Medical Center, the patients with the most favorable long-term prognosis have tumors <3 cm in size, with negative nodes at surgery, negative resection margins, have diploid tumor DNA content, and are younger (11).

Radiologic staging should therefore have a high positive predictive value for unresectability (11). Radiologists should concentrate their efforts in determining the T status of the tumor (i.e., the presence and extent of peripancreatic involvement T2, the presence of vascular involvement T3, and the presence of adjacent organ involvement T2 or T3). Detecting liver metastases, nodal disease, and carcinomatosis is also a goal of imaging, but, as will be discussed, is less successful even in centers of excellence.

For staging pancreatic carcinoma, in the best of hands, CT can predict tumor unresectability with an accuracy between 88 and 92% (6,12,13). However, CT is much less accurate in predicting resectability (45–72%). CT's greatest strength in differentiating resectable from unresectable lesions lies with its ability to detect extra pancreatic extension to adjacent arteries. The weakest aspect of CT lies with its relative inability to detect small hepatic metastasis, nodal disease, and subtle venous involvement, as well as carcinomatosis. Liver metastases >1.5–2 cm in size should be routinely detected by CT; unfortunately, up to one-third of metastatic lesions from pancreatic carcinoma are smaller (14). Up to 40% of patients with CT resectable tumors have peritoneal or small hepatic metastases at laparoscopy (14,15).

Detecting nodal metastases with CT is often impossible. There are five major node groups immediately draining the pancreas. Once these are involved, the porta hepatis, common hepatic, celiac, and proximal superior mesenteric groups are affected (9). Lastly, the periaortic, distal superior mesenteric, and other abdominal nodes can be involved. Because nodes in the first group are intimately associated with the pancreas, they are almost never visualized by CT. However, with progression to the porta hepatis, celiac, and mesenteric groups, CT is more able to detect disease. Unfortunately, one cannot rely on size as a criteria for nodal involvement, because normal size lymph nodes may contain tumor, and enlarged lymph nodes may be the result of inflammation or reactive hyperplasia (14).

As stated, the great strength of CT is the detection of extra pancreatic extension, specifically, the presence of arterial involvement (6–9,12,13,16–19). However, there are numerous reports in the surgical literature that question CT's ability to detect vascular disease, especially subtle mesenteric vein and portal venous involvement (20–26).

In the most recent CT series, angiography and CT showed equivalent or similar findings in 75%; CT showed vascular involvement not seen by angiography in 20%, and angiography showed vascular involvement missed by CT in only 5% *(6)*. Work by the same group continues to challenge the assertion in the surgical literature that angiography is necessary in the staging of these patients when CT shows no vascular involvement. They looked at the presence or absence of dilated pancreaticoduodenal veins in patients with pancreatic carcinoma. When dilated veins were not included in the evaluation, only 5/23 (22%) patients thought to be resectable by CT were surgically resectable. When the veins were included in the CT staging, six patients previously thought to be resectable were deemed unresectable, thus increasing the diagnostic accuracy for resectability to 29% (5/17) *(27)*.

A recent paper from M. D. Anderson showed that, with meticulous and focused technique, CT can detect venous involvement with a greater degree of accuracy than previously published *(12,13)*. Using 1.5-mm collimation (routine pancreatic scanning is generally performed using 3–5-mm collimation or slice thickness), when there was either a fat plane or normal pancreatic parenchyma between the tumor and the superior mesenteric or portal vein, the resectability rate was 95% (21/22 patients). When there was no fat plane or normal parenchyma between the tumor and the veins, CT was unreliable in predicting venous involvement. In the nine patients in whom the tumor was immediately adjacent to the vein, creating either a convex or concave impression, there was no vessel involvement in two, the tumor could be dissected off the vessel in three, the vein was resected in three, and the tumor was unresectable in one. One could argue, in cases in which the tumor was dissected off the vessel or in which the vein was resected, that the tumor was unresectable.

We are just beginning to discover the impact of spiral CT technology on staging pancreatic cancer. In the Johns Hopkins experience of 64 patients of potentially resectable tumors, the following was found: resectability accuracy 70% (95% CI, 59–81%); sensitivity for unresectability, 53%; specificity for resectability, 100% *(19)*. Unfortunately, 19/40 (47%) deemed resectable on spiral exam were unresectable. Spiral exams missed small, <10-mm hepatic metastases (8/19 [42%]) and subtle, portal or superior mesenteric venous involvement (7/19 [37%]).

One interesting observation in this series was the relatively high number of isoenhancing primary tumors using spiral technology. This was not a problem with older dynamic scanners capable of rapidly scanning a pancreas in 2 min, rather than the much faster rate of 20–30 s using spiral technology. Of the resected tumors, 14 were hypoattentuating and 10 were isoattentuating. The size and attenuation of the mass did not correlate with the enhancement characteristics. It is unclear whether isoenhancement is caused by early scanning in the arterial phase.

In the pancreatic CT literature published in the late 1970s and early 1980s *(28)*, using a nondynamic technique, isoehancement was a significant problem with approx 50% of tumors isoenhancing relative to the normal pancreas. Why is this problem of isoehancement of concern? If a tumor isoehances, and does not create mass-effect or obstruct or involve ducts or vessels, then the tumor will not be detected.

Recently, two centers have presented data on evaluating pancreatic carcinoma with a biphasic (pancreatic or arterial and hepatic or portal venous) scanning protocol. This involves two scanning sequences, one early in the arterial bolus phase of the contrast injection, and the other during the later portal venous phase. The experience to date is mixed, and more work is needed to determine the relative role of this technique *(29,30)*.

Lu et al. *(29)* did not detect isoehancing masses in any of the 27 patients evaluated with this spiral protocol.

Lastly, 3-D CT arteriography obtained from spiral CT data sets is now easier and does not require additional imaging time or contrast *(31–33)*. As stated before, however, this requires a workstation for postprocessing. Additionally, using current workstations, significant time (30–90 min) is required to sufficiently edit the data to obtain readable images. Nonetheless, as workstation virtual reality engine technology evolves with appropriate software, spiral CT-produced angiograms could easily replace angiography if a vascular map is necessary.

ANGIOGRAPHY

There are several papers in the surgical literature advocating the use of visceral angiography in the preoperative assessment of pancreatic carcinoma. Angiography is used to detect both arterial and venous involvement, as well as to provide a vascular map for the surgeon (especially in detecting arterial variants, such as a replaced right hepatic artery) *(20–26)*. In most cases, arterial involvement should be detected by a high-quality CT scan, even without CT angiography. In the previously cited CT series from Freeny et al. *(6)*, CT missed arterial involvement in only 3/60 cases. Venous involvement is often more difficult to detect with CT (*see* prior discussion). It is the author's opinion that, when there is subtle venous involvement, and CT is negative for that involvement, angiography will not detect the tumor extent either. The author also believes that surgeons who advocate the use of preoperative angiography base their recommendations on data using old CT technology. Fast, modern CT technology, with improved resolution, has markedly improved our ability to detect vascular disease, a fact supported by the most recent series *(6,12,13)*. Lastly, laparoscopic ultrasound may provide more information than CT and angiography in the assessment of vascular involvement *(34–36)*.

One other consideration in the angiography vs CT controversy is patient charge and cost *(37)*. Currently, the charge for a contrasted abdomen and pelvis CT examination at the Cleveland Clinic is approx $1400. If nonionic contrast media is used, the charge is $1650. The charge for an outpatient, two-vessel angiographic study, including recovery room use (recovery room used if an outpatient) and medications given, is $3500. Patient charge is not a reflection of cost, and certainly does not reflect current reimbursement of approx 50%.

At the Cleveland Clinic, the calculated costs of both CT and angiography are as follows: total direct, professional, and technical costs for an abdominal CT is approx $150 (assumes 35 min machine time and 17 min protocoling, reviewing, and interpreting time); if nonionic contrast media is used, the cost increases by $67); total direct, professional, and technical cost for an angiogram is approx $1100. Currently, we do not know the cost of a CT angiogram; however, it probably will not approach the cost of standard angiography, even when the cost of CT postprocessing is included.

MAGNETIC RESONANCE IMAGING

The experience with MRI in the detection and staging of adenocarcinoma of the pancreas is relatively preliminary. Historically, there have been few MRI machines capable of evaluating the pancreas using the appropriate pulse sequences. Several recent papers show MR superiority over CT, especially in the detection of small (<2 cm) pancreatic lesions *(38–45)*. The recent multi-institutional Radiology Diagnostic Oncology Group study *(46)* showed no significant difference between CT and conventional MR in staging for resectability (no breath-held, fast spin-echo, or rapid gradient-echo, contrasted exams performed).

The newer, faster, breath-hold MR sequences can now create images that are equivalent to CT quality. These sequences, in conjunction with contrast enhancement, may prove superior to CT. Further, pancreas-specific contrast agents are in the process of development and testing.

Currently, the great strength of MR over CT is in the detection of small intrahepatic metastases. If appropriate techniques can be developed so that the primary tumor and local extent could be assessed, then MR could be a tremendously powerful tool in the staging of this tumor. However, to the author's knowledge, there is no evidence that MR is superior in detecting small hepatic metastases in patients with pancreatic carcinoma.

Additionally, as with CT, MR angiography (MRA) can be performed. A recent preliminary report suggests that MR of the portal venous system is a reasonable screen for resectability; however, as with CT and other tests, MRA misses subtle venous disease that is unresectable *(47)*.

As with angiography, MR is costly. Despite significant decreases in imaging time with the fast sequences, upper abdominal MR still requires at least 35–40 min of machine time. Technologist familiarity with the scanning sequences is a significant problem at this institution. Sequence setup time is inappropriately long and cost is directly proportional to time spent on the machine. The charge for an MR abdominal case is approx $1100 (total professional and technical). The charge for Gd is $125. The total direct professional and technical cost for the same MR is approx $360 (Gd cost, $76; assumes 45 min machine time and 30 min of physician time protocoling, reviewing, and interpreting). Therefore, the cost of the MR is at least twice the cost of a CT. The only way MR cost will approach CT cost will be to reduce total machine time (15–20 min).

ULTRASOUND

Over the past 10 yr, there has been a virtual explosion of ultrasound technology. No longer is the radiologist or surgeon limited by a transabdominal approach. There are endoscopically adapted sonographic probes, probes for use in the operating room, and laparoscopy-adapted transducers, as well as transducers that can be placed at the end of an angiographic catheter for endovascular ultrasound.

In general, transabdominal ultrasound is much maligned in the United States as a method for the detection of pancreatic tumors. Much of this has to do with the body habitus of Americans (obesity is the sonographers bane), as well as with the fact that ultrasound is operator-dependent. However, given the proper operator and the proper patient, ultrasound should be able to detect tumors much smaller than by CT *(48)*. This requires a meticulous sonographer, a relatively thin patient and the liberal use of ingested water or methylcellulose to provide a sonographic window with which to visualize the pancreas. However, transabdominal ultrasound is not particularly sensitive in the detection of local extension, nodal disease, hepatic metastases, or carcinomatosis. Therefore, in general, transabdominal ultrasound is used as an initial screening examination in patients with obstructive jaundice. However, as previously stated, if the prior or pretest probability for malignant obstruction is high, a CT scan will generally yield more information *(1,2)*.

Endoscopic ultrasound (EUS) is a new, very accurate method in detecting focal abnormalities in the pancreas. However, like the other techniques discussed, cost is an important issue. It requires a skilled endoscopist/sonographer (may be the same individual), patient sedation, and recovery.

Perhaps the most exciting tool to be developed in the past several years is the adaptation of sonographic transducers to laparoscopic work. There are at least three papers in the literature supporting the use of laparoscopic ultrasound (LUS) in the staging of pancreatic carcinoma *(34–36)*. LUS is particularly good in detecting small hepatic metastases. Since laparoscopy is an excellent means of detecting unsuspected peritoneal disease, the most cost-effective method of pancreatic carcinoma staging may be laparoscopy followed by LUS in patients that have CT resectable lesions.

LUS has the greatest potential impact on the staging of pancreatic carcinoma, especially if it can be performed as an outpatient procedure. Patients could be initially staged with a well-performed spiral CT exam. If resectable on the basis of that exam (with or without a CT angiogram), the patient could proceed to a laparoscopic exam with ultrasound. If negative for peritoneal disease or intrahepatic metastases, then a formal laparotomy could be performed. This may be the most cost-efficient and effective approach.

SCINTIGRAPHY

Although most radiologists and surgeons do not think that nuclear medicine has any role in the diagnosis of pancreatic carcinoma, there are several centers now investigating scintigraphic techniques in detecting this tumor. The most prominent in the recent literature concerns F-18 fluorodeoxyglucose (FDG) positron emission tomography (PET). FDG is a glucose analog that is transported into cells and phosphorylated by hexokinase. It is unable to enter the glycolysis pathway and exits via glucose-6-phosphatase. In the normal cell, hexokinase activity equals the G-6-phosphatase activity. However, in a tumor cell, the hexokinase activity is much greater. Therefore, tumors retain more FDG than normal or inflammatory tissues. This is a new and promising agent; however, it is very expensive. Further, to precisely locate an area of increased uptake, this study must often be compared with a cross-sectional imaging technique such as CT or MR.

Early experience with FDG-PET for pancreatic carcinoma is encouraging *(49–51)*. There have been cases of lymph node and hepatic metastases detected with FDG and not with ultrasound or CT. However, there have also been false-positive and -negative FDG scans. Therefore, its current use continues to be investigational. This technique may be useful in patients with chronic pancreatitis, in whom a mass is identified by CT and or ultrasound. No consistent cross-sectional technique can differentiate an inflammatory mass from a tumor in patients with chronic pancreatitis. The technique may also be useful in patients who are CT-resectable, but who may have small hepatic metastases. As far as is known, FDG-PET has not detected subtle carcinomatosis.

As with MRI, cost issues become important with FDG-PET. PET facilities are very expensive both to start and run. Further, most nuclear medicine studies are expensive (cost, not change). If LUS develops to the point at which small liver lesions can be detected, and these procedures become more outpatient oriented (thus reducing in-hospital time and cost), then FDG-PET may not be cost-effective in patients with pancreatic carcinoma.

CT OR ULTRASOUND-GUIDED, PERCUTANEOUS BIOPSY

Image-guided biopsies of pancreatic lesions have been routinely performed for the past 10 yr with high accuracy. A variety of needles have been used, including "skinny needles" for fine-needle aspiration, cytopathologic examination, as well as larger hand-held or "gun"-directed needles for histologic core biopsies *(52–56)*. In a recent Mayo Clinic series (*N* = 211 CT-guided and 58 ultrasound-guided biopsies), CT had an accuracy of 86% and ultrasound 95% (ultrasound was used to biopsy larger masses). They used a variety of needle sizes, with cutting-type needles used for all biopsies, and the larger needles yielding more accurate results. Few complications resulted (a 1.1% major complication rate) *(56)*. Similar rates have been published for fine-needle aspiration biopsies of pancreatic carcinoma.

There is some concern in the surgical literature that percutaneous biopsy of pancreatic carcinoma can lead to malignant seeding of the needle tract or of the peritoneum *(57,58)*. This is based on a few case reports, as well as a report that multiple surgical biopsies can lead to rapid spread of intraabdominal disease *(59)*. This is further supported by a series published by Warshaw *(14)*. In his series, positive peritoneal washings were found in 30% of the operative patients. 75% of these patients had undergone a biopsy prior to surgery. However, this may not be relevant from an outcomes point of view. In a recent British series *(60)*, 170 patients with pancreatic carcinoma were followed for long-term outcome. One hundred nineteen had a pancreatic biopsy and the remainder did not. Thirteen percent had a fine-needle aspiration, 48% had an 18-gage cutting-biopsy procedure, 27% had an intraoperative biopsy, and 12% had an endoscopic procedure. There was no statistically significant difference in the survival time for the two groups.

It is the author's opinion that the benefits of image-guided percutaneous biopsy far outweigh the potential negatives from peritoneal seeding. However, every effort should be made to limit the number of passes into the pancreatic mass. Further, if proper technique is employed with 22 gage needles, and there is an experienced cytopathologist, fine-needle aspiration biopsy in this tumor should be preferred over a larger cutting biopsy.

Finally, cost issues again are becoming a greater force in medicine. A fine-needle aspiration biopsy is much less costly than even a laparoscopic guided biopsy. Ultimately, our goal in imaging this tumor will be to diagnose and stage appropriately, and to confirm that the staging is correct, with a fine-needle aspiration (i.e., the placement of the needle in an extrapancreatic site to prove nonresectability).

PANCREATIC CARCINOMA: IMPACT OF IMAGING ON PATIENT OUTCOME

Unfortunately, despite advances in image quality and technology, there is little evidence that these advances have altered the dismal outcome in patients with pancreatic carcinoma. When imaging detects a tumor, it is unresectable in the vast majority of patients. Despite advances in aggressive surgical and adjunct chemoradiation therapy *(61)*, in the largest series to date, only 36% of a heavily preselected population survives 3 yr *(11)*.

David Stephens of the Mayo Clinic (a noted abdominal radiologist with many years experience in diagnosing and staging pancreatic cancer) has recently written an editorial on CT staging of this tumor *(62)*. In this article, he quotes Gertrude Stein: "A difference in order to be a difference must make a difference." We have yet to see that imaging makes much of a difference in the long-term outcome of patients with this tumor. We need better ways of detecting the presence of the tumor before it is too late.

SUMMARY

The diagnosis and staging of pancreatic carcinoma starts with a well-performed, enhanced, dedicated CT of the pancreas and liver for both the detection of the tumor and the presence of extrapancreatic extension and distant metastases. It is the author's opinion that most cases of pancreatic carcinoma can be adequately staged as potentially resectable or unresectable on the basis of this examination alone. In cases in which vascular involvement is questioned, meticulous attention should be paid to the pancreaticoduodenal veins, as well as to the peripancreatic fat for subtle extension of tumor. If the patient is examined on a spiral scanner, CT angiography can be performed with relative ease with current off-line processors. CT continues to be limited in the detection of small hepatic metastases, peritoneal spread, lymph node involvement, and subtle venous disease. If a tumor is resectable based on CT criteria, the surgeon should proceed with a laparoscopic examination. If laparoscopy/peritoneal washing is negative for peritoneal spread, then LUs of the peripancreatic vessels and the liver should be performed. If all of these exams show a resectable tumor, then a formal laparotomy should commence.

For those patients who are CT unresectable, percutaneous biopsy remains the single most cost-effective method of confirming tumor presence.

REFERENCES

1. Arvan DA. Obstructive jaundice. In: Panzer RJ, Black BR, and Griner PF (eds). Diagnostic strategies for common medical problems. American College of Physicians, Philadelphia, 1991; pp. 131–140.
2. Frank BB. Clinical evaluation of jaundice: a guideline of the patient care committee of the American Gastroenterological Association. JAMA 1989; *262:*3031–3034.
3. Heiken JP, Brink JA, and Vannier MW. Spiral (helical) CT. Radiology 1993; *189:*647–656.
4. Johnson PT, Heath DG, Bliss DF, Cabral B, and Fishman EK. Three-dimensional CT: real-time interactive volume rendering. AJR 1996; *167:*581–583.
5. Freeny PC, Marks WM, Ryan JA, and Traverso LW. Pancreatic ductal adenocarcinoma: diagnosis and staging with dynamic CT. Radiology 1988; *166:*125–133.
6. Freeny PC, Traverso LW, and Ryan JA. Diagnosis and staging of pancreatic adenocarcinoma with dynamic computed tomography. Am J Surg 1993; *165:*600–606.

7. Megibow AJ, Zhou XH, Rotterdam H, Francis IR, Zerhouni EZ, Balfe DM, et al. Pancreatic adenocarcinoma: CT versus MR imaging in the evaluation of resectability-report of the radiology diagnostic oncology group. Radiology 1995; *195:*327–332.

8. Gulliver DJ, Baker ME, Cheng CA, Meyers WC, and Pappas TN. Malignant biliary obstruction: efficacy of thin-section dynamic CT in determining resectability. AJR 1992; *159:*503–507.

9. Megibow AJ. Pancreatic adenocarcinoma: designing the examination to evaluate the clinical questions. Radiology 1992; *183:*297–303.

10. Spiessl B, Beahrs OH, Hermanek P, Hutter RVP, TNM atlas: illustrated guide to the TNM/p TNM classification of malignant tumors, 3rd ed., 2nd revision, Scheibe O, Sobin LH, Wagner G (eds). Springer-Verlag, Berlin, 1992, pp. 132–139.

11. Yeo CJ, Cameron JL, and Lillemore KD. Pancreaticoduodenectomy for cancer of the head of the pancreas: 201 patients. Ann Surg 1995; *221:*721–733.

12. Loyer EM, David CL, Dubrow RA, Evans DB, and Charnsangevej C. Vascular involvement in pancreatic adenocarcinoma: reassessment by thin-section CT. Abdom Imaging 1996; *21:*202–206.

13. Fuhrman GM, Charnsangavej C, Abbruzzese JL, Cleary KR, Martin RG, Fenoglio CJ, and Evans DB. Thin-section contrast enhanced computed tomography accurately predicts the resectability of malignant pancreatic neoplasms. Am J Surg 1994; *167:*104–113.

14. Warshaw A and Fernández-Del Castillo C. Pancreatic carcinoma. N Engl J Med 1992; *326:*455–465.

15. Warshaw AL. Implications of peritoneal cytology for staging of early pancreatic cancer. Am J Surg 1991; *161:*26–30.

16. Megibow AJ, Bosniak MA, Ambos MA, and Beranbaum ER. Thickening of the celiac axis and/or superior mesenteric artery: a sign of pancreatic carcinoma on computed tomography. Radiology 1981; *141:*449–453.

17. Baker ME, Cohan RH, Nadel SN, Leder RA, and Dunnick NR. Obliteration of the fat surrounding the celiac axis and superior mesenteric artery is not a specific CT finding of carcinoma of the pancreas. AJR 1990; *155:*991–994.

18. Baker ME. Pancreatic adenocarcinoma: Are there pathognomonic changes in the fat surrounding the superior mesenteric artery? Radiology 1991; *180:*613–614.

19. Bluemke D, Cameron JI, Hruban R, Pitt H, Siegelman SS, Soyer P, and Fishman E. Potentially resectable pancreatic adenocarcinoma: spiral CT assessment with surgical and pathologic correlation. Radiology 1995; *197:*381–385.

20. Mackie CR, Lu CT, Noble HG, Cooper MB, Collins P, Block GE, and Moossa AR. Prospective evaluation of angiography in the diagnosis and management of patients suspected of having pancreatic cancer. Ann Surg 1979; *189:*11–17.

21. Jafri SZ, Aisen AM, Glazer GM, and Weiss CA. Comparison of CT and angiography in assessing resectability of pancreatic carcinoma. AJR 1984; *142:*525–529.

22. Rong GH and Sindelar WF. Aberrant peripancreatic arterial anatomy: considerations of performing pancreatectomy for malignant neoplasms. Am Surg 1987; *53:*726–729.

23. Warshaw AL, Gu Z, Wittenberg J, and Waltman AC. Preoperative staging and assessment of resectability of pancreatic cancer. Arch Surg 1990; *125:*230–233.

24. Dooley WC, Cameron JL, Pitt HA, Lillemoe KD, Yue NC, and Venbrux AC. Is preoperative angiography useful in patients with periampullary tumors? Ann Surg 1990; *211:*649–655.

25. Murugiah M, Windsor JA, Redhead DN, O'Neill JS, Suc B, Garden OJ, and Carter DC. The role of selective visceral angiography in the management of pancreatic and periampullary cancer. World J Surg 1993; *17:*796–800.

26. Biehl TR, Traverso W, Hauptmann E, and Ryan JA. Preoperative visceral angiography alters intraoperative strategy during the whipple procedure. Am J Surg 1993; *165:*607–612.

27. Hommeyer SC, Freeny PC, and Crabo LG. Carcinoma of the head of the pancreas: Evaluation of the pancreaticoduodenal veins with dynamic CT-potential for improved accuracy in staging. Radiology 1995; *196:*-223–238.

28. Ward EM, Stephens DH, and Sheedy PF. Computed tomographic characteristics of pancreatic carcinoma: an analysis of 100 cases. RadioGraphics 1983; *3:*547–565.

29. Lu DS, Vedantham S, Krasy RM, Kadell BM, Berger W, and Reber HA. Two-phase helical CT of pancreatic tumors: pancreatic versus hepatic phase enhancement of tumor, pancreas and vascular structures. Radiology 1996; *199:*697–701.

30. Choi BI, Chung MJ, Han JK, and Han MC. Spiral CT in the evaluation of pancreatic adenocarcinoma: relative value of arterial- and portal venous-phase scanning. Radiology 1995; *197(P):*245.

31. Fishman E, Wyatt SH, Ney DR, Kuhlman JE, and Siegelman SS. Spiral CT of the pancreas with multiplanar display. AJR 1992; *159:*1209–1215.

32. Rubin GD, Dake MD, Napel SA, McDonnell CH, and Jeffrey RB. Three-dimensional spiral CT angiography of the abdomen: initial clinical experience. Radiology 1993; *186:*147–152.

33. Winter TC, Freeny PC, Nghiem HV, Hommeyer SC, Barr D, Croghan AM, et al. Hepatic arterial anatomy in transplantation candidates: evaluation with three-dimensional CT arteriography. Radiology 1995; *195:*363–370.

34. Cuesta MA, Meijer S, Borgstein PJ, Mulder LS, and Sikkenk AC. Laparoscopic ultrasonography for hepatobiliary and pancreatic malignancy. Br J Surg 1993; *80:*1571–1574.

35. John TG, Greig JD, Crosbie JL, Miles WF, and Garden OJ. Superior staging of liver tumors with laparoscopy and laparoscopic ultrasound. Ann Surg 1994; *220:*711–719.

36. John TG, Greig JD, Carter DC, and Garden OJ. Carcinoma of the pancreatic head and periampullary region: tumor staging with laparoscopy and laparoscopic ultrasonography. Ann Surg 1995; *221:*156–164.

37. Alvarez C, Livingston EH, Ashley SW, Schwarz M, and Reber HA. Cost-benefit analysis of the work-up for pancreatic cancer. Am J Surg 1993; *165:*53–60.

38. Mitchell DG, Vinitski S, Saponaro S, Tasciyan T, Burk DL, and Rifkin MD. Liver and pancreas: improved spin-echo T1 contrast by shorter echo time and fat suppression at 1.5 T. Radiology 1991; *178:*67–71.

39. Semelka RC, Kroeker MA, Shoenut JP, Kroeker R, Yaffe CS, and Micflikier AB. Pancreatic disease: Prospective comparison of CT, ERCP, and 1.5-T MR imaging with dynamic gadolinium enhancement and fat suppression. Radiology 1991; *181:*785–791.

40. Vellet AD, Romano W, Bach DB, Passi RB, Taves DH, and Munk PL. Adenocarcinoma of the pancreatic ducts: comparative evaluation with CT and MR imaging of 1.5 T. Radiology 1992; *183:*87–95.

41. Gehl HB, Vorwerk D, Klose KC, and Günther RW. Pancreatic enhancement after low-dose infusion of Mn-DPDP. Radiology 1991; *180:*337–339.

42. Mitchell DG, Shapiro M, Schurict A, Barbot D, and Rosato FR. Pancreatic disease; findings of state-of-the-art MR images. AJR 1992; *159:*533–538.

43. Semelka RC and Ascher SM. MR imaging of the pancreas. Radiology 1993; *188:*593–602.

44. Gehl HB, Urhahn R, Bohndorf K, Klever P, Hauptmann S, Lodemann KP, et al. Mn-DPDP in MR imaging of pancreatic adenocarcinoma: initial clinical experience. Radiology 1993; *186:*795–798.

45. Toshifumi G, Matsui O, Kadoya M, Yoshikawa J, Miyayama S, Takashima T, et al. Small pancreatic adenocarcinomas: efficacy of MR imaging with fat suppression and gadolinium enhancement. Radiology 1994; *193:*683–688.

46. Megibow AJ, Zhou XH, Rotterdam H, Francis IR, Zerhouni EA, Balfe DM, et al. Pancreatic adenocarcinoma: CT versus MR imaging in the evaluation of resectability—report of the Radiology Diagnostic Oncology Group. Radiology 1995; *195:*327–332.

47. McFarland EG, Kaufman JA, Saini S, Halpern EF, Lu DSK, Waltman AC, and Warshaw AL. Preoperative staging of cancer of the pancreas: value of MR angiography vs. conventional angiography in detecting portal venous invasion. AJR 1996; *166:*37–43.

48. Campbell JP and Wilson SR. Pancreatic neoplasms: How useful is evaluation with US? Radiology 1988; *167:*341–344.

49. Bares R, Klever P, Hauptmann S, Hellwig D, Fass J, Cremerius U, et al. F-18 fluorodeoxyglucose PET in vivo evaluation of pancreatic glucose metabolism for detection of pancreatic cancer. Radiology 1994; *192:*79–86.

50. Stollfuss JC, Glatting G, Friess H, Kocher F, Beger HG, and Reske SN. 2-(fluorine-18)-fluoro-2-deoxy-D-glucose PET in detection of pancreatic cancer: value of quantitative image interpretation. Radiology 1995; *195:*339–344.

51. Inokuma T, Tamaki N, Torizuka T, Magata Y, Fuji M, Yonekura Y, et al. Evaluation of pancreatic tumors with positron emission tomography and F-18 fluorodeoxyglucose: comparison with CT and US. Radiology 1995; *195:*345–352.

52. Kocjan G, Rode J, and Lees WR. Percutaneous fine needle aspiration cytology of the pancreas: advantages and pitfalls. J Clin Pathol 1989; *42:*341–347.

53. Al-Kaisi N and Siegler EE. Fine needle aspiration cytology of the pancreas. Acta Cytol 1989; *33:*145–152.

54. Athlin L, Blind PJ, and Ångström T. Fine-needle aspiration biopsy of pancreatic masses. Acta Chir Scand 1990; *156:*91–94.

55. Parsons L and Palmer CH. How accurate is fine-needle biopsy in malignant neoplasia of the pancreas? Arch Surg 1989; *124:*681–683.

56. Brandt KR, Charboneau JW, Stephens DH, Welch TJ, and Goellner JR. CT and US guided biopsy of the pancreas. Radiology 1993; *187:*99–104.

57. Ferrucci JT, Wittenberg J, Margolies MN, and Carey RW. Malignant seeding of the tract after thin-needle aspiration biopsy. Radiology 1979; *130:*345–346.

58. Rashleigh-Belcher HJ, Russell RC, and Lees WR. Cutaneous seeding of pancreatic carcinoma by fine-needle aspiration biopsy. Brit J Radiol 1986; *59:*183–185.

59. Weiss SM, Skibber JM, Mohiuddin M, and Rosato FE. Rapid intra-abdominal spread of pancreatic cancer. Arch 1985; *120:*415–416.

60. Balen FG, Little A, Smith AC, Theis BA, Abrams KR, Houghton J, et al. Biopsy of inoperable pancreatic tumors does not adversely influence patient survival time. Radiology 1994; *193:*753–755.

61. Lillemoe K. Current management of pancreatic carcinoma. Ann Surg 1995; *221:*133–148.

62. Stephens DH. Pancreatic adenocarcinoma: editorial commentary. Abdom Imaging 1996; *21:*207–210.

9

Diagnosis and Staging of Pancreatic Cancer

The Role of Laparoscopy

Margaret Schwarze and David W. Rattner

INTRODUCTION

Patients with adenocarcinoma of the pancreas have a dismal prognosis. Only 3% of all patients with this tumor survive for 5 yr *(1)*. However, resection of pancreatic cancer in selected patients can lead to 5-yr survival rates of 20%, as well as prolongation of median survival for those who recur *(2,3)*. A key task in managing patients with pancreatic cancer is to efficiently determine which patients may benefit from a therapeutic intervention, and which patients are unlikely to receive either significant palliation or chance of cure from a potentially morbid therapy.

It is useful to categorize pancreatic cancer patients into three broad groups: first, the fortunate 10–20% with resectable tumors; second, the small group with locally advanced disease whose survival can be lengthened by radiotherapy *(4)*; and third, patients who have metastatic disease upon presentation and who comprise the largest group. Historically, surgeons have justified the morbidity of a laparotomy in patients with pancreatic cancer as the only avenue to a potentially curative resection or as the "best" palliation of jaundice. Because of the excellent results with modern large-bore biliary endoprostheses, it is hard to justify palliative surgical biliary bypass, which has a 19% mortality rate, with an average survival of 5.4 mo postoperatively *(1)*. Advances in preoperative imaging, diagnostic laparoscopy, and laparoscopic ultrasound can identify nearly all patients with locally advanced and metastatic disease. Thus, surgery with palliative intent is only necessary for those patients with duodenal obstruction. Conversely, surgery with curative intent, i.e., pancreaticoduodenectomy, can be undertaken following an appropriate staging evaluation, with resectability rates of 80–95% *(5,6)*.

RATIONALE FOR LAPAROSCOPY
IN STAGING PANCREATIC CANCER

Pancreatic cancer tends to spread to the peritoneum and liver more than any other gastrointestinal tumor, but the primary tumor is relatively small. These metastatic im-

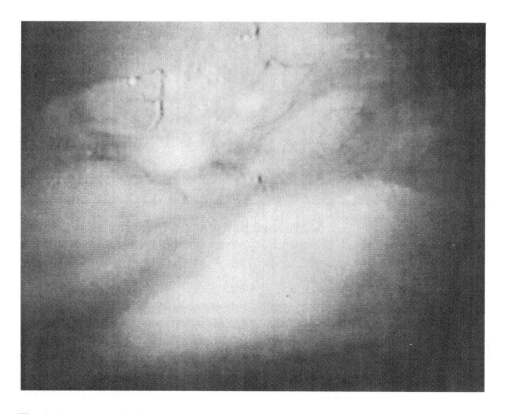

Fig. 1. Laparoscopic view of a small peritoneal implant, which is typical of pancreatic cancer. This patient had an apparently resectable 2-cm tumor of the head of the pancreas visualized on CT scan, with no apparent liver or peritoneal metastases.

plants are often too small to be detected by CT scans and other preoperative imaging modalities (Fig. 1). Prior to the use of laparoscopy at The Massachusetts General Hospital, only 23% of patients undergoing attempted therapeutic laparotomy proved to be resectable, and metastatic disease was frequently found. In 1985, Warshaw found such implants in 14/40 patients with negative preoperative metastatic evaluations *(7)*. Furthermore, 88% of patients with negative findings at laparoscopy went on to have definitive therapy (i.e., resection or intraoperative radiotherapy) at the time of laparotomy. In 1988, Cuschieri validated Warshaw's findings *(8)*. Of 73 patients with pancreatic cancer, 51 patients were thought suitable for laparotomy after an initial staging evaluation (which did not include CT scanning). These 51 patients then underwent laparoscopy in which 42/51 (82%) had findings of metastatic disease, rendering them unresectable. Laparoscopy correctly identified 42 of 43 patients with metastatic disease. The remaining eight patients went on to receive definitive therapy. In 1991, a study by Brady et al. *(9)* examined 25 patients with suspected hepatic and peritoneal malignancy that was not demonstrable on CT scans. Forty-eight percent of these patients were found to have metastatic disease at laparoscopy, usually consisting of minute peritoneal implants.

Warshaw and Gu *(6)* reported further experience with laparoscopy in 1990, with a cohort of 88 patients whose diagnostic workup included CT, MRI, laparoscopy, and

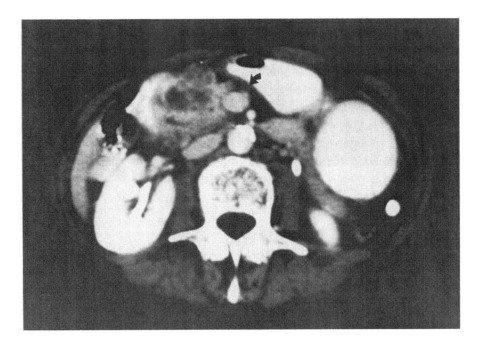

Fig. 2. Abdominal CT scan demonstrating a large, but potentially resectable, pancreatic cancer. Note that the superior mesenteric vein appears to be free of the tumor (arrow). When laparoscopy was performed, multiple peritoneal nodules (1–5 mm) were identified and confirmed by biopsy to be metastatic adenocarcinoma. This patient was treated with an endoscopically placed biliary stent.

angiography. Among 47 patients felt to be resectable on the basis of preoperative imaging studies, 23 patients were found to have metastatic disease, of which 22 were diagnosed laparoscopically. Even in retrospect, dynamic CT was able to identify only 2 out of 23 cases of metastatic disease found at laparoscopy, and MRI held similar results. This study demonstrated the limitations of CT to identify metastases of <1 cm in the liver or peritoneum, compared to laparoscopy, which was able to identify small metastases in 22 out of 23 cases, for a 96% detection rate. A follow-up study by Fernandez et al. *(10)* in 1995 concurred with earlier results, with laparoscopic specificity of 100% and sensitivity of 93%. With their staging protocol, Warshaw and colleagues were able to improve the resectability rate of patients from 23 to 78%. This does not indicate more aggressive surgery, but instead indicates the elimination in advance of most patients with tumors that are unresectable.

Some groups claim that accurate staging of pancreatic cancer can be obtained with thin-section dynamic CT scanning alone. Freeny et al. *(11)* report the accuracy of CT in predicting resectability is 72% (which is substantially greater than the figure of 45% for CT without angiography reported by Warshaw), and, for predicting unresectability, 100%. Furthermore, they report that among those patients found to have unresectable disease diagnosed primarily at laparotomy, none were excluded from surgery on the basis of small liver or peritoneal metastasis *(11)*. This experience has not been duplicated in the authors' practice (Fig. 2).

Recently, Conlon et al. *(5)* have elevated the use of laparoscopy to be the key modality for determining resectability in patients whose CT scans show no evidence of metastatic disease. In contrast to the technique used by previous authors, Conlon et al. used a multiport technique, with more extensive exposure and dissection around the pancreas, lesser sac, and superior mesenteric vein. This allowed not only detection of metastatic disease, but also determination of portal vein and other vascular involvement. With this technique, they reported a diagnostic accuracy of 91%. Only 67/115 patients undergoing laparoscopy were felt to be resectable, and continued to laparotomy. Of these 67 patients, six patients had disease that had been understaged laparoscopically (five patients had hepatic metastases and one patient had portal vein involvement not found at laparoscopy). Thus, a correct assessment of resectability was made in 61/67 (91%) patients.

CYTOLOGY

A number of studies have examined the value of peritoneal cytology obtained by saline lavage at the time of laparoscopy *(10,12–14)*. Occasionally, malignant cells may be found in the peritoneum in the absence of visible metastases. Although such cells are more commonly found in patients with gross metastatic disease, their presence in the absence of visible metastases is an ominous prognostic indicator, and serves to emphasize the point that pancreatic cancer sheds malignant cells into the peritoneal cavity early and commonly. Negative cytology, on the other hand, does not necessarily predict a good prognosis.

Among 16 patients at Massachusetts General Hospital (over the past 10 yr) with positive peritoneal cytology in the absence of visible metastatic tumor, who appeared to be resectable on the basis of imaging and laparoscopic findings, none could ultimately be resected with clear margins *(10,12)*. This experience has been confirmed by Lei, who reported in 1994 *(13)* that 100% of patients with positive cytology were unresectable and survival at 6 mo was 0%. The M. D. Anderson experience also found that positive peritoneal cytology occurred rarely (5% of patients), and, although one of four patients with malignant cells in the peritoneal lavage underwent resection, that patient developed metastases within 8 mo of surgery *(14)*. Thus, cytologic examination of peritoneal washings provides only a small amount of additional information regarding prognosis or resectability. Most patients with positive cytology already have intraabdominal metastases evident at the time of laparoscopy, and nearly a third have extrapancreatic vascular invasion *(12)*.

TECHNIQUE

The method originally popularized by Warshaw *(7)* consists of a systematic inspection of the pelvis, abdomen, and diaphragmatic and peritoneal surfaces via two ports. All procedures are performed under general anesthesia, usually on an outpatient basis. After establishing a pneumoperitoneum, the laparoscope is introduced into the peritoneal cavity through an infraumbilical port. A second trocar is then placed in the right upper quadrant. Five hundred cc saline are instilled into the peritoneal cavity, and the patients placed sequentially in Trendelenburg position, reverse Trendelenburg position, and rotated to both the right and left. The irrigant is then aspirated for cytologic analysis. Using an irrigator, probe, or blunt grasper, all surfaces of the liver are carefully inspected and palpated with the instrument. The diaphragmatic surfaces and upper abdominal viscera are then examined. It is important to elevate the transverse colon, thus exposing the root of the mesentery, because the presence of tumor or implants in this location is a sign of unresectability. Finally, the patient is placed in steep Trendelenburg and the bowel swept out of the pelvis, so that the pelvic recesses of the peritoneal cavity, a common site of early peritoneal seeding, can be visualized. The retrogastric space is not routinely examined. All suspicious metastatic lesions are biopsied under direct vision, using biopsy forceps. Liver lesions can also be biopsied with a true-cut needle placed percutaneously and guided into the suspicious lesion via laparoscopic visualization. If the examination is negative, the port sites are closed and the remainder of the staging work-up is completed as described in the next section.

Conlon et al. *(5)* have expanded the procedure to include evaluation of the lesser sac and retrogastric space, as well as evaluation of the portal and superior mesenteric vein. Conlon's technique uses a four-port approach, as well as a 30° laparoscope. The patient is placed in Trendelenburg position with 10° of left lateral tilt, so that the left lateral segment of the liver and the right lower lobe of the liver, including its anterior and lateral surfaces, can be examined, as well as the hilus and foramen of Winslow. The degree of Trendelenburg is then decreased and lateral tilt reversed for identification of the ligament of Treitz and inspection of the mesocolon and mesocolic vein. Next, the gastrohepatic omentum is incised to examine the caudate lobe of the liver, the vena cava, and the celiac axis. Inspection of the lesser sac also includes sampling of celiac, portal, and perigastric lymph nodes. Of the 115 patients in the original report, 108 (94%) had complete laparoscopic examination.

ADDED VALUE OF LAPAROSCOPIC ULTRASOUND

The added value of laparoscopic ultrasound (LUS) is primarily in its ability to diagnose portal vessel involvement and deep hepatic metastasis, which can be missed by routine laparoscopy *(15)*. In 1993, Murugiah et al. *(16)* were able to demonstrate that LUS could improve the diagnostic accuracy of laparoscopy alone. In their series, two of 12 patients with suspected pancreatic malignancy, and a negative preoperative evaluation, had lesions detected by LUS that were not visible by routine laparoscopy. More recently, Hann et al. *(17)* have used LUS to assess portal vein involvement in cases in which equivocal vascular involvement was seen on CT scans. In a series of 24 patients, peripancreatic vasculature was visualized in 22 patients, and encasement identified in 12/22. In the authors' experience, most cases of vascular involvement have been apparent from either CT scans or preoperative arteriograms. Unfortunately, a normal appearance of the portal vein on LUS has not always guaranteed resectability, because the superior mesenteric vein may be involved by disease in the uncinate process, which is more difficult to evaluate.

A variety of LUS probes are commercially available. Straight probes are easier to work with initially, because orientation of the ultrasound beam is perpendicular to the probe, and therefore less confusing to the surgeon. Flexible tip probes, however, allow better visualization of the liver. When a liver lesion is identified, it may be difficult to biopsy, since the biopsy needle must be in the plane of the ultrasound scan. Newer probes, which combine a transducer with a biopsy needle, should help overcome this problem. To visualize the pancreas and peripancreatic vasculature, the probe is placed

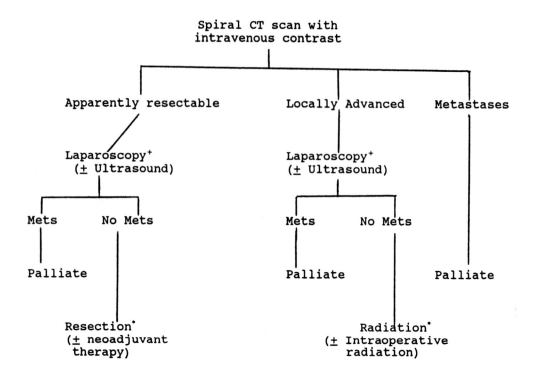

Fig. 3. An algorithm for evaluating patients with pancreatic cancer. Palliation of jaundice is generally accomplished with an endoscopically placed biliary stent. The only role for surgery in palliation is to relieve duodenal obstruction.

through a right-sided port and placed directly on the pancreas. This will often afford a sagittal view of the portal vein. For a complete examination, however, the probe should also be placed through an inferiorly placed port to obtain a coronal view of the veins. Peripancreatic and celiac lymph nodes can also be readily identified with LUS, although caution must be taken in assuming metastatic disease on the basis of size alone, since many patients will have pancreatitis secondary to either obstruction by the tumor or recent endoscopic procedures.

STAGING WORKUP FOR PANCREATIC CANCER

Appropriate use of thin-section, contrast-enhanced CT scans and laparoscopy can streamline evaluation of patients with pancreatic cancer, and optimize resource utilization. For patients who have symptoms suspicious for pancreatic malignancy, the first-line test should be spiral CT with oral and intravenous contrast. This will demonstrate the presence of tumor and the extent of its involvement, including its potential for vascular encasement and metastatic disease. For patients who appear to have localized disease, laparoscopy should be the next procedure, before committing the patient to a laparotomy. A more extensive evaluation of the lesser sac and mesenteric vasculature, as described by Conlon et al. *(5)* is important if one relies on the laparoscopy to determine resectability. If a less extensive evaluation is performed, angiography may identify some patients with vascular involvement unappreciated by CT scan. For patients who are not scheduled to receive preoperative radiotherapy or neoadjuvant protocols, proceeding directly to laparotomy, if laparoscopy is favorable, is appropriate. However, if a course of preoperative radiation is planned, laparoscopy should be planned as a separate outpatient procedure, and performed prior to beginning the course of radiation. Furthermore, collection of peritoneal cytology may provide additional prognostic information. If laparoscopic ultrasonography is available, it is likely to improve the accuracy of staging in experienced hands. By using this sequence of procedures, nontherapeutic laparotomies and unnecessary use of radiation can be prevented (Fig. 3).

REFERENCES

1. Warshaw AL and Fernandez del-Castillo C. Pancreatic carcinoma. N Engl J Med 1992; *326:*455–465.
2. Conlon KC, Klimstra DS, and Brennan MF. Long-term survival after curative resection for pancreatic ductal adenocarcinoma: clinicopathologic analysis of 5 year survivors. Ann Surg 1996; *223:*273–279.
3. Fernandez-del Castillo C, Rattner DW, and Warshaw AL. Standards for pancreatic resection in the 1990s. Arch Surg 1995; *130:*295–300.
4. Moertel CG, Frytak S, Hahn RG, et al. Therapy of locally unresectable pancreatic carcinoma: a randomized comparison of high dose (6000 rads) radiation alone, moderate dose radiation (4000 rads + 5-fluorouracil), and high dose radiation + 5-fluorouracil: The Gastrointestinal Tumor Study Group. Cancer 1981; *48:*1705–1710.
5. Conlon KC, Dougherty E, Klimstra DS, Coit DG, Turnbull ADM, and Brennan MF. The value of minimal access surgery in the staging of patients with potentially resectable peripancreatic malignancy. Ann Surg 1996; *223:*134–140.
6. Warshaw AL, Gu Z, Wittenberg J, and Waltman AC. Preoperative staging and assessment of resectability of pancreatic cancer. Arch Surg 1990; *125:*230–233.
7. Warshaw AL, Tepper JE, and Shipley WU. Laparoscopy in the staging and planning of therapy for pancreatic cancer. Am J Surg 1985; *151:*76–80.
8. Cuschieri A. Laparoscopy for pancreatic cancer: Does it benefit the patient? Eur J Surg Oncol 1988; *14:*41–44.
9. Brady PG, Peebles M, and Goldschmid S. Role of laparoscopy in the evaluation of patients with suspected hepatic and peritoneal malignancy. Gastrointest Endosc 1991; *37:*27–30.
10. Fernandez-del Castillo C, Rattner DW, and Warshaw AL. Further experience with laparoscopy and peritoneal cytology in the staging of pancreatic cancer. Br J Surg 1995; *82:*1127–1129.
11. Freeny PC, Traverso LW, and Ryan JA. Diagnosis and staging of pancreatic adenocarcinoma with dynamic computed tomography. Am J Surg 1993; *165:*600–606.
12. Warshaw AL. Implications of peritoneal cytology for staging of early pancreatic cancer. Am J Surg 191; *161:*26–30.
13. Lei S, Kini J, Kim K, and Howard JM. Pancreatic cancer cytologic study of peritoneal washings. Arch Surg 1994; *129:*639–642.
14. Leach SD, Rose JA, Lowy AM, et al. Significance of peritoneal cytology in patients with potentially resectable adenocarcinoma of the pancreatic head. Surgery 1995; *118:*472–478.

III
Treatment

10

Standard Forms of Pancreatic Resection

Peter W. T. Pisters, Jeffrey E. Lee, and Douglas B. Evans

INTRODUCTION

As experience has increased in surgical referral centers, the published morbidity and mortality rates for pancreaticoduodenectomy have declined. Surgeons have focused on how to perform the operation safely, but less attention has been given to which patients are the most suitable candidates for pancreatectomy, or to such fundamental oncologic issues as the definition and status of microscopic surgical margins, the anatomic distribution of regional lymph node metastases, and patterns of tumor recurrence and their implications for site-specific therapeutic intervention. In contrast to surgery for adenocarcinoma of the esophagus, stomach, or colorectum, pancreaticoduodenectomy requires complete reconstruction of the upper gastrointestinal tract, including reanastomosis of the pancreas, bile duct, and stomach. The magnitude of the operation and its associated morbidity often result in a lengthy period of recovery. For patients who experience early tumor recurrence, quality survival time may be quite brief, because the time of surgical recovery merges with the time of symptomatic tumor recurrence.

Therefore, our current and future challenge is to more clearly define:

1. which patients should undergo major pancreatic resection;
2. the oncologic importance of the extent of regional lymphadenectomy; and
3. the appropriate use of adjuvant therapy to maximize quality survival time.

This chapter will focus on the Western experience with pancreaticoduodenectomy for adenocarcinoma of the pancreatic head, with specific emphasis on the oncologic rationale for the current diagnostic and therapeutic approach to this disease.

ASSESSMENT OF RESECTABILITY

Computed tomography (CT) and laparoscopy are two of the most important contemporary studies used in the staging and assessment of resectability of pancreatic adenocarcinoma.

Computed Tomography

Significant improvements in CT technology over the past decade have enhanced physicians' ability to image the pancreas and retroperitoneum. These include the development of dynamic scanning, in which contrast material is administered intravenously by automatic injector, and helical CT scanning, in which the shorter scan time permits the use of various slice thicknesses (3–5 mm) and pitch factors (1–2) to cover the entire pancreas and liver during the proper phase of contrast enhancement. Helical scanning permits the entire pancreas to be imaged during the bolus phase of intravenous contrast enhancement, when maximal enhancement of the normal pancreatic parenchyma occurs. This approach maximizes the differences in density between the enhancing normal pancreatic parenchyma and the relatively hypodense tumor mass.

When parenchymal lesions are large, the hypodense area is usually apparent during both the bolus and delayed phases of intravenous contrast enhancement. However, when tumors are small, do not change the contour of the pancreas, or are not accompanied by secondary signs (biliary obstruction), they can generally be detected only during the bolus phase of contrast enhancement. It is therefore imperative that CT scans be done during the bolus phase, so that the density difference between the tumor and the pancreatic parenchyma is at its maximum.

These subtle but important aspects of the technical performance of CT, combined with the lack of clear, objective radiographic criteria for resectability, have led to highly variable radiographic resectability rates in the published literature. However, when thin-section CT is performed during the bolus phase of contrast enhancement and the scans are evaluated by experienced physicians, the accuracy of radiographic prediction of resectability exceeds 80% *(1)*. The objective CT criteria for resectability include the absence of extrapancreatic disease, a patent superior mesenteric–portal vein (SMPV) confluence, and no direct tumor extension to the celiac axis or superior mesenteric artery (SMA) (Figs. 1–3). The accuracy of high-quality CT in predicting unresectability is well established *(2,3)*.

When the objective radiographic criteria outlined above were applied to a series of 145 patients referred to The University of Texas M. D. Anderson Cancer Center for presumed or biopsy-proven periampullary cancer, only 42 patients fulfilled these specific criteria for resectability *(1)*. Thirty-seven (88%) of the 42 patients were able to undergo pancreaticoduodenectomy. Only five patients (12%) were found to have unresectable tumors at laparotomy (two patients with locally advanced disease, one patient with a positive regional lymph node, one patient with a 3-mm liver metastasis, and one patient with a tumor implant on the visceral peritoneum of the small bowel mesentery). Final pathologic evaluation of the retroperitoneal margin of resection was used to confirm the accuracy of these specific radiographic criteria in predicting resectability. No patient had a grossly positive margin of resection, and only five (20%) of 25 patients with adenocarcinoma of pancreatic head origin were found to have a microscopic focus of adenocarcinoma at the retroperitoneal margin. This was despite the fact that many patients had undergone a previous nontherapeutic laparotomy prior to referral and nine patients required resection of the superior mesenteric vein (SMV) or the SMPV confluence because of local extension of tumor.

In the absence of extrapancreatic disease, the relationship of the low-density tumor mass to the superior mesenteric artery (SMA) and celiac axis is the main focus of preoperative imaging studies. The goal of both the pancreatic surgeon and the radiologist in assessing resectability is the accurate prediction of the likelihood of obtaining a negative retroperitoneal margin of resection. It is imperative that all clinical studies that

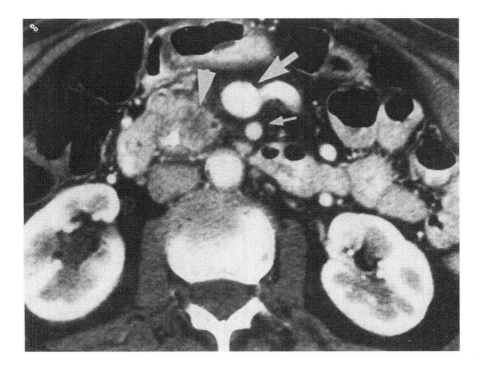

Fig. 1. Contrast-enhanced CT scan demonstrating a resectable adenocarcinoma of the pancreatic head (arrowhead). Note the normal fat plane between the tumor and both the superior mesenteric artery (small arrow) and the superior mesenteric vein (large arrow). The intrapancreatic portion of the common bile duct contains a stent, which was endoscopically placed for biliary drainage.

evaluate the accuracy (sensitivity and specificity) of any preoperative imaging modality in assessing resectability correlate the radiographic findings with the microscopic margins of excision, i.e., the end point for analysis should not be whether the tumor was resected, but whether the tumor was resected with negative surgical margins. The lack of accurate pathologic assessment of pancreaticoduodenectomy specimens (i.e., no assessment or an imprecise definition of the retroperitoneal margin) is of major concern in the interpretation of the large body of literature on staging prior to pancreaticoduodenectomy.

Endoscopic Retrograde Cholangiopancreatography

If a low-density mass is not seen on CT scans, patients with extrahepatic obstructive jaundice undergo diagnostic and therapeutic endoscopy with endoscopic retrograde cholangiopancreatography (ERCP). This allows for direct examination of the ampulla, and when endoscopically identified periampullary lesions are seen, biopsy can be performed. For patients with strictures apparent on ERCP, brushings of the strictures can often be obtained for cytologic diagnosis. To minimize the risk of cholangitis in patients who undergo diagnostic ERCP in the setting of extrahepatic biliary obstruction, endoscopic stents are routinely placed. Endoscopic stent placement should also be per-

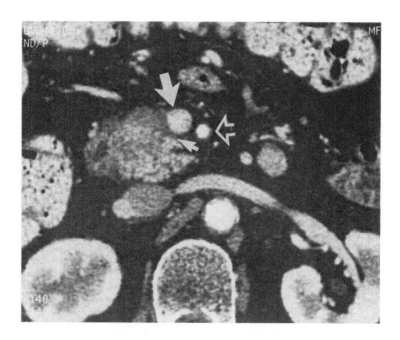

Fig. 2. Contrast-enhanced CT scan demonstrating a resectable adenocarcinoma of the pancreatic head (small arrow), with loss of the normal fat plane between the tumor and the superior mesenteric vein (large arrow). Pancreaticoduodenectomy would commonly require segmental resection of the superior mesenteric vein. Note the normal fat plane between the tumor and the superior mesenteric artery (open arrow).

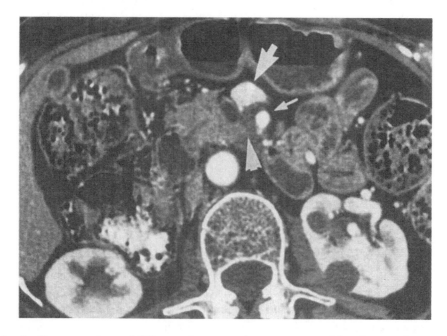

Fig. 3. Contrast-enhanced CT scan demonstrating an unresectable adenocarcinoma of the uncinate process of the pancreas (arrowhead). Note the loss of the normal fat plane between the tumor and the posterior wall of the superior mesenteric vein (large arrow) and the lateral wall of the superior mesenteric artery (small arrow).

formed in patients who present with biliary obstruction and are enrolled in preoperative multimodality-therapy protocols. In the absence of preoperative protocols, endoscopic examination of the periampullary area may not be absolutely necessary in patients who present with extrahepatic biliary obstruction and a low-density mass (in the region of the pancreatic head) on CT, and who meet the above radiographic criteria for resectability.

Staging Laparoscopy

Laparoscopy has been used in patients with radiographic evidence of nonmetastatic pancreatic cancer to detect extrapancreatic tumor not visualized on preoperative CT scans. This approach has been employed to further limit the use of laparotomy to patients with localized disease. Studies by Cuschieri and Fernandez-del-Castillo *(4,5)* have demonstrated the utility of diagnostic laparoscopy in detecting occult liver and peritoneal metastases not visualized on preoperative CT scans. However, both of these studies included patients with radiographic evidence of locally advanced disease that was not amenable to surgical resection. As expected, with the more locally advanced nature of these patients' disease, there was a greater yield of occult positive findings at laparoscopy. In contrast, when laparoscopy was limited to patients who fulfilled strict radiographically defined (high-quality, thin-section CT) criteria for resectability, Fuhrman and colleagues *(1)* could not confirm the diagnostic value of routine preoperative laparoscopy.

The reported utility of laparoscopy in published studies is directly related to the extent of local disease and the point in the diagnostic sequence at which laparoscopy is applied. If diagnostic laparoscopy is performed early in the evaluation of the patient with extrahepatic biliary obstruction (prior to contrast-enhanced helical CT), it will have a higher overall yield of positive findings. For example, a recent study that concluded that laparoscopy and laparoscopic ultrasonography were highly effective in assessing resectability of pancreatic cancers did not employ CT in all patients prior to laparoscopy *(6)*. Moreover, only 19 of 38 (50%) patients with pancreatic cancer had resectable disease at laparotomy, with most of the patients with unresectable disease having locally advanced disease—a finding that is usually evident on high-quality CT scans.

A larger study recently reported from Memorial Sloan-Kettering Cancer Center (MSKCC) involved 115 patients with peripancreatic tumors thought to be resectable based on CT scans *(7)*. All patients underwent a careful laparoscopic examination, including inspection of the lesser sac and biopsy of celiac, portal, or perigastric lymph nodes. Unresectable disease was found in 41 of 108 (38%) evaluable patients at laparoscopy. Sixty-one of the remaining 67 patients (91%) underwent pancreatic resection, although it was not stated whether the margins of resection were positive or negative. Overall, only 53% of the initial 115 patients underwent resection, suggesting that the prelaparoscopic CT scans were of inferior quality; in fact, most scans were obtained prior to referral to MSKCC. Further, laparoscopic evaluation suggested vascular encasement in 14 patients. Assuming the technical ability to safely resect the SMPV confluence, tumor adherence to the SMV or SMPV should not represent a contraindication to resection (even if not discovered until surgery). Tumor invasion of the SMA or proximal celiac axis can be accurately assessed with high-quality CT, but can be seen at surgery only following pancreatic transection; thus, evaluation of arterial invasion or encasement is an unrealistic expectation of laparoscopy. The recent report from MSKCC *(7)*, taken together with the existing body of literature on staging laparoscopy for pancreatic cancer, suggests that if laparoscopy is used only in patients with localized, potentially resectable disease defined by strict objective radiographic criteria, it will have a much lower rate of overall positive findings. This issue is important in the evaluation of the emerging body of literature on staging laparoscopy in pancreatic cancer.

Routine laparoscopy certainly may prevent unnecessary laparotomy in an occasional patient with presumed radiographically localized, potentially resectable pancreatic cancer. However, no data are available with which to evaluate the cost-effectiveness of the routine use of diagnostic laparoscopy in patients who fulfill objective radiographic criteria for resectability, using contemporary imaging techniques. Laparoscopy is certainly favored over laparotomy in patients who have equivocal radiographic findings, such as small hypodense regions in the hepatic parenchyma, which are suspicious for hepatic metastases, but are not amenable to percutaneous biopsy, or who have evidence of ascites or other CT findings suspicious for carcinomatosis. Further studies to evaluate the true incidence of clinically significant positive laparoscopic findings influencing the overall therapeutic management of patients whose tumors meet objective radiographic criteria for resectability will be required to support the routine use of diagnostic laparoscopy in this patient population.

Angiography

The more widespread application of contrast-enhanced, helical CT scanning has eliminated the role for routine preoperative angiography in patients with pancreatic cancer. Angiography does not provide sufficient anatomic detail to define the relationship between the tumor and the superior mesenteric vessels, as is provided by high-quality, contrast-enhanced CT. The major stated justification of routine preoperative angiography is that it allows for identification of mesenteric vessel encasement and aberrant hepatic arterial anatomy, minimizing the risk of iatrogenic injury. However, neoplastic encasement of the superior mesenteric or celiac vessels, which is so extensive that it causes angiographic abnormalities, is always identifiable on high-quality, contrast-enhanced CT. Furthermore, aberrant hepatic arterial anatomy can also frequently be identified on routine axial CT images, or can be appreciated intraoperatively at the time of portal dissection. Angiography should therefore be reserved for selected patients who have undergone previous biliary bypass involving the common bile duct. In such cases, angiography prior to reoperation in the porta hepatis may minimize the risk of iatrogenic injury during the portal dissection, when there is extensive scarring from a previous biliary procedure *(8)*.

EXTENT OF RESECTION

Regional Pancreatectomy vs Standard Pancreaticoduodenectomy

Regional pancreatectomy for adenocarcinoma of the pancreatic head, unlike standard pancreaticoduodenectomy, involves removal of lymphatic tissue to the left of the celiac axis and SMA, with circumferential skeletonization of these vessels. Regional pancreatectomy, as performed in the United States and Japan, assumes that a wider lymphadenectomy will increase rates of long-term patient survival. However, evidence for this is lacking. In oncologic surgery, there are three reasons to remove lymph nodes: staging of disease, local tumor control, and patient cure. In general, lymph node metastases are believed to be a marker of systemic disease, and, for solid tumors, we rarely associate local-regional lymphadenectomy with cure of the disease. Exceptions to this philosophy remain controversial, and are largely limited to diseases such as malignant melanoma, medullary carcinoma of the thyroid, and gastrinoma associated with multiple endocrine neoplasia type 1. Three principal concerns about the use of regional pancreatectomy for adenocarcinoma of the pancreatic head are: the high morbidity and mortality of the procedure *(9–11)*; the long-term complications related to poor gastrointestinal function, which lead to weight loss and chronic debilitation *(12–15)*, and the application of such an extensive local-regional therapy, with its associated sequelae, to a disease with such a dominant site of distant organ metastasis (liver). In patients who survive the operation, skeletonization of both sides of the celiac axis and SMA deinnervates the proximal gastrointestinal tract, resulting in rapid gastrointestinal transit and chronic nutritional depletion. Dissection to the left of the SMA and celiac axis with the intent of removing possible micrometastatic disease within lymph nodes remains of unproven benefit in patients with adenocarcinoma of the pancreatic head.

Criticism of regional pancreatectomy should not be misinterpreted as advocating an inadequate operative procedure to the right of the SMA; there is equal lack of justification for performing an incomplete retroperitoneal dissection at the time of pancreaticoduodenectomy by not removing all tissue to the right of the SMA, or by leaving tumor on the posterior or lateral aspect of the SMV. An adequate pancreaticoduodenectomy requires paracaval soft tissue resection, dissection along the periadventitial plane of the proximal SMA, and may require the use of venous resection in patients with isolated involvement of the SMV or SMPV confluence in the absence of tumor extension to the SMA. Three technical maneuvers of great controversy in the performance of standard pancreaticoduodenectomy (Fig. 4) include the extent of paracaval soft-tissue resection, the scope of the retroperitoneal vascular dissection, and the role of pylorus preservation.

Kocher Maneuver and Paracaval Soft-Tissue Resection

The authors' approach to pancreaticoduodenectomy involves an extended Kocher maneuver, which is not widely performed in the Western surgical community. This maneuver is performed by medial mobilization of the lymphatic tissue overlying the medial aspect of the right renal hilus, to encompass the medial portion of Gerota's fascia, as well as the soft tissues overlying the inferior vena cava and origin of the proximal left renal vein (Fig. 5). The oncologic rationale for this extended Kocher maneuver is based on the high incidence of lymph node positivity in the posterior pancreaticoduodenal region, as first reported in the pathologic studies of Cubilla et al. *(16)* and confirmed in subsequent studies *(17–19)*. This dissection adds little time to the operation, and may decrease the risk of local recurrence within the retroperitoneum, which is a dominant site of tumor recurrence in the absence of multimodality therapy *(1,8,20)*. Clearly, efforts to improve local control are unlikely to result in major improvements

Clockwise Resection

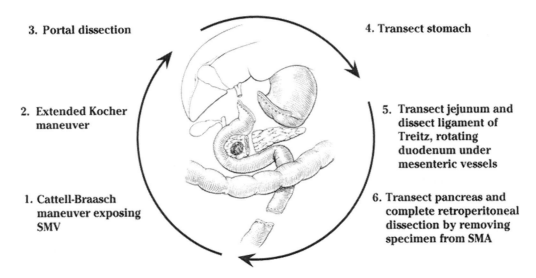

3. Portal dissection

4. Transect stomach

2. Extended Kocher maneuver

5. Transect jejunum and dissect ligament of Treitz, rotating duodenum under mesenteric vessels

1. Cattell-Braasch maneuver exposing SMV

6. Transect pancreas and complete retroperitoneal dissection by removing specimen from SMA

Fig. 4. Six surgical steps of pancreaticoduodenectomy. Used with permission from ref. *8.*

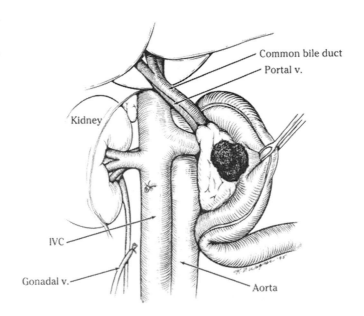

Fig. 5. Illustration of step 2 in the performance of pancreaticoduodenectomy. An extended Kocher maneuver has been performed with division of the gonadal vein. Note the extension of the Kocher maneuver to the left lateral border of the aorta. IVC, inferior vena cava.

in survival duration, but may alter patterns of recurrence and thereby improve the quality of survival for patients with resectable pancreatic cancer.

Many surgeons also use the Kocher maneuver to allow assessment of the relationship of the tumor to the SMA by palpation (Fig. 6). However, this method of assessment of this critical tumor–vessel relationship is imprecise, because the three-dimen-

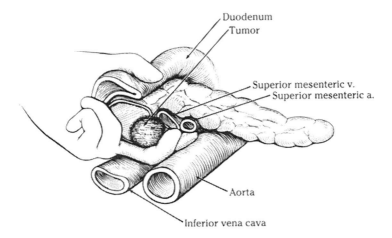

Duodenum
Tumor

Superior mesenteric v.
Superior mesenteric a.

Aorta

Inferior vena cava

Fig. 6. Intraoperative palpation to determine the relationship of the tumor to the mesenteric vessels at the time of the Kocher maneuver. The tumor is palpated with the left hand. The difficulty in assessing the tumor–vessel relationship by palpation emphasizes the critical importance of preoperative high-quality, contrast-enhanced CT scans. Used with permission from ref. *33*.

sional relationship of the tumor to the SMA is extremely difficult to discern by palpation. The dense mesenteric neural plexus surrounding the SMA at this level, and the desmoplastic peritumoral response often associated with a sclerotic adenocarcinoma, make accurate assessment by palpation impossible. Intraoperative assessment of the relationship of the tumor to the SMA, which is often measured only in millimeters, can be performed only by dissection in the periadventitial plane along the SMA. This vascular dissection cannot be performed until after gastric and pancreatic division, at which point the surgeon has already committed to resection. Thus, no form of intraoperative palpation can evaluate the tumor–SMA relationship precisely enough that the surgeon may proceed with gastric and pancreatic transection with reasonable expectation of negative gross and microscopic retroperitoneal margins along the SMA (Fig. 7). Therefore, decision-making regarding local tumor resectability, namely, the relationship of the tumor mass to the superior mesenteric vessels, should be made on the basis of preoperative thin-section, contrast-enhanced CT. If state-of-the-art preoperative imaging is combined with the use of objective radiographic criteria for operation, the incidence of positive-margin resections will be minimized *(17)*.

The oncologic significance of obtaining a negative retroperitoneal margin at the time of pancreaticoduodenectomy cannot be overstated. The median survival among patients undergoing pancreaticoduodenectomy with a positive margin of resection is approx 9 mo (Table 1; *21–26*). Although the overall morbidity and mortality rates for the procedure have declined, the period required to recover near-normal gastrointestinal function is usually a minimum of 4–6 wk in the absence of significant perioperative complications. Given the fact that patients who receive palliative 5-fluorouracil-based chemoradiation without surgery (for more locally advanced disease) have a median survival that is comparable to that of patients who have had resection with positive margins, it is difficult to find objective data to support a policy of palliative resection.

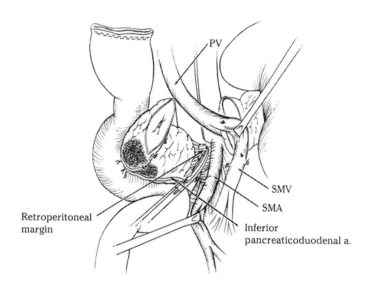

Fig. 7. Illustration of the final step in resection of the specimen. Medial retraction of the superior mesenteric–portal vein confluence facilitates dissection of the soft tissues adjacent to the lateral wall of the proximal SMA. The retroperitoneal margin is defined as the soft-tissue margin directly adjacent to the proximal 3–4-cm of the SMA. This margin is identified by the surgeon immediately upon specimen removal, and evaluated by the surgeon and pathologist (in the adjoining pathology suite) by microscopic examination of a 2–3-mm full-face (en-face) section of the margin. The inferior pancreaticoduodenal artery is identified at its origin from the SMA, ligated, and divided. PV, portal vein; SMV, superior mesenteric vein. Used with permission from ref. *1*.

Retroperitoneal Vascular Dissection

The retroperitoneal dissection along the SMPV confluence and SMA represents the most important technical step when performing pancreaticoduodenectomy. This is because of the tendency of pancreatic adenocarcinoma to extend into the extrapancreatic retroperitoneal soft tissues and nerve sheaths adjacent to the right side of the SMA. In addition, larger, more medially located lesions within the head of the gland will often be inseparable from or pathologically invading the SMPV confluence. The pancreatic surgeon should have a clear understanding of the oncologic significance of the periarterial dissection and should have a technical strategy for dealing with tumor adherence to the SMV or SMPV confluence.

Tumor involvement of the SMV and SMPV confluence is considered by most Western surgeons to be a contraindication to pancreaticoduodenectomy. However, reports of venous resection at the time of pancreaticoduodenectomy often involve patients with arterial involvement suggesting retroperitoneal tumor extension that could not be completely resected *(27,28)*. In contrast, isolated involvement of the SMPV confluence without radiographically evident involvement of the SMA can be managed intraoperatively with resection of the involved segment of vein and vascular reconstruction. Detailed evaluation of patients requiring venous resection and reconstruction reveals a long-term outcome that is comparable to that of similarly staged patients not requiring vascular

Table 1
Median Survival for Patients Who Underwent Surgical
Resection for Adenocarcinoma of the Pancreas and Were
Found to Have a Positive Margin of Resection

Ref. (year)	*N*	Margin	Median survival (mo)
Tepper *(21)* (1976)	17[a]	G/M	8
Trede *(22)* (1990)	54	G/M	10
Whittington *(23)* (1991)	19	G	[b]
Willett *(24)* (1993)	37	G/M	11
Nitecki *(25)* (1995)	28	G	9
Yeo *(26)* (1995)	58	G/M	10

G, grossly positive margin; M, microscopically positive margin.
[a] All patients also had positive regional lymph nodes.
[b] Two patients alive at 18 mo of follow-up.
(Adapted with permission from ref. *17*.)

resection *(29,30)*. Thus, isolated involvement of the SMPV confluence is an anatomic issue that requires a technical strategy, but does not represent an adverse prognostic factor precluding potentially curative resection. This is in contrast to neoplastic extension to the wall of the SMA (Fig. 3). Patients with tumor extension to the SMA are unable to undergo resection with a negative retroperitoneal margin. This fundamental distinction between tumor involvement of the SMV or SMPV confluence and involvement of the SMA is critical. Attempted resection of locally advanced tumors that extend to the SMA will result in a positive margin of resection; such patients have a short survival, whether operated upon in the West (Table 1) or in Japan *(14,31)*.

Tumor adherence to the SMV or SMPV confluence is usually suspected preoperatively from contrast-enhanced helical CT scans *(32)*. Intraoperatively, following pancreatic transection, the tumor is found to be inseparable from the lateral wall of the SMV or SMPV confluence, which prevents dissection of the confluence from the adjacent pancreatic head and uncinate process. This, in turn, prevents medial mobilization of the SMPV confluence, which is necessary to expose the SMA to allow dissection of the specimen from the right lateral wall of this artery (final step in tumor resection). This can be managed by division of the splenic vein and exposure of the SMA medial to the SMPV confluence. Dividing the splenic vein also provides sufficient mobility and adequate length of uninvolved vein for a tension-free primary anastomosis between the SMV and portal vein after segmental venous resection (Fig. 8). It may be optimal, however, to preserve splenic (and inferior mesenteric) venous return where possible, to minimize the risk of postoperative sinistral portal hypertension after splenic vein ligation. If the SMPV confluence is preserved, it is difficult to mobilize a satisfactory length of vein to facilitate a tension-free primary anastomosis, unless the segment of resected vein is limited to <2 cm (Fig. 9). Consequently, if the SMPV confluence is preserved, interposition grafting is required. An internal jugular vein interposition graft provides a

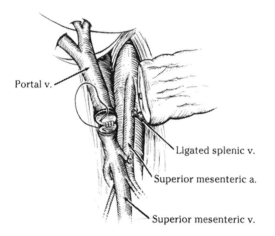

Fig. 8. Illustration of the final step in pancreaticoduodenectomy when segmental venous resection is required. In preparation for segmental resection of the superior mesenteric vein, the splenic vein has been divided and the superior mesenteric artery identified. The retroperitoneal dissection is completed by dissecting the specimen free from the lateral wall of the artery. The tumor is then attached only by the superior mesenteric–portal venous confluence, which is excised with the specimen. Reconstruction is performed with an end-to-end anastomosis of the portal vein and the superior mesenteric vein. Used with permission from ref. *33*.

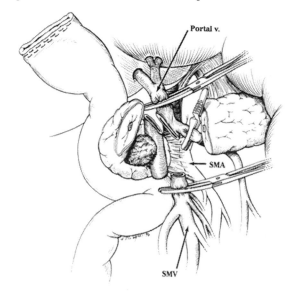

Fig. 9. Illustration of the final step in pancreaticoduodenectomy when segmental venous resection is performed with splenic vein preservation. The SMA is clamped to provide inflow occlusion prior to venous resection and reconstruction. SMV, superior mesenteric vein.

convenient, readily accessible, and appropriately sized graft for the SMV and portal vein (Fig. 10). The technique for this has been outlined in detail elsewhere. *(32,33).*

The dissection along the SMA is of critical oncologic significance for the reasons outlined above. Two specific issues warrant comment. First, this dissection should occur in the immediate periadventitial plane along the SMA. The SMA is readily identi-

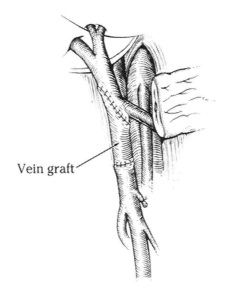

Vein graft

Fig. 10. Illustration of the authors' preferred method of reconstruction of the superior mesenteric–portal vein confluence using an internal jugular vein interposition graft (vein graft).

fiable within a 3–4-mm dense sheath of neural tissue located deep and medial to the SMV. The periadventitial plane is identified and dissection proceeds cephalad along the right anterolateral surface of the SMA, separating the perivascular soft tissues from the artery. This ensures the maximal retroperitoneal margin and also minimizes the risk of iatrogenic vascular injury. This latter point is particularly important, because iatrogenic injury to the SMA, or major bleeding from the friable superior and inferior pancreaticoduodenal branches, can occur if dissection occurs through an imprecise plane in the lateral soft tissues to the right of the SMA. Second, the SMA may be injured once the specimen is completely freed from the SMV/portal vein and lateral traction is applied to the specimen; at this point in the dissection, the SMA is often pulled or bowed out to the right, where it is vulnerable to injury unless dissection proceeds under direct vision of the artery (Fig. 11).

Pylorus Preservation

Preservation of the antral pyloroduodenal segment, in combination with pancreaticoduodenectomy, was first described by Traverso and Longmire in 1978 *(34)*. Since then, increasing numbers of pancreatic surgeons have employed this modification of the procedure, particularly for patients with benign disease or small periampullary lesions. Proponents of the technique argue that preservation of the antral pyloric pump mechanism results in improved long-term upper gastrointestinal function, with associated salutary nutritional sequela *(26,35,36)*. Physiologic studies demonstrate that pylorus preservation decreases intestinal transit time, lessens diarrhea (steatorrhea), normalizes glucose metabolism, and improves postoperative weight gain *(37,38)*. Critics of this modification counter that the reported improvements in gastrointestinal nutritional function are small, if any, and that they come at the expense of an increased in-

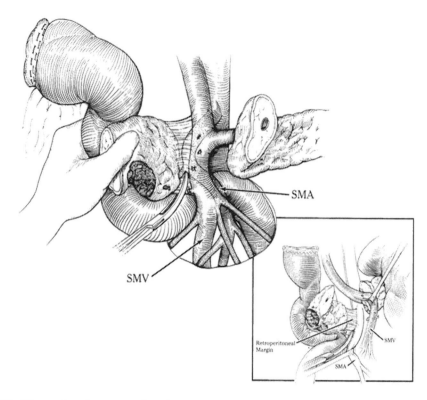

Fig. 11. Illustration demonstrating the potential for arterial injury during the final step in pancreaticoduodenectomy, if the retroperitoneal dissection is performed without direct visualization of the lateral wall of the SMA. Lateral traction on the specimen can cause lateral displacement of the proximal SMA, making arterial injury possible. In contrast (*see* insert), complete medial mobilization of the superior mesenteric–portal vein confluence and direct visualization of the SMA will avoid iatrogenic arterial injury and allow the performance of a more complete retroperitoneal dissection. SMV, superior mesenteric vein.

cidence of delayed gastric emptying in the early postoperative period. Moreover, leaving a distal segment of stomach and duodenum may compromise the margin of excision and prevent adequate peripyloric lymphadenectomy, thereby compromising any survival benefit of the operation. Published data to date involve retrospective comparisons that have yielded mixed results (*39–41*). Most pancreatic surgeons agree that pylorus preservation should not be performed for patients with bulky tumors of the pancreatic head, duodenal tumors involving the first or second portions of the duodenum, or lesions with grossly positive pyloric or peripyloric lymph nodes.

The technique for pylorus-preserving pancreaticoduodenectomy is identical to that for standard pancreaticoduodenectomy, except in the approach to the antrum, pylorus, and duodenum. Pylorus preservation involves not only proximal division of the gastrointestinal tract beyond the pylorus, but, more important, preservation of sufficient blood supply to the proximal duodenum, and preservation of vagal innervation to the antrum and pylorus. Therefore, caution must be exercised in the portal dissection to

Table 2
Survival of Patients with Pancreatic Adenocarcinoma Who Underwent Pancreaticoduodenectomy (Western Experience)

Ref. (year)	No.	Follow-up (mo)	Median survival (mo)	Estimated 5-yr survival (%)
Trede *(22)* (1990)	133	–	–	24
Cameron *(42)* (1991)	81	–	12.7	21
Whittington *(23)* (1991)	72	–	15–16	–
Roder *(39)* (1992)	53	24	12	6
Bakkevold *(43)* (1993)	83	–	11.4	–
Geer *(44)* (1993)	146	28	18	24
Willett *(24)* (1993)	72	11	–	13
Tsao *(35)* (1994)	27	30	18	6.6
Zerbi *(45)* (1994)	90	16	12/19[a]	–
Allema *(46)* (1995)	67	–	–	15
Yeo *(26)* (1995)	201	12	15.5	21
Nitecki *(25)* (1995)	174	22[b]	17.5	6.8
Staley *(17)* (1996)	39	19	19	19

[a] Received adjuvant intraoperative radiation therapy.
[b] Mean.

avoid unnecessary division of the right gastric artery or injury to the nerves of Laterget. This fundamental technical difference in the pylorus-preserving procedure is essential to facilitate a well-vascularized duodenal anastomosis, and to avoid postoperative gastroparesis.

RESULTS OF WESTERN EXPERIENCE WITH PANCREATICODUODENECTOMY

Table 2 *(17,22–26,35,39,42–46)* outlines the long-term results of recent large series of patients undergoing pancreaticoduodenectomy for pancreatic adenocarcinoma. The median survival ranges consistently between 13 and 19 mo, with 5-yr actuarial survival rates of approx 20%. Postoperative adjuvant chemoradiation has been shown to improve survival rates over pancreaticoduodenectomy alone (Table 3; *26,47–49*). Foo and colleagues *(49)* have reported a very favorable median survival of 23 mo for selected patients who received chemoradiation following pancreatectomy and Yeo and colleagues *(30)* reported a median survival of 20 mo in 56 patients treated with combined-modality therapy, compared to 12 mo in a concurrent nonrandomized cohort of 22 patients treated with pancreaticoduodenectomy alone. However, postoperative adjuvant therapy studies are prone to selection bias, since patients usually offered protocol-based therapy are those with more favorable performance status, who recovered rapidly from uncomplicated surgery. Recent data suggest that perioperative complications or slow postoperative recovery may prevent at least 25% of patients from receiving planned postoperative adjuvant therapy *(51)*.

Table 3
Recent Chemoradiation Studies in Patients with Resectable Pancreatic Cancer

Ref. (year)	No. patients[a]	EBRT dose (Gy)	Chemotherapy agent(s)	Median survival (mo)
Postoperative (adjuvant)				
Kalser *(47)* (1985)	21	40	5-FU	20
Surgery alone	22	–	–	11
GITSG *(48)* (1987)	30	40	5-FU	18
Whittington *(43)* (1991)	28	45–63	5-FU, Mito-C	16
Foo *(49)* (1993)	29	35–60	5-FU	23
Yeo *(26)* (1995)	56	>45	5-FU	20
Surgery alone	22	–	–	12
Preoperative (neoadjuvant)				
Hoffman *(51)* (1995)	23	50.4	5-FU, Mito-C	17
Staley *(17)* (1996)	39	30–50.4	5-FU	19

EBRT, external-beam radiation therapy; 5-FU, 5-fluorouracil; mito, mitomycin C.
All patients underwent a pancreatectomy with curative intent.

Chemoradiation, when given prior to pancreaticoduodenectomy, has been shown to alter patterns of treatment failure compared to surgery alone or other multimodality treatment regimens *(17)*. Staley and colleagues *(52)* recently reported on a cohort of 39 patients treated with preoperative 5-fluorouracil-based chemoradiation, followed by pancreaticoduodenectomy and intraoperative electron-beam radiation therapy. Twenty-nine of the 39 patients (74%) developed recurrence. In contrast to historical data, the majority of recurrences were in distant sites. The liver was the most frequent site of recurrence, with liver metastases constituting a component of initial treatment failure in 53% of patients (69% of all patients who had recurrences). Isolated local or peritoneal recurrences occurred in only four (10%) patients. Despite this major improvement in local-regional tumor control, the overall gain in median survival was modest (Table 2), because liver metastases were such a dominant site of recurrent disease. These data suggest that major improvements in long-term survival for patients who have pancreatic adenocarcinoma will require development of more effective systemic therapy. Therefore, future local-regional treatment strategies should strive to minimize the toxicity, treatment time, and cost of chemoradiation and surgery, while maintaining therapeutic efficacy.

The inability of surgeons to objectively define resectability preoperatively (with non-invasive imaging studies), standardize surgical technique, and prospectively assess pathologic margins of resection are largely responsible for the small amount of data that exists on the use of multimodality therapy for this disease. Variability in patient selection, operative technique, and specimen analysis make questions regarding adjuvant therapy impossible to answer. The future development of multi-institution phase III trials will depend on our ability to standardize these critical variables in the surgical management of patients with pancreatic cancer.

REFERENCES

1. Fuhrman GM, Charnsangavej C, Abbruzzese JL, Cleary KR, Martin RG, Fenoglio CJ, et al. Thin-section contrast-enhanced computed tomography accurately predicts the resectability of malignant pancreatic neoplasms. Am J Surg 1994; *167:*104–111.

2. Freeny PC, Traverso LW, and Ryan JA. Diagnosis and staging of pancreatic adenocarcinoma with dynamic computed tomography. Am J Surg 1993; *165:*600–606.

3. Warshaw AL, Gu ZY, Wittenberg J, and Waltman AC. Preoperative staging and assessment of resectability of pancreatic cancer. Arch Surg 1990; *125:*230–233.

4. Fernandez-del-Castillo C, Rattner DW, and Warshaw AL. Further experience with laparoscopy and peritoneal cytology in the staging of pancreatic cancer. Br J Surg 1995; *82:*1127–1129.

5. Cuschieri A. Laparoscopy for pancreatic cancer: does it benefit the patient? Eur J Surg Oncol 1988; *14:*41–44.

6. Bemelman WA, de Wit LT, van Delden OM, Smits NJ, Obertop H, Rauws EJ, et al. Diagnostic laparoscopy combined with laparoscopic ultrasonography in staging of cancer of the pancreatic head region. Br J Surg 1995; *82:*820–824.

7. Conlon KC, Dougherty E, Klimstra DS, Coit DG, Turnbull AD, and Brennan MF. The value of minimal access surgery in the staging of patients with potentially resectable peripancreatic malignancy. Ann Surg 1996; *223:*134–140.

8. Tyler DS and Evans DB. Reoperative pancreaticoduodenectomy. Ann Surg 1994; *219:*211–221.

9. Fortner JG, Kim DK, Cubilla A, Turnbull A, Pahnke LD, and Shils ME. Regional pancreatectomy: en bloc pancreatic, portal vein and lymph node resection. Ann Surg 1977; *186:*42–50.

10. Nagakawa T, Konishi I, Ueno K, Ohta T, Akiyama T, Kayahara M, et al. Surgical treatment of pancreatic cancer. The Japanese experience. Int J Pancreatol 1991; *9:*135–143.

11. Sindelar WF. Clinical experience with regional pancreatectomy for adenocarcinoma of the pancreas. Arch Surg 1989; *124:*127–132.

12. Dresler CM, Fortner JG, McDermott K, and Bajorunas DR. Metabolic consequences of (regional) total pancreatectomy. Ann Surg 1991; *214:*131–140.

13. Hiraoka T. Extended radical resection of cancer of the pancreas with intraoperative radiotherapy. Baillieres Clin Gastroenterol 1990; *4:*985–993.

14. Nagakawa T, Konishi I, Ueno K, Ohta T, Akiyama T, Kanno M, et al. The results and problems of extensive radical surgery for carcinoma of the head of the pancreas. Jpn J Surg 1991; *21:*262–267.

15. Nagakawa T, Kurachi M, Konishi K, and Miyazaki I. Translateral retroperitoneal approach in radical surgery for pancreatic carcinoma. Jpn J Surg 1982; *12:*229–233.

16. Cubilla AL, Fortner J, and Fitzgerald PJ. Lymph node involvement in carcinoma of the head of the pancreas area. Cancer 1978; *41:*880–887.

17. Staley CA, Lee JE, Cleary KR, Abbruzzese JL, Fenoglio CJ, Rich TA, et al. Preoperative chemoradiation, pancreaticoduodenectomy, and intraoperative radiation therapy for adenocarcinoma of the pancreatic head. Am J Surg 1996; *171:*118–124.

18. Kayahara M, Nagakawa T, Kobayashi H, Mori K, Nakano T, Kadoya N, et al. Lymphatic flow in carcinoma of the head of the pancreas. Cancer 1992; *70:*2061–2066.

19. Nagakawa T, Kobayashi H, Ueno K, Ohta T, Kayahara M, and Miyazaki I. Clinical study of lymphatic flow to the paraaortic lymph nodes in carcinoma of the head of the pancreas. Cancer 1994; *73:*1155–1162.

20. Evans DB, Lee JE, Pisters PWT. Pancreaticoduodenectomy (Whipple Operation) and total pancreatectomy for cancer. In: Nyhus LM, Baker RJ and Fischer JF (eds), Mastery of surgery, Little Brown, Boston, MA, 1997; pp. 1233–1249.

21. Tepper J, Nardi G, and Sutt H. Carcinoma of the pancreas: review of MGH experience from 1963 to 1973. Analysis of surgical failure and implications for radiation therapy. Cancer 1976; *37:*1519–1524.

22. Trede M, Schwall G, and Saeger HD. Survival after pancreatoduodenectomy. 118 consecutive resections without an operative mortality. Ann Surg 1990; *211:*447–458.

23. Whittington R, Bryer MP, Haller DG, Solin LJ, and Rosato EF. Adjuvant therapy of resected adenocarcinoma of the pancreas. Int J Radiat Oncol Biol Phys 1991; *21:*1137–1143.

24. Willett CG, Lewandrowski K, Warshaw AL, Efird J, and Compton CC. Resection margins in carcinoma of the head of the pancreas. Implications for radiation therapy. Ann Surg 1993; *217:*144–148.

25. Nitecki SS, Sarr MG, Colby TV, and van Heerden JA. Long-term survival after resection for ductal adenocarcinoma of the pancreas. Is it really improving? Ann Surg 1995; *221:*59–66.

26. Yeo CJ, Cameron JL, Lillemoe KD, Sitzmann JV, Hruban RH, Goodman SN, et al. Pancreaticoduodenectomy for cancer of the head of the pancreas. 201 patients. Ann Surg 1995; *221:*721–731.

27. Allema JH, Reinders ME, van Gulik TM, Van Leeuwen DJ, de Wit LT, Verbeek PC, et al. Portal vein resection in patients undergoing pancreatoduodenectomy for carcinoma of the pancreatic head. Br J Surg 1994; *81:*1642–1646.

28. Roder JD, Stein HJ, and Siewert JR. Carcinoma of the periampullary region: who benefits from portal vein resection? Am J Surg 1996; *171:*170–175.

29. Harrison LE, Klimstra DS, and Brennan MF. Isolated portal vein involvement in pancreatic adenocarcinoma. A contraindication to resection? Ann Surg 1996; *224:*342–349.

30. Leach SD, Lee JE, Charnsangavej C, Cleary KR, Lowy AM, Fenoglio CJ, Pisters PWT, and Evans DB. Patient survival following pancreaticoduodenectomy with resection of the superior mesenteric-portal vein confluence adenocarcinoma of the pancreatic head. Br J Surg, in press.

31. Takahashi S, Ogata Y, and Tsuzuki T. Combined resection of the pancreas and portal vein for pancreatic cancer. Br J Surg 1994; *81:*1190–1193.

32. Fuhrman GM, Leach SD, Staley CA, Cusack JC, Charnsangavej C, Cleary KR, et al. Rationale for en bloc vein resection in the treatment of pancreatic adenocarcinoma adherent to the superior mesenteric–portal vein confluence. Ann Surg 1996; *223:*154–162.

33. Cusack JC, Jr., Fuhrman GM, Lee JE, and Evans DB. Managing unsuspected tumor invasion of the superior mesenteric–portal venous confluence during pancreaticoduodenectomy. Am J Surg 1994; *168:*352–354.

34. Traverso LW and Longmire WP, Jr. Preservation of the pylorus in pancreaticoduodenectomy. Surg Gynecol Obstet 1978; *146:*959–962.

35. Tsao JI, Rossi RL, and Lowell JA. Pylorus-preserving pancreaticoduodenectomy. Is it an adequate cancer operation? Arch Surg 1994; *129:*405–412.

36. Grace PA, Pitt HA, and Longmire WP. Pylorus preserving pancreaticoduodenectomy: an overview. Br J Surg 1990; *77:*968–974.

37. Crucitti F, Doglietto G, Bellantone R, Miggiano GA, Frontera D, Ferrante AM, et al. Digestive and nutritional consequences of pancreatic resections. The classical vs the pylorus-sparing procedure. Int J Pancreatol 1995; *17:*37–45.

38. Kozuschek W, Reith HB, Waleczek H, Haarmann W, Edelmann M, and Sonntag D. A comparison of long term results of the standard whipple procedure and the pylorus preserving pancreaticoduodenectomy. J Am Coll Surg 1994; *178:*443–453.

39. Roder JD, Stein HJ, Huttl W, and Siewert JR. Pylorus-preserving versus standard pancreaticoduodenectomy: an analysis of 110 pancreatic and periampullary carcinomas. Br J Surg 1992; *79:*152–155.

40. Sharp KW, Ross CB, Halter SA, Morrison JG, Richards WO, Williams LF, et al. Pancreatoduodenectomy with pyloric preservation for carcinoma of the pancreas: a cautionary note. Surgery 1989; *105*:645–653.

41. Patel AG, Toyama MT, Kusske AM, Alexander P, Ashley SW, and Reber HA. Pylorus-preserving Whipple resection for pancreatic cancer. Is it any better? Arch Surg 1995; *130*:838–842.

42. Cameron JL, Crist DW, Sitzmann JV, Hruban RH, Boitnott JK, Seidler AJ, et al. Factors influencing survival after pancreaticoduodenectomy for pancreatic cancer. Am J Surg 1991; *161*:120–124.

43. Bakkevold KE and Kambestad B. Long-term survival following radical and palliative treatment of patients with carcinoma of the pancreas and papilla of Vater—the prognostic factors influencing the long-term results. A prospective multicentre study. Eur J Surg Oncol 1993; *19*:147–161.

44. Geer RJ, and Brennan MF. Prognostic indicators for survival after resection of pancreatic adenocarcinoma. Am J Surg 1993; *165*:68–72.

45. Zerbi A, Fossati V, Parolini D, Carlucci M, Balzano G, Bordogna G, et al. Intraoperative radiation therapy adjuvant to resection in the treatment of pancreatic cancer. Cancer 1994; *73*:2930–2935.

46. Allema JH, Reinders ME, van Gulik TM, Koelemay MJ, Van Leeuwen DJ, de Wit LT, et al. Prognostic factors for survival after pancreaticoduodenectomy for patients with carcinoma of the pancreatic head region. Cancer 1995; *75*:2069–2076.

47. Kalser MH and Ellenberg SS. Pancreatic cancer. Adjuvant combined radiation and chemotherapy following curative resection. Arch Surg 1985; *120*:899–903.

48. Gastrointestinal Tumor Study Group. Further evidence of effective adjuvant combined radiation and chemotherapy following curative resection of pancreatic cancer. Cancer 1987; *59*:2006–2010.

49. Foo ML, Gunderson LL, Nagorney DM, McLlrath DC, van Heerden JA, Robinow JS, et al. Patterns of failure in grossly resected pancreatic ductal adenocarcinoma treated with adjuvant irradiation +/−5 fluorouracil. Int J Radiat Oncol Biol Phys 1993; *26*:483–489.

50. Hoffman JP, Weese JL, Solin LJ, et al. Preoperative chemoradiation for patients with resectable pancreatic adenocarcinoma: an Eastern Cooperative Oncology Group (ECOG) phase II study. Proc Am Soc Clin Oncol 1995; *14*:201.

51. Spitz FR, Abbruzzese JL, Lee JE, Pisters PWT, Lowy AM, Fenoglio CJ, et al. Preoperative and postoperative chemoradiation strategies in patients treated with pancreaticoduodenectomy for adenocarcinoma of the pancreas. J Clin Oncol 1997; 15:928–937.

52. Evans DB, Abbruzzese JL, and Rich RA. Cancer of the pancreas. In: DeVita VT Jr, Hellman S, and Rosenberg SA (eds), Cancer: principles and practice of oncology, 5th ed., Lippincott, Philadelphia, PA, 1997; pp. 1054–1087.

11

Extended Radical Whipple Resection for Cancer of the Head of the Pancreas

Operative Procedure and Results in Our Institution

F. Hanyu, T. Imaizumi, M. Suzuki, N. Harada, T. Hatori, and A. Fukuda

INTRODUCTION

Despite advances in diagnostic procedures, early detection of pancreatic cancer is still rare in most cases. Therefore, surgical therapy is often performed in advanced cases of invasive ductal adenocarcinoma of the pancreas, and the long-term prognosis is poor. The 5-yr survival rate of pancreatic cancer is reported to be 3.5–25% in Western countries (1–9). The 1993 annual report of registered cases of pancreatic cancer in Japan (10) showed that the 5-yr survival rate was 17.5% after curative surgery, which is much lower than that in other cancers of the gastrointestinal tract. In the early years of the authors' department, a standard operation was performed only to remove the main tumor; therefore, the resection rate was low and surgical treatment was often noncurative. Reflecting on the poor results, and inspired by Fortner's report on regional pancreatectomy (11), this department introduced the extended radical Whipple resection in 1978 (12). Depending on the extent of cancer invasion, major vessels including the portal vein, lymph nodes, and nerve plexuses were resected en bloc in order to improve the radicality of surgery. There are now 11 5-yr survivors after trial and error. This paper reports on this operative procedure for invasive ductal adenocarcinoma of the pancreatic head, and the postoperative results achieved in this department.

OPERATIVE PROCEDURES

At present, extended pancreatoduodenectomy (PD) is a basic treatment for invasive ductal adenocarcinoma of the pancreatic head in this department. The operative procedure consists of en bloc resection of veins in the portal system, regional lymphadenectomy in more than D2 groups, and extra pancreatic nerve plexuses (13) dissection.

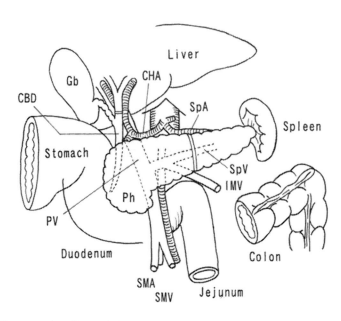

Fig. 1. The resection lines of the pancreas and the bile duct. The resection line of the pancreas is designed 2–3 cm caudal to the origin of the splenic artery (resection of head and body of the pancreas). The bile duct is divided on the hepatic side of the junction of the hepatic triad, that is, at the level of the common hepatic duct. Ph, pancreatic head; Gb, gall bladder; CBD, common bile duct; SMA, superior mesenteric artery; CHA, common hepatic artery; SpA, splenic artery; PV, portal vein; SMV, superior mesenteric vein; IMV, inferior mesenteric vein; SpV, splenic vein.

Essential points of the resection and dissection technique are as follows: In extended PD, the pancreas is resected 2–3 cm left of the origin of the splenic artery. While holding the four major vessels (the portal trunk, proper hepatic artery, and superior mesenteric artery and vein) and splenic artery with tapes, the dorsal pancreatic artery is ligated and divided. The superior border of the pancreas is adequately elevated to the tail. Along with dissection of the posterior surface of the pancreas from the superior border, dissection is also performed from the inferior side. When dissection of the superior mesenteric artery and vein is completed from the periphery to the root, the inferior mesenteric vein can be separated upward on the left side of the superior mesenteric artery. The splenic vein is identified and the pancreatic tail is elevated from the inferior mesenteric and splenic veins. Assuming a resection line 2–3 cm left of the origin of the splenic artery, two marking threads are placed at the superior and inferior borders of the pancreas. After resection of the pancreas, including the duct, with a sharp knife, bleeding sites at the cut ends are treated with electrocoagulation or nonabsorbable penetrating sutures, and not with a mattress suture or a fish-mouth suture. Frozen sections from the entire pancreatic stump, with a 5–6 mm thickness, are examined during surgery. When histological diagnosis suggests residual lesions, a further resection is added (Fig. 1).

Following pancreatic resection, lymph nodes and nerve plexuses located around the celiac artery and over the root of the superior mesenteric artery are sharply dissected

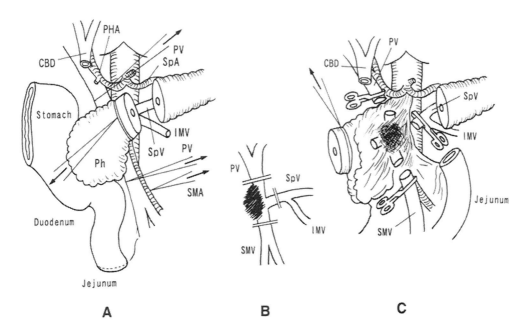

Fig. 2. Combined resection of the portal veinous system. Holding the portal trunk and superior mesenteric vein with tapes (**A**), the portal trunk, including the spleno–portal junction, superior mesenteric vein, and splenic vein, are clamped (**B**) and resected (**C**). Ph, pancreatic head; CBD, common bile duct; SMA, superior mesenteric artery; PHA, proper hepatic artery; SpA, splenic artery; PV, portal vein; SMV, superior mesenteric vein; IMV, inferior mesenteric vein; SpV, splenic vein.

by exposing the arterial wall from the left to the anterior surface. Since the pancreatic head and portal vein are still fixed to the superior mesenteric artery with the pancreatic plexus, however, further dissection of lymph nodes is difficult at this stage. The portal trunk, superior mesenteric vein, and splenic vein are clamped with a forceps, and divided. The superior mesenteric artery is not clamped. No specific portal shunts are created (Fig. 2). After resection of veins of the portal system, the pancreatic plexus becomes visualized as a cord-like structure running from the superior mesenteric artery to the right, by lifting the pancreatic head and duodenum with the left hand. The superior mesenteric artery is exposed and lifted with a tape, to dissect lymph nodes and plexuses. When the inferior pancreaticoduodenal artery is ligated and sectioned at the root, *en bloc* resection of the tumor in the pancreatic head is performed with the portal vein, retroperitoneal connective tissue, extra pancreatic nerve plexuses, and lymph nodes attached.

Reconstruction of the portal vein is performed by uninterrupted end-to-end anastomosis with a 5-0 Prolene three-point traction. An uninterrupted reverted suture is performed from the left border of the anterior venous wall. After completion of suturing the anterior wall, the vascular forceps is turned around at 180 degrees to expose the posterior venous wall. The posterior wall is then sutured by the same technique. The growth-factor suture is finally applied to the connected vein. During anastomosis, the venous cavity should be washed repeatedly with heparinized saline. Systemic admin-

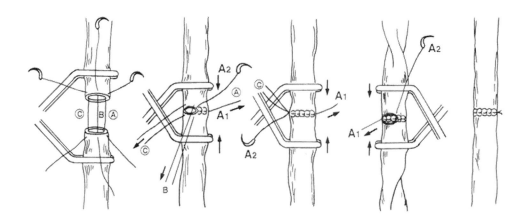

Fig. 3. Reconstruction of the portal vein (end-to-end anastomosis). Reconstruction of the portal vein is performed by end-to-end anastomosis with a three-point suture (**A, B, C**). The A2 thread is used to suture the anterior venous wall from the left (B thread) to the right (C thread). After completion of suturing the anterior wall, the vascular forceps is turned around at 180 degrees to expose the posterior venous wall. The posterior wall is then sutured by the same technique. The growth-factor suture is finally applied to the connected vein by using threads A1 and A2.

istration of heparin is not required. No specific shunts are created in the portal vein (Fig. 3). After reconstruction of the portal vein, additional dissection of extrapancreatic nerve plexuses, celiac ganglions, and paraaortic lymph nodes is performed, if necessary.

Figure 4 shows the resected state after extended PD, dissection of the retroperitoneal nerve plexuses and D2 lymph nodes, and resection of the portal vein. The retroperitoneal tissue is completely dissected, and remaining cord-like structures of aorta, inferior vena cava, celiac artery system, superior mesenteric artery, and portal venous system are visualized. The portal trunk and superior mesenteric vein are connected by end-to-end anastomosis, and the splenic vein and superior mesenteric vein are connected by end-to-side anastomosis. Although Child's method is usually used as a reconstructive procedure after PD, we recently follow Traverso's method *(14)* in which the entire stomach and pyloric ring are preserved.

RESULTS

Resectability

From January 1968 to December 1995, 1212 patients with pancreatic cancer were treated at this department. Among them, 364 patients underwent surgery for cancer of the pancreatic head (resectability, 47%) (Table 1). In 316 of the 364 patients (87%), the tumor was histologically diagnosed as invasive ductal adenocarcinoma. Based on the Japanese staging classification *(13)*, 4 patients (1%) had stage I disease, 4 (1%) stage II, 68 (22%) stage III, and 240 (76%) stage IV. Therefore, 98% of cases were classified as advanced cancer. A similar result was obtained by using the Union Internationale Contre Le Cancer (UICC) staging classification *(15)* (Table 2). Extended radical resection was performed in 249 patients (pancreatoduodenectomy in 227, and

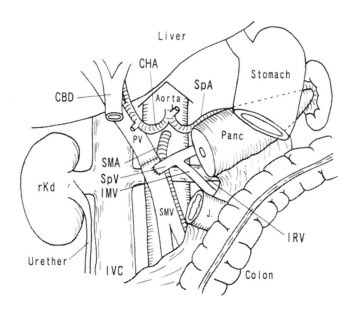

Fig. 4. Resected state after extended radical PD for cancer of the pancreatic head. Following dissection of retroperitoneal nerve plexuses and D2 lymph nodes, reconstruction of the portal vein has been performed. The retroperitoneum is completely dissected, and remaining cord-like structures of the aorta, the inferior vena cava, the celiac artery, the superior mesenteric artery, and the portal venous system are visualized. The portal trunk and superior mesenteric vein are connected by end-to-end anastomosis, and the splenic vein and superior mesenteric vein are connected by end-to-side anastomosis. CBD, common bile duct; Panc, residual pancreatic body and tail; J, jejunum; rKd, right kidney; SMA, superior mesenteric artery; CHA, common hepatic artery; SpA, splenic artery; PV, portal vein; SpV, splenic vein; IVC, inferior vena cava; IRV, left renal vein.

Table 1
Resectability for Pancreatic Cancer

	Patients	Resection
Pancreas head	769	364 (47%)
Pancreas body and tail	361	116 (32%)
Entire pancreas	82	0 (0%)
Total	1212	480 (40%)

Table 2
Comparison Between UICC Staging and Japanese Staging for Pancreatic Cancer

TNM classification		Japanese classification	
Stage	Patients	Stage	Patients
I	42 (13%)	I	4 (1%)
II	18 (6%)	II	4 (1%)
III	236 (75%)	III	68 (22%)
IV	20 (6%)	IVa	189 (60%)
		IVb	51 (16%)

Table 3
Operative Procedures for Invasive Ductal Adenocarcinoma of the Pancreatic Head[a]

Whipple operation	294	Extended	227
		Standard	67
Total pancreatectomy	22	Extended	22

[a] Procedure performed in extended operation; extended lymphadenectomy, 220 (88%); Retroperitoneal tissue dissection, 195 (78%); Resection of portal venous system, 172 (69%); Resection of arterial system, 11 (4%).

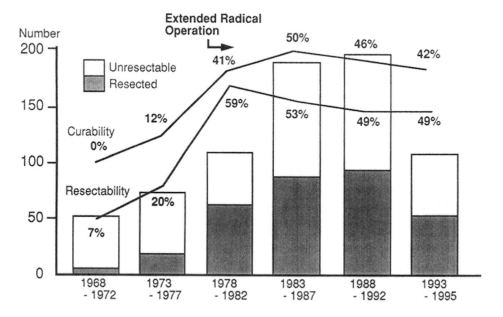

Fig. 5. Changes in resectability and curability for the invasive ductal adenocarcinoma of the head of the pancreas.

total pancreatectomy in 22). Lymph nodes in the D1 and D2 groups or more were dissected in 220 patients. Combined resection of the retroperitoneal nerve plexuses, portal venous system, and major arteries were performed in 195, 172, and 11 patients, respectively (Table 3). The resectability for cancer of the pancreatic head had been 7–20% before the introduction of extended radical resection, but it was about 50% over the past 5 yr. The curability has also been improved dramatically, from 10 to 40–50% (Fig. 5).

Morbidity and Mortality

The morbidity and mortality rates of extended radical PD were 20 and 4%, respectively. There were no significant differences in the percentages between extended radical PD and the standard operation (morbidity 22%, mortality 12%). Therefore, the ex-

Table 4
Morbidity, Mortality, and Early Postoperative
Complications After PD for Invasive Ductal Adenocarcinoma
of the Pancreatic Head

	Extended ($n = 249$)	Standard ($n = 67$)
Morbidity[a]	49 (20%)	15 (22%)
Mortality	10 (4%)	8 (12%)

[a] Morbidity: Leakage of pancreaticojejunostomy, 7%; intraabdominal hemorrhage, 2%; intraabdominal abscess, 2%; leakage of choledocojejunostomy, 1%; vascular obstruction, 1%; GI tract hemorrhage, 1%; biliary hemorrhage, 0.4%.

tended procedure did not increase the risk of PD. Postoperative complications of extended radical PD were 7% in leakage of the pancreaticojejunostomy, and 2% in intra-abdominal bleeding and in intra-abdominal abscess; however, the incidence of leakage at the pancreaticojejunostomy was similar after the two operative procedures. In patients who underwent combined portal resection, the morbidity and mortality rates were 23 and 5%, respectively. These figures are not significantly higher than those in patients who did not undergo combined portal resection (13 and 3%, respectively). Therefore, combined portal resection did not increase the risk of PD. Complications associated with pancreaticojejunal and vascular anastomoses have decreased recently. We have encountered no operative death after surgery over the last 5 yr (Table 4).

Survival Rate and 5-Yr Survivors

Long-term results of PD were evaluated with the cumulative survival curve. The 1-, 3-, and 5-yr survival rates were 41, 10 and 8% in the standard operation group, and 42, 13, and 9% in the extended radical PD group, respectively. There were no significant differences between the two groups. Long-term results of PD were also evaluated in terms of curability by surgery. The 1-, 3-, and 5-yr survival rates in patients who underwent surgery of curability A or B were 81 (52%), 24 (14%), and 24 (12%), and the 1- and 3-yr survival rates were 34 and 1% in patients who underwent surgery of curability C (noncurative surgery), respectively.

The 3- and 5-yr survival rates in patients with no lymph node metastasis, and who had extended radical operation were 29–24%, and were better than those of patients with positive lymph node (6–6%). No significant difference was seen in the survival rates between patients with positive lymph node in group 1 and patients in groups 2 and 3. Five-yr survivors were seen even in the patients with positive lymph node in groups 1, 2, and 3. Among the patients with positive lymph nodes, no relation was seen between the grade of positive lymph node and the survival rates. In 53% of patients who underwent portal vein resection, direct invasion of cancer was noted in the pv1–pv3 areas. However, long-term results in the portal resection group were related to curability of operation, and not to the extent of cancer invasion. When curative surgery was performed, good long-term survival was expected, even in cases of extensive invasion to the wall of the portal vein (Table 5). Surgery was curative (curability A or B) in all 11 5-yr survivors of cancer of the pancreatic head. Extended radical PD was performed in

Table 5
Survival Rates for Invasive Ductal Adenocarcinoma
of the Pancreatic Head in Relation to Grades of Portal
Invasion (1968–1995)

	Survival rates		
	1 yr (%)	3 yr (%)	5 yr (%)
Standard operation ($n = 67$)	41	10	8
Extended operation ($n = 227$)	42	13	9
Curability A ($n = 46$)	82	24	24
Curability B ($n = 68$)	52	14	12
Curability C ($n = 113$)	34	1	0
$n(0)$ ($n = 45$)	77	29	24
$n(+)$ ($n = 182$)	38	6	6
$n_1(+)$ ($n = 143$)	45	7	7
$n_2(+)$ ($n = 35$)	41	5	5
$n_3(+)$ ($n = 4$)	50	25	25
pv0 ($n = 132$)	59	13	11
pv1 ($n = 22$)	53	–	–
pv2 ($n = 41$)	29	0	0
pv3 ($n = 32$)	35	13	13

10 patients, with one exception (Case 10). Portal resection was combined in four patients (Cases 2,5,9,11). Tumor invasion to the portal vein was observed in the pv2 (Case 9) and pv3 (Cases 2,11). Extrapancreatic nerve plexus invasion was found in three patients (Cases 4,9,11). Three patients (Cases 2,7,11) had lymph node metastasis of n2 or more. Pathological diagnosis was tubular adenocarcinoma in 10 cases (6 moderately differentiated type, 3 well-differentiated type, 1 poorly differentiated type) and papillary adenocarcinoma in one case. One patient (Case 1) is alive at a maximum of 16.6 yr, and five patients have survived more than 10 yr (Cases 1–5). Two of these five patients (Cases 2,5) underwent combined portal resection. One patient (Case 11) died of hepatic metastasis 5 yr after surgery, when metastasis to the #16 lymph node was found. Two patients (Cases 3,9) died of pneumonia and malnutrition. The other eight patients are well and alive at present (Table 6).

DISCUSSION

Pancreatoduodenectomy, which was first completed by Whipple *(16)* in 1935, has been modified by several surgeons *(17,18)*, and is now the most fundamental operation for periampullary cancer. Because of advances of intraoperative and postoperative management, the risk of this operative procedure has decreased. However, the majority of cases of pancreatic cancer are surgically treated in an advanced stage, although useful diagnostic methods have been developed. With the conventional operative procedure, the resection rate is low and long-term results are extremely poor. In the Japanese history of surgery for pancreatic cancer, resection of only the main lesion was

Table 6
Long-Term Survivors of Invasive Ductal Adenocarcinoma of the Pancreatic Head (11 Cases)

| Case | Age | Sex | Japanese classification | | | | | | | Procedure | Curability | Outcome (yr) |
			Stage	Histology	ts	rp	pv	pl	n			
1	67	M	III	Mod.	2	0	0	−	1	Ext.	A	16.6, alive
2	51	M	IVb	Pap.	4	2	3	−	3	Ext. + PV	B	11.8, alive
3	67	M	II	Poor	2	0	0	−	1	Ext.	A	11.3, died
4	70	M	III	Well	1	1	0	+	1	Ext.	A	11.0, alive
5	54	M	III	Mod.	3	0	0	−	0	Ext. + PV	A	10.3, alive
6	72	M	IVa	Mod.	1	2	0	−	0	Ext.	B	9.4, alive
7	57	M	III	Mod.	1	0	0	−	2	Ext.	B	9.2, alive
8	55	M	III	Mod.	2	0	0	−	0	Ext.	A	8.2, alive
9	50	M	IVa	Well	3	2	2	+	0	Ext. + PV	B	7.5, died
10	63	M	I	Mod.	1	0	0	−	0	Stn.	A	6.9, alive
11	72	M	IVb	Well	1	2	3	+	2	Ext. + PV	B	5.0, died

Pap., papillary adenocarcinoma; Well, well-differenciated adenocarcinoma; Mod., moderately differentiated adenocarcinoma; Poor, poorly differenciated adenocarcinoma.

Ext., extended radical Whipple operation; PV, portal venous system resection; Stn, standard Whipple operation.

performed, and lymph node or plexus dissection was not conceived of until the late 1970s. The operative procedure was not well established and postoperative long-term results were miserable in those years. Then, Moore et al. *(19)* and McDermott *(20)* reported combined portal resection and Fortner *(11)* advocated regional pancreatectomy. Japanese surgeons were inspired by their papers and began to introduce new operative procedures for pancreatic cancer *(21)*.

As a surgical challenge to pancreatic cancer, the authors have performed combined dissection of the surrounding organs and major vessels, as well as total pancreatectomy, since the early years of the department, where they succeeded in total pancreatectomy in 1971, pancreatoduodenectomy associated with resection and reconstruction of the portal vein and hepatic artery in 1972, and total pancreatectomy associated with resection and reconstruction of the superior mesenteric artery and vein in 1978. Even when surgery was performed successfully, however, the standard operation consisted of noncurative resection of lesions without dissection of lymph nodes or plexuses. Therefore, long-term results were so poor that most patients died within a half year, or at a maximum of 3 yr, after surgery. Most cases of advanced pancreatic cancer showed invasion to the portal vein, which was regarded as nonresectable. Even when resection of portal invasion was attempted in such cases, residual tumor recurred at the surface of the portal vein. Residual cancer frequently appeared in the retroperitoneum, and metastasized lymph nodes and pancreatic stump. Such residual tumors were the main cause of noncurative surgery. Reflecting on the poor results, we introduced extended radical PD in 1978 to improve surgical curability. Systemic dissection of extended lymph nodes and plexuses and *en bloc* resection of the portal vein, which should be regarded as an intrapancreatic vessel, were the basic concept of extended radical PD. As a result, the resectability for cancer of the pancreatic head has recently been improved from 7–20% to about 50%. The curability has also been improved dramatically from 10% to nearly 50% *(12,22)*. The morbidity and mortality rates did not increase after the introduction of extended radical PD. Postoperative complications of extended radical PD were associated with retroperitoneal tissue dissection and vascular resection. However, the incidence of leakage at the pancreaticojejunal anastomosis was similar after extended radical PD and after the standard operation. There were no significant differences in the morbidity and mortality rates between extended radical PD and the standard operation; therefore, the extended procedure did not increase the risk of PD. There were no significant differences in long-term results and the cumulative survival rate between the extended radical PD group and standard operation group. Long-term survivors underwent curative surgery in both groups. Extended radical PD was performed and found to be curative (curability A or B) in 10 5-yr survivors of cancer of the pancreatic head.

It has been thought that lymph node metastasis strongly influenced the prognosis of the carcinoma of the pancreas. Nitecki et al. *(2)* reported that patients without lymph node metastases had greater 5-yr survival than patients with at least one lymph node metastasis (14 vs 1%, $p < 0.001$). Crist et al. *(7)* also reported that the actuarial 5-yr survival rate was 48% for the patients with negative lymph nodes, and 1% for the patients with one or more positive lymph nodes ($p < 0.05$). On the other hand, Gall et al. *(23)* reported that extended lymphadenectomy did not improve 5-yr survival rates in patients with pancreatic cancer. In the authors' series of extended operations, 5-yr survival rate in patients with negative lymph node was 24%, and it was 6% in patients with positive nodes, but long-term survivors were seen in patients with positive lymph node in groups 1, 2, and 3. No significant difference was seen between the grade of the lymph node metastasis and the survival rate. Those data suggest that long-term survivors after extended radical operation in this series could be obtained by not only lymph node dissection, but also wide dissection of the retroperitoneal tissue and the nerve plexus. Crist et al. *(7)* also wrote that long-term survival is possible even in patients with positive lymph nodes. Long-term results in the portal resection group were related to curability of operation, rather than to the extent of cancer invasion.

Among the patients who received the portal vein resection, no relation was seen between the grade of the tumor invasion to the wall of the portal vein and the survival rates, but long-term survival was possible if curative resection could be performed. The authors' thought that the portal system was one of the intrapancreatic vessels, and was resected without exposure of the tumor. In this series, the 3- and 5-yr survival rates were 8 and 5%, respectively, and the survival rates were favorable and were similar to those in Ishikawa's report *(24)*. Some reports in Western countries, however, claim that the portal vein resection for pancreatic cancer can improve neither the rates of curative resection nor survival rates and it is only a palliative procedure *(25,26)*.

An early diagnosis of pancreatic cancer is the most important for the improvement of therapeutic results. At present, however, the majority of cases are in an advanced stage at diagnosis and extended radical operation plays an important role in the curative therapy for this condition. We introduced extended radical PD to achieve a good resectability. As a result, a number of patients who underwent curative surgery have survived for a long period of time. On the other hand, in cases of extremely advanced cancer, curative surgery is impossible because of local residual tumors, which is the limitation of extended radical PD. Other therapeutic methods should be recommended for these cases. Diagnostic imaging methods, such as computed tomography and selective abdominal angiography, are essential for an accurate evaluation of pancreatic cancer, to decide the indication of surgical intervention *(22)*. In the prospect of therapy for pancreatic cancer, we are in a rational phase *(27)* in which surgical therapy with extended radical PD is the principal choice, and the extent of cancer is carefully evaluated with various imaging methods before surgery.

SUMMARY

The authors report the operative procedure of extended radical pancreatoduodenectomy (PD), the most fundamental surgery for cancer of the pancreatic head, and introduce therapeutic results in the 28-yr history of this department. To improve postoperative results, it is important that the extent of cancer is carefully evaluated with radiological methods to decide the indication of extended radical operation performed as curative surgery.

REFERENCES

1. Gudjonsson B. Cancer of the pancreas, 50 years of surgery. Cancer 1987; *50:*2284–2303.
2. Nitecki SS, Sarr MG, Colby TV, and van Deerden JA. Long-term survival after resection for ductal adenocarcinoma of the pancreas. Ann Surg 1995; *221:*59–66.
3. Wade TP, El-Ghazzawy AG, Virgo KS, and Johnson FE. The Whipple resection for cancer in U.S. Department of Veterans Affairs Hospitals. Ann Surg 1995; *221:*241–246.
4. Grace PA, Pitt HA, Tompkins RK, DenBeaten L, and Longmire WP, Jr. Decreased morbidity and mortality after pancreatoduodenectomy. Am J Surg 1986; *151:*141–149.
5. Andersen HB, Baden H, Brahe NEB, and Burcharth F. Pancreaticoduodenectomy for periampullary adenocarcinoma. J Am Cell Surg 1994; *179:*545–552.
6. Allema JH, Reinders ME, van Gulik TM, Koelemay MJ, van Leewen DJ, de Wit LT, Gouma DJ, and Obertop H. Prognostic factors for survival after pancreaticoduodenectomy for patients with carcinoma of the pancreatic head region. Cancer 1995; *75:*2069–2076.
7. Crist DW, Sitsmann JV, and Cameron JL. Improved hospital morbidity, mortality, and survival after the Whipple procedure. Ann Surg 1987; *205:*358–365.
8. Fernandez-del Gastillo F, Rattner DW, and Warshaw AL. Standards for pancreatic resection in the 1990s. Arch Surg 1995; *130:*295–300.
9. Trade M, Schwall G, and Saeger H. Survival after pancreatoduodenectomy: 118 consecutive resections without an operative mortality. Ann Surg 1990; *211:*447–458.
10. The Pancreatic Cancer Registry of the Japan Pancreas Society. Annual report of registered cases of pancreatic cancer in Japan (in Japanese), 1993.
11. Fortner JG. Regional resection of cancer of the pancreas, a new surgical approach. Surgery 1973; *73:*307–320.
12. Hanyu F, Suzuki M, and Imaizumi T. Whipple operation for pancreatic carcinoma: Japanese experience. In: Beger HG, Buchler MW, and Malfertheiner P. (eds), Standards in pancreatic surgery. Springer-Verlag, Berlin, 1993; pp. 646–653.
13. Japan Pancreas Society. General rules for cancer of the pancreas, (3rd ed.) Kanehara Shuppan, Tokyo (in Japanese), 1986.
14. Traverso LW and Longmire WP. Presentation of the pylorus in pancreaticoduodenectomy. Surg Gynecol Obstet 1978; *146:*959–962.
15. TNM Atlas. Springer-Verlag, Berlin, 1992; pp. 132–139.
16. Whipple AO, Parsons WB, and Mullins CR. Treatment of carcinoma of the ampulla of Vater. Ann Surg 1935; *102:*763–779.
17. Cattell RB. Resection of the pancreas. Dissection of special problem. Surg Clin North Am 1943; *23:*753–766.

18. Child CGM. Pancreaticojejunostomy and other problems associated pancreas. Ann Surg 1944; *119:*845–855.
19. Moore GE, Sako Y, and Thomas LB. Medical pancreaticoduodenectomy with resection and reanastomosis of the superior mesenteric vein. Surgery 1951; *30:*1–4.
20. McDermott WV Jr. A one-stage pancreatoduodenectomy with resection of the portal vein for carcinoma of the pancreas. Ann Surg 1952; *136:*1012–1017.
21. Nagakawa T, Kurachi M, Konishi K, and Miyazaki I. Translateral retroperitoneal approach in radical surgery for pancreatic carcinoma. Jap J Surg 1982; *12:*229–233.
22. Hanyu F and Imaizumi T. Extended radical surgery for carcinoma of the head of the pancreas. In: Beger HG, Buchler MW, and Schoenberg MH, (eds), Cancer of the pancreas. Universitatsverlag Ulm GmbH, Ulm, 1996; pp. 389–395.
23. Koeckerrling F, Kessler H, Hermanek P, and Gall FP. The role of lymph node dissection in the treatment of ductal carcinoma of the pancreas. In: Beger HG, Buchler MW, Schoenberg MH (eds), Cancer of the pancreas. Universitatsverlag Ulm GmbH, Ulm, 1996; pp. 403–408.
24. Ishikawa O, Ohhigashi H, and Imaoka S. Preoperative indications for extended pancreatectomy for locally advanced pancreas cancer involving the portal vein. Ann Surg 1992; *215:*231–236.
25. Allema JH, Reinders ME, van Gulik TM, van Leeuwen DJ, De Wit LTh, Verbeek PCM, and Gouma DJ. Portal vein resection in patients undergoing pancreatoduodenectomy for carcinoma of the pancreatic head. Br J Surg 1994; *81:*1642–1646.
26. Launois B, Franci J, Bardaxoglou E, Ramee MP, Paul JL, Mallendant Y, and Campoin JP. Total pancreatectomy for ductal adenocarcinoma of the pancreas with special reference to resection of the portal vein and multicentric cancer. World J Surg 1993; *17:*122–127.
27. Porter RA. Carcinoma of the pancreaticoduodenal area, operability and choice of procedure. Ann Surg 1958; *148:*711–724.

12

Extended Pancreatic Resection for Carcinoma of the Pancreas

Tatsushi Naganuma and Yoshifumi Kawarada

INTRODUCTION

The frequency of occurrence of cancer of the pancreas has been steadily increasing in both sexes in Japan, as in Western countries, and pancreatic carcinoma is now the fourth leading cause of cancer deaths in Japan.

In Japan, extended surgery and super-extended surgery have been performed to treat pancreatic cancer, in an attempt to achieve radical curativeness, but the diagnosis of pancreatic cancer is usually made too late for curative resection. Local recurrence and recurrence in the form of early hematogenous hepatic metastasis develop quite often, and the results of such treatment are still poor (1).

In Western countries, recently, some papers have documented both improved operative results and better long-term survival rates for patients treated by pancreatic resection (2–7). Therefore, the present study reviews the therapeutic outcome of resection of pancreatic cancer in this department, according to the General Rules for Cancer of the Pancreas (8), and assesses the value of extended resection.

In addition, the authors review the pancreatic cancer treatment results of the Pancreatic Cancer Registry Committee of the Japan Pancreas Society, including a search of the literature, and assess the best approach to the surgical treatment of pancreatic cancer at the present time.

SUBJECTS AND METHODS

Surgery was performed in 164 of the 184 cases of invasive pancreatic ductal carcinoma encountered at the surgical department of Mie University, during 20-yr period from September 1976 to August 1996 (eight cases of cystadenocarcinoma and three cases of pancreatic intraductal carcinoma have been excluded), and resection was performed in 82 (50%). The 164 patients who underwent surgery consisted of 126 patients with cancer of the head of the pancreas and 38 patients with cancer of the body or tail. The 82 patients who underwent resection were divided as follows: 11 patients underwent standard operations (pancreatectomy stopping at D1 lymph node dissection) in the early pancreatic surgery period until April 1981, and 71 patients underwent extended surgery (pancreatectomy associated with D2 lymph node dissection or vascular combined resection) in the late pancreatic surgery period from May 1981 onward, we conducted a comparative assessment of resection rates, surgical procedures, portal vein combined resection, curative resection rates, and outcome in the resected cases.

Performance status *(9)* was assessed 1 yr postoperatively in live cases without recurrence after surgery as the index of quality of life (QOL).

Stage classification of the 126 surgical cases of pancreatic head cancer into surgical stages according to the Classification of Pancreatic Cancer, Japan Pancreas Society, First English Edition (1996) *(10)*, yielded the following: stages I and II, 4 cases; stage III, 16 cases; stage IVa, 47 cases, and stage IVb, 59 cases, indicating that the 106 stage IV cases constituted the overwhelming majority (84.1%). Actuarial survival rates were assessed by comparing the nonresection cases and the resection cases according to type of resection and curability in the 62 stage IV patients (58.4%) without liver metastasis, extraperitoneal or other types of distant metastasis, or peritoneal dissemination. In addition, in July 1994, we started performing biliary bypass operations with antrectomy *(11)* or gastric partition *(12)* in stage IV cases in which there was judged to be no hope of curative resection, even by performing extended resection. We also compared results of treatment and QOL in these patients with those undergoing pancreatoduodenectomy (PD), which resulted in noncurative resection.

The X2 test was used to perform the statistical analyses. The Kaplan-Meyer method was used for actuarial survival rates, and the Cox-Mantel method was used to test for significant differences. The cumulative survival rates have been calculated by the actuarial method.

GENERAL RULES FOR CANCER OF THE PANCREAS *(8,10)*

The General Rules for Cancer of the Pancreas use degree of peripancreatic extension (T), liver metastasis (H), lymph node metastasis (N), and distant metastasis to other organs outside the abdominal cavity (M) as factors comprising the degree of pancreatic cancer progression; invasion of the pancreatic capsule anteriorly (S), invasion of the tissue in contact with the posterior aspect of the pancreas (RP), invasion of the intrapancreatic bile duct (CH), invasion of the duodenal wall (DU), invasion of the portal vein (PV), and invasion of the arterial system (A) have been adopted as factors governing T.

Thus, criteria similar to those of the Union Internationale Contre le Cancer (UICC) TNM classification *(13)* were adopted for T-factor in terms of degree of peripancreatic extension, and, even among the T1 lesions, small pancreatic cancers (TS1), with a tumor diameter of 2 cm or less, were distinguished as T1a. In the case of lymph node classification, on the other hand, the Japan N factor classification (slight modifications according to assigned lymph node group) used up until now was adopted (Fig. 1).

Stage IV was divided into stages IVa and IVb. Stage IVa consisted of P0, H0, M0 cases that were T1 and N3 (+), T2 and N2 (+), or T3 and N1; stage IVb consisted of P-, H-, or M-positive cases that were T2 and N3 (+) or T3 and N2 (+).

In the present study, surgical radical curativeness in the resected cases were divided into curability A (no residual tumor), curability B (high probability of cure), and cur-

A

	Po Ho Mo				P1,2,3/H1,2,3 or M1
	N0	N1	N2	N3	
T1a Tumor size $\leqq$ 2.0cm S0+RP0+PV0+A0+DU0+CH0,1	I	II	III	IVa	IVb
T1b Tumor size $\geqq$ 2.0cm S0+RP0+PV0+A0+DU0+CH0,1	II	II	III		
T2 Regardless of tumor size One or more positive factor(s) among S1, RP1, PV1, A1, DU1,2,3 CH2,3	III	III	IVa		IVb
T3 Regardless of tumor size One or more positive factor(s) among S2,3, RP2,3, PV2,3, A2,3	IVa				

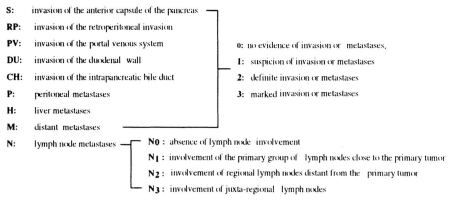

S:	invasion of the anterior capsule of the pancreas
RP:	invasion of the retroperitoneal invasion
PV:	invasion of the portal venous system
DU:	invasion of the duodenal wall
CH:	invasion of the intrapancreatic bile duct
P:	peritoneal metastases
H:	liver metastases
M:	distant metastases
N:	lymph node metastases

0: no evidence of invasion or metastases,
1: suspicion of invasion or metastases
2: definite invasion or metastases
3: marked invasion or metastases

N0 : absence of lymph node involvement
N1 : involvement of the primary group of lymph nodes close to the primary tumor
N2 : involvement of regional lymph nodes distant from the primary tumor
N3 : involvement of juxta-regional lymph nodes

1) These staging are expressed with capital letter for macroscopic findings and with small letter for microscopic findings including additional factors : intrapancreatic lymphatic vessel invasion (**ly**), vascular invasion (**v**), neural invasion (**ne**)

2) Surgical stage classification is expressed with capital letter as "Surgical Stage" and conclusive stage classification comprising of microscopic factors is expressed with small letter as "conclusive stage".
According to General Rules for the Study of Pancreatic Cancer (The 4th Edition, 1993) by Japan Pancreas Society

B

	M0		M1
	N0	N1	
T1 Limited to pancreas T1a $\leq$ 2cm Tab > 2cm	I	III	IV
T2 Invasion to duodenum,bile duct and peripancreatic tissue	I	III	IV
T3 Invasion to stomach,spleen,colon and large vessels	II	III	I V

N0: No regional lymph node metastasis

N1: Regional lymph node metastasis

M0: No distant metastasis

M1: Distant metastasis

Fig. 1. (A) Classification of pancreatic cancer, Japan Pancreas Society (*10*). **(B)** UICC TNM classification of carcinomas of the pancreas.

ability C (definite residual tumor), based on the Rules for Pancreatic Cancer, and cases in which curability A or B was possible were classified as curative resection.

RESULTS

Comparison of Therapeutic Outcome of Extended Surgery and Standard Operation

Resection Rate, Surgical Procedure, and Curative Resection Rate

Pancreatectomy was performed in 82 of our 164 pancreatic cancer patients; the resection rate was significantly higher ($p < 0.05$) in the 130 patients in the later period who underwent extended surgery (54.6%) than in the 34 early-period patients in whom the standard operation was performed (32.4%).

The surgical procedure used to treat cancer of the head of the pancreas was pancreatoduodenectomy (PD) in 40 patients and total pancreatectomy (TP) in 23 patients, with PD being performed more often in both the early period and the late period. Distal pancreatectomy (DP) was employed to treat all of the patients with cancer of the body or tail of the pancreas in both the early period and the late period. Portal vein combined surgery was performed in 29 of the 82 patients (35.4%) who underwent pancreatectomy, and all were late-period extended surgery patients.

There were 48 curative resection cases in which curability A or B was performed (58.5%) among the 82 pancreatic cancer resection patients, and the curative resection rate was significantly higher (67.7%) in the extended surgery cases than in the standard operation cases (9.1%; $p < 0.05$).

Among the cases treated by extended resection, the curative resection rate of the 29 patients who underwent portal vein resection (PVR [+]) was 64.3%, vs 71.8% in the 42 cases without portal vein resection (PVR [−]).

Postoperative Morbidity and Mortality

The postoperative morbidity and mortality of the 11 patients who underwent standard resection were 18.2 and 0%, respectively, as opposed to 14.9 and 1.4%, respectively, in the 71 patients who underwent extended resection; the difference between the two groups was not significant.

Pancreatic fistulas were observed as a postoperative complication in three cases, after extended resection alone. All of the patients improved in response to conservative management, except one patient who died as a result of complication by multiple organ failure (MOF), secondary to anastomotic leakage of the colonic reconstruction after partial resection of colon and total gastrectomy, in addition to total pancreatectomy (Table 1). There was no difference in morbidity or mortality according to type of operation, or whether the patients underwent portal vein resection.

Surgical Procedure and Outcome

The postpancreatectomy actuarial survival rates were significantly higher in the 71 patients who underwent extended surgery (1-, 3-, and 5-yr rates of 48.7, 21.4, and 12.8%, respectively) than in the 11 patients treated by the standard operation (27.3, 9.1, and 0%, respectively) (Table 2).

Moreover, when actuarial survival rates in the 71 patients who underwent extended surgery were compared according to whether they had undergone portal vein resection

Table 1
Complications of Pancreatic Resection in First Department of Surgery, Mie University, and Other Authors

	Author, dates (ref.)					
	Mie		Crist et al., 1987 *(3)*	Trede et al., 1990 *(2)*	Castillo et al., 1995 *(21)*	Saito 1995 *(22)*
Complications	1976–1991	1991–1996	1981–1986	1985–1989	1991–1994	1994
No. of Pts.	11	71	47	118	231	493
% with complications	18.2	14.1	37.0	18	34.8	NA[a]
Pancreatic fistula	–	4.2	12.8	7.6	7.5	9.3
Gastric outlet obstruction	–	–	31.9	–	6.9	–
GI hemorrhage	9.1	1.4	6.4	3.4	–	1.2
Intraabdominal hemorrhage	–	–	2.1	1.7	–	3.7
Abscess	9.1	2,8	4.3	1.7	4.3	3.4
Wound infection	9.1	5.6	12.8	–	–	–
Renal failure	–	–	6.4	–		2.2
Cardiopulmonary events	–	1.4	8.5	–	2.1	2.2
Enterocutaneous fistula	–	1.4	–	–		–
Biliary fistula	–	1.4	6.4	2.5	3.7	1.8
Sepsis	–	1.4	10.6	–	2.1	NA[a]
Cholangitis	–	1.4	–	–	1.8	
Mortality	0	1.4	2.1	0	0.4	2.0

[a] NA: Not available.

Table 2
Actuarial Survival Rates in Relation to Type of Resection in First Department of Surgery, Mie University

	No.	Actuarial survival rate (%)			
Type of resection	of pts.	1-Yr	3-Yr	5-Yr	Longest survival
Standard operation	11	27.3	9.1	0[a]	
PD	5	20.0	20.0	0[a]	4 yr 10 mo (Dead)[b]
TP	4	50.0	0	0[a]	1 yr 8 mo (Dead)[b]
DP	2	0	0	0[a]	6 mo (Dead)[b]
Extended operation	71	48.7	21.4	12.8	
PD	35	48.2	19.4	15.5	12 yr (Dead)[c]
TP	19	52.9	17.6	11.8	9 yr 6 mo (Dead)[d]
DP	17	41.7	27.8	0	3 yr 4 mo (Alive)
Total	82	44.9	17.9	12.0	

[a] $P < 0.01$.
[b] Died of recurrence.
[c] Died of pneumonia.
[d] Died of chronic lung disease.

Table 3
Actuarial Survival Rates According to Stage and Type of Resection in First Department of Surgery, Mie University

Stage	No. of pts.	Type of resection (no. of pts.)	Actuarial survival rate (%)			
			1-Yr	3-Yr	5-Yr	
I and II	5	Std. op. (0)	–	–	–	
		Exd. op. (5)	100	100	100	
III	16	Std. op. (2)	100	50.0	0	$P < 0.1$
		Exd. op. (14)	83.9	38.4	25.6	
IVa	34	Std. op. (5)	20.0	0	0	$P < 0.05$
		Exd. op. (26)	46.6	14.0	7.0	
IVb	27	Std. op. (4)	0	0	0	n.s.
		Exd. op. (23)	18.2	0	0	

Std. op., standard operation; Exd. op., extended operation.

(PVR [+]) or not (PVR [−]), the actuarial survival rates were found to be significantly higher in the 29 PVR (+) patients (1-, 3-, and 5-yr survival rates of 56.1, 33.1, and 24.8%, respectively; $p < 0.05$) than in the 42 PVR (−) patients (35.7, 3.6, and 0%, respectively). Furthermore, the longest survival time in the PVR (+) cases, both PD and TP patients, was 23 mo, with all of the patients dying within 2 yr. One of the patients in whom DP was performed, however, is alive at 40 mo.

Comparison of Cumulative Survival Rates According to Surgical Stage

A comparison of outcome according to surgical stage in patients treated by the standard operation and extended resection showed no stage I or II patients treated by the standard operation, and a 5-yr survival rate of 100% in the five patients treated by extended surgery. In stage III, the 5-yr survival rate was higher in the 14 patients who underwent extended resection (25.6%) than in the two patients who underwent the standard operation (0%). In stage IVa, the survival rates were significantly higher in the 29 patients who underwent extended resection (1-, 3-, and 5-yr rates of 46.6, 14.0, and 7.0%, respectively; $p < 0.05$) than in the five patients who underwent the standard operation (20.0, 0, and 0%).

In stage IVb, on the other hand, the 1-yr survival rate in the four patients who underwent the standard operation was 0%, as opposed to 1- and 3-yr survival rates of 18.2 and 0% among the 23 patients treated by extended resection, but the differences between the groups were not significant (Table 3).

Performance Status in Survivors Without Recurrence 1 Yr After Surgery

Examination of performance status in survivors without recurrence 1 yr after surgery according to type of resection revealed performance status of 0 in 6 of the 12 (50%) PD cases. There was only one grade 0 case (12.5%) among the eight TP cases, and the one grade 2 case (12.5%) and two grade 3 cases (25%) accounted for a total of 37.5%. All three DP cases were grade 0. The difference between the standard and the extended resections was not significant (Fig. 2).

	Performance status (Grade) *				
	0	1	2	3	4
PD (n=13)	● ○ ○ ○ ○ ○	● ○ ○ ○ ○	○		
TP (n=8)	○	● ○ ○ ○	○	● ○	
DP (n=3)		○ ○ ○			

Fig. 2. Postoperative performance status in the First Department of Surgery, Mie University. *F/U < 1 yr without recurrence and/or distant metastasis after surgery. Grades: 0, fully ambulatory and symptom free; 1, fully ambulatory with symptoms; 2, in bed <50% of the day; 3, in bed >50% of the day; 4, confined to bed all day. ● Standard resection cases; ○ extended resection cases.

Surgical Procedure and Actuarial Survival Rate of Pancreatic Head Cancer, Stage IV Without H, M, P

Surgical Procedure and Outcome

Among the 106 stage IV patients with cancer of the pancreatic head, 62 had no intraoperative evidence of liver metastasis (H), distant metastasis (M), or peritoneal dissemination (P). The 1-, 3-, and 5-yr actuarial survival rates in those in whom curative resection was possible were 66.7, 0, and 0%, respectively, in the three standard resection cases, vs 52.2, 8.7, and 4.3% in the extended resection cases. Among the noncurative resection cases, there were no 1-yr or more survivors among either the five standard resection cases or the 10 extended resection cases, and there were no 1-yr or more survivors among the 20 cases not treated by resection.

The actuarial survival rate was significantly higher ($p < 0.01$) in the extended resection curative cases than in the extended resection noncurative cases and the nonresection cases, but it was not significantly different from the nonresection survival rate in either the standard resection or extended resection noncurative cases (Fig. 3).

Postoperative Results of Palliative PD and Biliary Bypass with Antrectomy or Gastric Partition

There have been six cases treated by biliary bypass operations with antrectomy or gastric partition since 1994 (group 1) and 11 PD cases without curative resection (group 2). When the time of nasogastric tube (NG tube) removal and intolerance of oral feeding persisting more than 8 d after surgery, i.e., delayed gastric emptying, complication rate, hospital stay, and survival period, were compared between group I and group II, the duration of NG tube insertion was found to be shorter in group I than in group II, but the incidences of postoperative morbidity were not significantly different (16.7 and 27.2%, respectively) (Fig. 4; Table 4). The two patients in group II both had a pancreatic fistula and improved in response to conservative therapy. Prognosis was compared between two groups; hospital stay was definitely longer in Group II than group I. From the viewpoint of the length of stay at home and QOL, no difference between the two groups could be found.

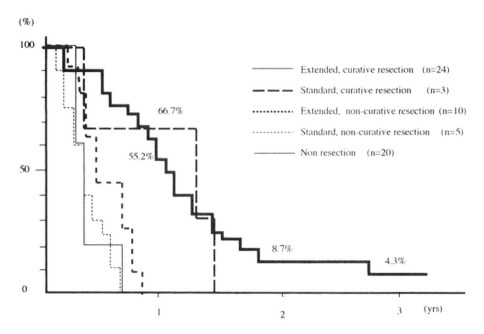

Fig. 3. Actuarial survival rates according to type of operation and curability in the First Department of Surgery, Mie University (stage IV cases of pancreatic head cancer, without P,H,M).

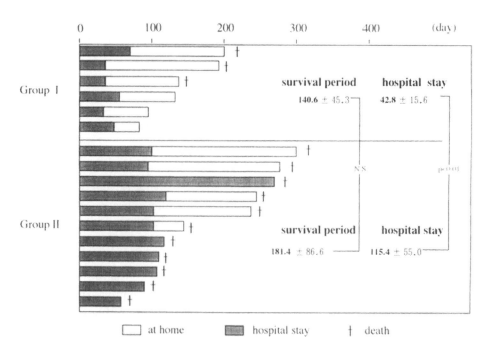

Fig. 4. Survival period and hospital stay in stage IV pancreatic cancer in the First Department of Surgery, Mie University.

Table 4
Clinical Results and Survival in Stage IV of Pancreatic Cancer in First Department of Surgery, Mie University

	Group I Biliary bypass with antrectomy or gastric partition[a]	Group II PD (noncurative)[a]
No. of patients	6	11
Removal of NG tube (d)	4.8 ± 1.7	16.5 ± 10.2
Rate of delayed gastric emptying (%)	16.7	100
Morbidity (%)	16.7	27.2
Hospital stay (d)	42.8 ± 15.6	115.4 ± 55.0
Survival period (d)	140.6 ± 45.3	181.4 ± 86.6

[a] $p < 0.01$.

DISCUSSION

In 1968, Howard *(14)* reported 41 consecutive PDs without operative mortality. In 1973, Fortner *(15)* advocated regional pancreatectomy as a means of treating cancer of the pancreatic head area, and, although it attracted the interest of surgeons worldwide for a time, because super-extended resection does not have any life-prolonging effect, and because of quality of life considerations, except in a few institutions, it is now hardly used at all to treat pancreatic cancer in Western countries, and the pancreatic cancer resection rates are 5–30% *(16–18)*. In 1987, Gudjonsson *(19)* came to the pessimistic conclusion that the tremendous effort toward curative resection of pancreatic cancer over the previous 50 yr had been to no avail, and in 1989 Sindelar *(20)* of the United States National Cancer Institute performed regional pancreatectomy to treat 20 pancreatic cancer patients and concluded that the procedure was followed by a great number of complications and was not an effective operation in terms of survival.

On the other hand, thanks to improvements in surgical technique and postoperative management during the past 30 yr, the 20–40% operative mortality in the 1960s decreased to 10–12% in the 1970s, and it has recently fallen to 5% at centers with considerable experience in performing pancreatic surgery *(16–18)*. Pancreatic fistula, in particular, has decreased markedly. Castillo et al. *(21)* of Massachusetts General Hospital have reported that the mortality rate for pancreatectomy for pancreatic cancer 20 yr ago was a high 20%, with a low 5-yr survival rate of only 5%, but that, according to recent data, the surgical mortality rate is only 5%, and the anticipated 5-yr survival rate is 20%. Moreover, in Germany, Trede et al. *(2)* have reported a better outcome, with no surgical deaths, in their patients who underwent extended resection.

According to reports of Pancreatic Cancer Registry cases, operative mortality was 2.0% (10 cases) among the 493 patients who underwent pancreatic resection, and pancreatic fistula was observed in 46 of them (9.3%) *(22)*; (Table 1). Hanyu et al. *(23)* and Ishikawa et al. *(24)* reported no increases in morbidity and mortality as a result of performing extended resection, compared with standard resection, and the results in this department also showed no increases in morbidity or mortality when extended resection was performed (Table 1).

In Japan, on the other hand, the resection rate was 24.5% in 1981, when national tabulations based on the Pancreatic Cancer Registry were begun, but by 1994 had risen to 43.5% *(22)*. The reason for this, in addition to the rise in number of cases of pancreatic cancer discovered in stages in which it is still resectable, because of recent diagnostic advances, appears to be the positive attitude toward cancer resection in Japan. Thus, the value of extended resection in the treatment of pancreatic cancer needs to be reassessed.

Although referred to as "extended resection," the procedure varies from institution to institution. In Japan, however, the most commonly performed extended resection procedure involves dissection of up to at least the D2 lymph nodes, with partial or complete removal of the nerve plexus around the superior mesenteric artery. Portal vein resection, and so on, is also sometimes performed, and we perform the procedure in a similar manner.

First, in regard to lymphadenectomy, it is well known that pancreatic cancer gives rise to a high rate of lymph node metastasis. Most lymph node metastasis involves the first group of lymph nodes, but the frequency of metastasis to the second group of lymph nodes is 5–20% *(25)* (Fig. 6).

Ishikawa et al. *(24)* compared survival rates in early-period D1 surgery, from 1971 to 1981, and late-period D2 surgery, from 1981 to 1983, and reported much better results for D2 surgery (3- and 5-yr cumulative survival rates of 38 and 28%, respectively) than D1 surgery (13 and 9%, respectively), and, according to their 1996 report, the cumulative 5-yr survival rate after D2 surgery was 26% *(26)*.

The authors also obtained a significantly higher resection rate and postoperative actuarial survival rate in this department, as a result of performing extended resection associated with D2 lymph node dissection, from May 1981 onward, than by the standard operation employed prior to that time (Table 2).

Consequently, dissection of at least two groups of lymph nodes is now considered necessary in Japan to improve the outcome, even when the pancreatic cancer is small *(27,28)*.

It is important to bear in mind, when deciding whether to perform partial or complete dissection of the plexus around the superior mesenteric artery, that total resection is complicated by highly intractable diarrhea, and postoperative QOL is very poor. This department usually only performs hemicircular dissection of the plexus around the superior mesenteric artery on the right side.

Next, regarding combined resection of the portal vein or superior mesenteric artery, the fact that there are high rates of invasion of the portal vein, superior mesenteric artery, and common hepatic artery in pancreatic cancer is considered the reason for often being unable to resect them.

According to reports of Pancreatic Cancer Registry cases in Japan up until 1994, combined resection of the portal vein was performed in 21.9% of the cases and combined arterial resection in 4% *(22)*; in this department, combined resection of the portal vein was performed in 29 of the 82 (35.4%) patients who underwent pancreatic cancer resection. Takahashi et al. *(29)* reported five patients with a 5-yr or longer survival among cases of combined portal vein resection, with one patient who underwent combined celiac artery resection surviving for 3 yr 5 mo; but they stated that the outcome of patients with a high degree of portal vein invasion, extending into the lumen, was death within 1 yr in every case, and reported that aggressive resection is not indicated in cases in which preoperative portal phlebography has shown evidence of total constriction of the portal vein. Similarly, Ishikawa et al. *(30)* and Nakao et al. *(31)* also reported a correlation between preoperative portal phlebography findings and outcome, claiming that the outcome was particularly poor when complete occlusion of the portal vein was observed.

When we compared the actuarial survival curves for the 71 patients treated by extended resection, according to whether they had undergone portal vein resection (29 patients) or not (42 patients), we found that the patients who had not undergone portal resection had significantly longer survival times, and that all of the patients who had undergone TP and PD, combined with portal vein resection, had died within 2 yr. However, one patient who under went DP has survived 3 yr 4 mo. Hanyu et al. *(23)* reported obtaining 5-yr or longer survivals in four cases in which they observed tumor invasion of the portal vein and performed combined portal vein resection. If curative resection proves to be possible, we feel that choosing portal vein resection will be very meaningful.

According to the reports of various investigators, the results of combined resection of the superior mesenteric artery remain very poor *(15–20)*.

Next, when we reviewed the types of pancreatectomy in the resected cases, according to the results of surgical procedures to treat carcinoma of the pancreas in the Pancreatic Cancer Registry in Japan, we found that TP had been performed in 730 cases (14.4%), PD in 3,117 cases (61.4%), DP in 1,090 cases (21.7%), and so on. The use of TP has been decreasing annually, with percentages for the above procedures in 1994 of 5.0, 64.1, and 25.7%, respectively; the figures reported for 1994 include 20.8% for PD, which consisted of pylorus-preserving pancreatoduodenectomy (PpPD) *(22)*.

The basis for recommending TP as a procedure for the treatment of cancer of the head of the pancreas lies in being able to resect discontinuous invasion toward the tail, multiple foci, or even lymph node metastases toward the tail area. However, the fact that no improvement in outcome was obtained as a result of TP, and the fact that patient quality of life (QOL) deteriorates because of the diabetes, loss of pancreatic exococrine function, and so on, which inevitably follow TP, have led to its abandonment in most institutions *(32,33)*. Many of the TP patients in the present study also had high performance status grades (Fig. 2), and QOL was poor. We also think that TP should be avoided as much as possible.

On the other hand, since the paper on PpPD by Traverso and Longmire in 1978 *(34)*, there have been reports from many institutions of favorable postoperative outcome in the treatment of cancer of the papilla and cancer of the lower biliary tract, and, recently, PpPD has come to be used to treat early cancer of the pancreas. Although Braasch et al. *(35)* reported no difference in outcome between PpPD and PD in pancreatic cancer, Roder et al. *(36)* compared the postoperative results of conventional PD and PpPD in 53 cases of cancer of the head of the pancreas, and reported better long-term outcome after PD. Based on the results in the pancreatic registry cases in Japan, because lymph node metastasis to the infrapyloric nodes is found in 9% of the cases *(19)*, and so on, there is still controversy concerning the application of this procedure to the treatment of cancer of the head of the pancreas. Nevertheless, because PpPD results in better QOL than PD, the number of institutions actively performing PpPD has been increasing in Japan, as well *(29,37,38)*.

Table 5
Resection Rates and Actuarial 5-Yr Survival Rates of Pancreas Head Carcinoma

Author (ref.)	Year of publication	No. of resected cases	Resection rate (%)	Actuarial 5-yr survival rate (%)	No. of survivors for more than 5 yr
Nakase et al. *(39)*	1975	332	18.3	3.0	6
Ishikawa et al. *(24)*	1988	59	–	28.0[a]	2
Tsuchiya et al. *(58)* (8 institutions)	1989	220	43.7	7.7	11
Manabe et al. *(43)*	1989	83	37.0	33.4[b]	5
Nakao et al. *(47)*	1994	101	66.0	4.3	2
Matsuno et al. *(44)*	1994	65	21.5	2.1	2
Hanyu et al. *(46)*	1994	328	48.0	10.0	13
Takahashi et al. *(29)*	1995	149	59.0	9.0	10
Nagakawa et al. *(41)*	1996	78	50.3	35.9[c]	10
The authors	1996	62	48.4	11.8	6

[a] D2 LN dissection cases.
[b] Radical pancreatoduodenectomy cases.
[c] Pathologically curative resection cases.

Based on the above findings, to determine whether a real improvement in the outcome of pancreatic cancer had been achieved, the authors searched the literature for changes in postoperative survival rates in cancer of the head of the pancreas, and found that, according to the data compiled from 57 major Japanese institutions by Nakase et al. *(39)* in 1975, the outcome of pancreatic cancer resection in Japan had a 5-yr survival rate of 3%, with six cases of 5-yr survival among 230 patients. Extended operations and multidisciplinary therapy came to be performed later, and, although relatively good outcomes were obtained in 28.0–35.9% *(24,40–43)*, according to the results for cases in which radically curative operations had been possible, overall the figure was about 10% for almost all institutions *(44–47)*, no matter where, and there were no more than about 10 5-yr survival patients at any single institution (Table 5).

In Western countries, on the other hand, there were no more than 144 5-yr-survival cases (35%) among 1400 cases of pancreatic cancer resection in a survey report by Gudjonssonn *(19)*, and, in another report, the 5-yr survival rate was slightly less than 10% *(48–51)*. Recently, however, some institutions have reported 5-yr survival rates exceeding 10–20% *(2–7)*, although the number of institutions is small. According to a recent report by Yeo et al. *(5)* at the Johns Hopkins Medical Institutions in 1995, the actuarial 5-yr survival for all 201 resected cases was 21%, and, with 3-yr survival rates for pancreatic cancer resection of 14% in the 1970s, 21% in the 1980s, and 36% for the 1990s, the rates have been improving decade by decade, and this has been accompanied by improvement in outcome. However, they have not been performing extended resection. They report 11 patients with at least 5 yr of survival among 201 cases of pancreatic cancer resection, which are almost the same results as achieved in Japan, where extended resection has been actively performed. These results have surprised surgeons around the world, however, they refer to actuarial rather than actual survival rates.

Table 6
Total Number and Survivor of Pancreatic Cancer

Author (ref.)	Institution	Years covered	Total number	Survivors %
Wade et al. *(50)*	Veteran Administration Hospital	1975–1984	3938	15 (0.3)[a]
Warren et al. *(53)*	Lahey Clinic	1942–1971	1380	13 (0.9)[a]
Cameron et al. *(4)*	Johns Hopkins Hospital	1969–1990	1328	11 (0.8)[b]
Yeo et al. *(5)*	Johns Hopkins Hospital	1970–1994	201 (Resected cases)	11 (5.4)
Nitecki et al. *(48)*	Mayo Clinic	1981–1991	1740	10 (0.5)
Geer et al. *(6)*	Memorial Sloan Kettering Hospital	1983–1990	799	10 (1.3)
Hannoun et al. *(54)*	Hospital Saint Antoine	1970–1990	920	10 (1.1)[b]
Baumel et al. *(55)*	148 French hospitals	1982–1988	4676	15 (0.3)
Tannapfel et al. *(56)*	Friedrich-Alexander University	1972–1987	334 (Operation cases)	10 (2.9)[b]
Gall et al. *(51)*	University of Erlangen/Nurnberg	1969–1987	587	16 (3.2)
Kümmerle et al. *(57)*	University of Mainz	1964–1982	782	10 (1.2)
Trede et al. *(2)*	University of Heidelberg	1985–1989	605	11 (1.8)
Manabe et al. *(43)*	Kyoto University	1969–1987	425	10 (2.3)[b]
Tsuchiya et al. *(58)*	441 institutions	1966–1983	3315	35 (1.1)
Takahashi et al. *(29)*	Tochigi Cancer Center	1974–1992	253	10 (4.0)
Hanyu et al. *(23)*	Tokyo Woman's Medical College	1968–1993	1088	15 (1.4)
Nagakawa *(41)*	Kanazawa University	1973–1994	229 (Operation cases)	10 (4.4)
The authors	Mie University	1976–1996	184	6 (3.3)

[a] Including other periampullary carcinoma.
[b] This data was not described.

On the other hand, when the reports of institutions with at least 10 5-yr survivors were summarized based on Gudjonsson's 1995 tabulation *(52)*, and the total of more than 300 pancreatic cancers in almost all of the reports were used as subjects, it was found that most reports were on a total number of more than 300 cases of pancreatic cancer, and that the 5-yr or more survival rate was only 0.3–4.4% *(46–54)*. In the reports by Gall et al. *(51)*, Trede et al. *(2)*, Manabe et al. *(43)*, Tsuchiya et al. *(58)*, Takahashi et al. *(29)*, Hanyu et al. *(46)*, and Nagakawa *(41)*, which included the results of extended resection, the 5-yr or more survival rates were no more than 1.1–4.4%. The results in this department showed six 5-yr or more survivors (3.3%) out of a total of 184 pancreatic cancer patients. Eleven 5-yr or more survivors were also reported by Yeo et al. *(5)*, but the total number of pancreatic cancer patients was not mentioned (Table 6).

Table 7
Prognostic Factors of Pancreatic Cancer

Tumor extension (refs.)	Operative factor (refs.)	Histological and biological factor (refs.)
Stage *(26,60,61)*	Curability *(60–62)*	Histology *(6)*
Tumor size *(5,39,59–63)*	Blood transfusion *(5,61)*	Lymph node meta *(3,26,32,59–61)*
Lymph node meta	Pylorus preserving *(5)*	Blood vessel invasion *(4,32,59,60)*
(5,26,32,59–61)		
Perivascular *(26)*	Surgical margin *(5,7)*	Perineural invasion *(40)*
Blood vessel *(4,32,59,60)*		DNA *(5,61,62)*
PV invasion *(26)*		G1-tumor cell differentiation *(61)*
Serosal invasion *(48,60)*		Tumor S fraction *(61)*
		c-erbB3 *(60,64)*
		Ki-67 *(60,64)*
		Tenascin *(60,64)*

Conversely, as shown in Table 7, a variety of biological factors, such as DNA analysis, are now being reported as prognostic factors for long-term survival after pancreatic resection, in addition to tumor extension, including tumor size and stage, and operative factors such as curability (Table 7; *3–7,26,32,48,59–64*). Yeo et al. *(5)* have also cited improvements in operative technique in recent years, along with diploid tumor DNA content, tumor diameter <3 cm, negative node status, negative resection margins, and so on, as the strongest predictors of long-term survival, but they did not discuss differences in the distribution of these factors in their patients in individual decades.

An assessment of Pancreatic Cancer Registry patients in Japan showed that the outcome of pancreatic cancer was relatively good in patients with TS1 and NO lesions, but very poor in patients with TS2 or higher lesions, and in those who already have lymph node metastasis (Fig. 5; *22*).

The classification of tumor in particular stage must accurately evaluate tumor extension and correctly reflect the prognosis. The General Rules for Cancer of the Pancreas were first published in Japan in 1980, and are now being widely used. They were revised in 1993 *(8)*, however, and an English translation was published in 1996 *(10)*. The result was that T category, as tumor extension, now resembles the UICC classification *(13)*. The lymph node group classification, on the other hand, has been revised based on the notion that lymph nodes included in ordinary pancreatic head resection or distal pancreatectomy be referred to as N1, taking into account outcome and lymph flow viewed from the standpoint of frequency of lymph node metastasis, based on the results of an analysis of 11,317 cases compiled by the Pancreatic Cancer Registry in Japan from 1981 to 1990 (Fig. 6). The greatest difference between the Japanese classification and the UICC classification is how to deal with the para-aortic lymph nodes. While the para-aortic lymph nodes are classified as "other than N1" (regional node metastasis) in the UICC classification, the lymph nodes from the celiac trunk to the trunk of the inferior mesenteric artery (16a2, 16b1) are classified as N2 in the General Rules for Cancer of the Pancreas (Fig. 1).

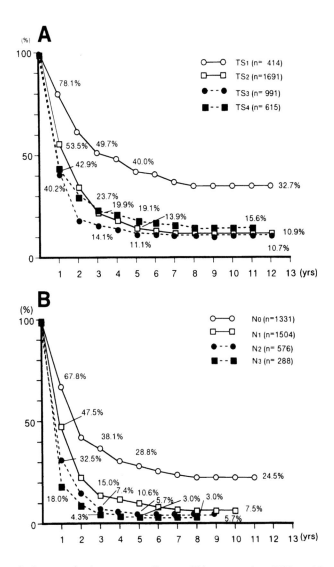

Fig. 5. Cumulative survival rate according to **(A)** tumor size (TS) and lymph node involvement (N). From the Japan Pancreas Society (1994; *22*).

In the Pancreatic Cancer Registries in Japan in 1993 and 1994 *(22,65)*, after the revision of the General Rules for Cancer of the Pancreas, it was found that, among the 1,241 operated cases whose stage classification had been registered, there were 771 stage IV cases (62.1%) and only 71 stage I cases (5.7%), figures relatively consistent with the findings in clinical settings (Table 8).

When the outcome of resected cases of pancreatic cancer in our own department was then compared according to surgical stage and whether standard resection or extended resection had been performed, the outcome after extended resection was significantly better than after standard resection in stage III and stage IVa patients, but the outcome in stage IVb patients was poor, even when extended resection was performed, and no difference in outcome from standard resection was found (Table 3).

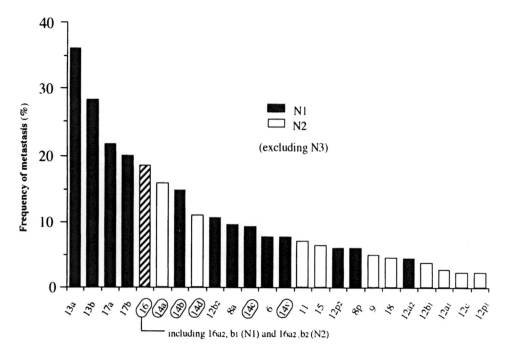

Fig. 6. Frequency of lymph node metastasis of resected pancreatic head carcinomas (excluding mucinous cystadenocarcinoma and islet cell carcinoma). A review of 11,317 cases of pancreatic carcinoma in Japan *(24)*.

Table 8
Surgical Stage and Operation Procedure of Pancreatic Cancer in Japan[a]

Stage	Resection	Palliative operation	Celiotomy	Total (%)
I	71	0	0	71 (5.7)
II	133	4	0	137 (11.0)
III	243	15	4	262 (21.1)
IV	394	302	75	771 (62.1)
Total	493	321	42	1241 (100)

[a] (By the Japan Pancreas Society, 1993 and 1994) *(22,64).*

Recent data in the Pancreatic Cancer Registry in Japan show that pancreatic resection was performed in almost all cases from stage I to stage III. A review of the operative procedures in the 771 stage IV cases revealed that pancreatic resection was performed in 394 cases (51.5%), but that palliative operations had been performed in 302 cases (39.2%) and celiotomy in 75 (9.7%) (Table 8; *22,65*). Thus, selecting the operative procedure and deciding whether to perform extended resection in Stage IV cases need to be discussed.

In the past, extended resection was actively performed in the pursuit of radicality and in the hope of improving outcome in the treatment of advanced cancer, such as stage IV, in many institutions in Japan. However, recently, more consideration is being given to patients' postoperative QOL.

In the present study, performance status was maintained 1 yr postoperatively, and QOL was favorable in nonrecurrent cases, even when extended resection was performed, but QOL in patients with residual tumor and early postoperative recurrence was considered poor.

Ishikawa et al. reported that even when extended resection was performed, if tumor diameter was more than 4 cm, there was no nodal involvement beyond the N1 lesion, and bilateral portal vein invasion was present, 1-yr or more survival could not be expected, and QOL was poor. They claimed that extended resection was not indicated in such patients.

In contrast, in the recent trend toward reexamining resection for pancreatic cancer in Western countries, there have been scattered papers recommending palliative pancreatic resection in locally advanced cancer, claiming that a life-prolonging effect can be achieved compared to palliative pancreatic resection, even if it ultimately proves to be noncurative resection *(66–70)*.

When the authors then examined the operative procedures and survival rates in the 62 stage IV pancreatic head cancer patients in this department, with no intraoperative evidence of liver metastasis, distant metastasis, or peritoneal dissemination, they discovered that the outcome was significantly more favorable in those who underwent curative resection by extended resection than in the noncurative resection cases and the nonresection cases. However, there was no difference in survival rate in the cases that ended in noncurative resection, compared to the nonresection cases (Fig. 3).

For this reason the authors have been performing biliary bypass with antrectomy *(11)* or gastric partition *(12)* in stage IV patients in this department since July 1995, whenever there was judged to be no hope of curative resection, even by performing extended resection (group I). When their surgical results were assessed in comparison with stage IV patients in whom PD was performed, and which ended in noncurative resection (group 2), the authors found that, although there were no significant differences between the groups in postoperative morbidity or survival duration, oral feeding was started significantly sooner and hospital stay was significantly shorter in group 1 than in group 2, and QOL was more favorable in group 1 than in group 2 (Fig. 4; Table 4).

Based on the above assessment, at least in stage IV patients in whom noncurative resection that would leave cancer behind is foreseen, since PD itself is very difficult as a technique, it appears necessary to rigorously choose whether to perform PD.

Accordingly, when deciding on the method of treatment in stage IV patients, it is necessary to judge carefully whether curative resection is desirable, even in stage IVa cases.

Thus, there are many stage IV patients in whom no improvement is achieved by performing extended surgery. This seems to be the current state of affairs regarding extended operations in the treatment of pancreatic cancer. Great strides in diagnosis and the development of effective adjuvant therapy are anticipated in the future.

CONCLUSION

Based on the above findings, it appears that extended resection should not be performed on all advanced surgical stage IV patients, and that surgical procedures should be selected, taking quality of life into consideration, for patients with surgical stage IVb lesions or patients in whom curability B or better operations cannot be expected, even through surgical stage IVa.

REFERENCES

1. Kawarada Y, Nemoto A, and Mizumoto R. Surgical treatment for carcinoma of the head of the pancreas. In: Takada T (eds), New frontiers in hepato-biliary-pancreatic surgery, Bangkok Medical, Bangkok, 1993; pp. 196–199.
2. Trede M, Schwall G, and Saeger HD. Survival after pancreatectomy: 118 consecutive resections without an operative mortality. Ann Surg 1990; *211:*447–458.
3. Crist DW, Sitzmann JV, and Cameron JL. Improved hospital morbidity, mortality, and survival after the Whipple procedure. Ann Surg 1987; *206:*358–365.
4. Cameron JL, Crist DW, Sitzmann JV, et al. Factors influencing survival after pancreaticoduodenectomy for pancreatic cancer. Am J Surg 1991; *161:*120–125.
5. Yeo CH, Cameron JL, Lillemoe KD, Sitzmann JV, Hruban RH, Goodman SN, et al. Pancreaticoduodenectomy for cancer of the head of the pancreas: 201 patients. Ann Surg 1995; *221:*721–733.
6. Geer RJ and Brennan MF. Prognostic factors for survival after resection of pancreatic adenocarcinoma. Am J Surg 1993; *165:*68–73.
7. Wilette CG, Lewandrowsky K, and Warshaw AL. Resection margins in carcinoma of the head of the pancreas: implications for radiation therapy. Ann Surg 1991; *214:*648–656.
8. Japan Pancreas Society. General rules for the study of pancreatic cancer, 4th ed, Kanehara, Tokyo, 1993 (in Japanese).
9. World Health Organization. Handbook for reporting results of cancer treatment, WHO, Geneva, 1979.
10. Japan Pancreas Society. Classification of pancreatic cancer, 1st ed. Kanehara, Tokyo, 1996.
11. Lucas CE, Ledgerwood AM, Saxe JM, Bender JS, and Lucas WF. Antrectomy, a safe and effective bypass for unresectable pancreatic cancer. Arch Surg 1994; *129:*795–799.
12. Slim K, Pezet D, Riff Y, and Chipponi J. Antral exclusion as an adjunct to palliative gastrojejunostomy for cancer of the pancreas. Press Med 1996; *25:*674–676 (in French).
13. (Hermanek P, Sobin LH eds) UICC TNM classification of malignant tumours, 4th ed., 2nd revision, Springer, Berlin, 1992.
14. Howard JM. Pancreatico-duodenectomy: forty-one consecutive Whipple resections without and operative mortality. Ann Surg 1968; *168:*629–640.
15. Fortner JG. Regional resection of cancer of the pancreas: a new surgical approach. Surgery 1973; *73:*658–662.
16. Ashley SW and Reber HA. Surgical management of exocrine pancreatic cancer. In: Go VLW, (eds), The pancreas: biology, pathobiology, and disease, 2nd ed., Raven, New York 1993; pp. 913–929.
17. Warshaw AL. Pancreatic carcinoma. New Eng J Med 1992; *326:*455–465.
18. Warshaw AL and Swanson RS. What's new in general surgery; pancreatic cancer in 1988. Ann Surg 1988; *208:*541–553.
19. Gudjonsson B. Cancer of the pancreas: 50 years of surgery. Cancer 1992; *60:*2284–2303.
20. Sindelar WF. Clinical experience with regional pancreatectomy for adenocarcinoma of the pancreas. Arch Surg 1989; *124:*127–132.
21. Castillo CF, Rattner DW, and Warshaw AL. Standards for pancreatic resection in the 1990s. Arch Surg 1995; *130:*295–300.
22. Saito Y. The annual report of pancreatic cancer. Pancreatic Cancer Register Committee, Japan Pancreas Society 1994. Suizo 1995; *10:*535–564. (in Japanese)
23. Hanyu F, Suzuki M, and Imaizumi T. Whipple operation for pancreatic carcinoma: Japanese experience. In: Beger HG et al. (eds), Standards in pancreatic surgery, Springer-Verlag, Berlin 1993; pp. 647–653.
24. Ishikawa O, Ohhigashi H, Sasaki Y, Kabuto T, Fukuda I, Furukawa H, Imaoka S, and Iwanaga T. Practical usefulness of lymphatic and connective tissue clearance for the carcinoma of the pancreas head. Ann Surg 1988; *208:*215–220.

25. Saito Y. The annual report of pancreatic cancer. Pancreatic Cancer Register Committee 1991; 1981–1990, Japan Pancreas Society (in Japanese).

26. Ishikawa O. Surgical technique, curability and postoperative quality of life in an extended pancreatectomy for adenocarcinoma of the pancreas. Hepato-gastroenterology 1996; 320–325.

27. Noguchi T, Vaidya P, and Kawarada Y. Surgical treatment and prognostic factors in TS1 carcinoma of the pancreas. J Hep Bil Pancr Surg 1995; *2:*376–383.

28. Satake K, Nishikawa H, Yokomatsu H, Kawazoe Y, Kim KS, Haku A, and Umeyama K. Surgical curability and prognosis for standard versus extended resection for T1 carcinoma of the pancreas. Surg Gynecol Obstet 1992; *175:*259–265.

29. Takahashi S, Ogata Y, Miyazaki H, Maeda D, Murai S, Yamataka K, and Tsuzuki T. Aggressive surgery for pancreatic duct cell cancer: feasibility, validity, limitations. World J. Surg 1995; *19:*653–660.

30. Ishikawa O, Ohigashi H, Iamoka S, Furukawa H, Sasaki Y, Fujita M, Kuroda C, and Iwanaga T. Preoperative indications for extended pancreatectomy for locally advanced pancreas cancer involving the portal vein. Ann Surg 1991; *215:*231–236.

31. Nakao A, Harada A, Nonami T, Kaneko T, Inoue S, and Takagi H. Clinical significance of portal invasion by pancreatic head carcinoma. Surgery 1995; *117:*50–55.

32. Ozaki H. Modern surgical treatment of pancreatic cancer. Int J Pancreatol 1994; *16:*121–129.

33. van Heerden JA, Mcilrath DC, Ilstrup DM, and Weiland LH. Total pancreatectomy for ductal adenocarcinoma of the pancreas. An update. World J Surg 1988; *12:*668–662.

34. Traverso LM and Longmire WP. Preservation of the pylorus in pancreaticoduodenectomy. Surg Gynecol Obstet 1978; *146:*959–962.

35. Braasch JW, Rossi RL, Watkins EJR, Deziel DJ, and Winter PF. Pyloric and gastric preserving pancreatic resection. Ann Surg 1986; *204:*411–418.

36. Roder JD, Stein HJ, Huttle W, and Siewert JR. Pylorus preserving versus standard pancreticoduodenectomy: an analysis of 110 pancreatic and periampullary carcinoma. Br J Surg 1992; *79:*152–155.

37. Suzuki T, Hamanaka Y, Shinagawa Y, Wadamori K, Iizuka N, Tanaka A, and Ueno T. Pylorus-preserving pancreatoduodenctomy in Japan: history and present status. J Hep Bil Pancr Surg 1994; *4:*379–384.

38. Takada T. Pylorus-preserving pancreato-duodenectomy: Technique and indications. Hepato-gastroenterology 1993; *40:*422–425.

39. Nakase A, Matsumoto Y, Uchida K, and Honjo I. Surgical treatment of cancer of the pancreas and the periampullary region: cumulative results in 57 institutions in Japan. Ann Surg 1977; *185:*52–57.

40. Nagakawa T, Konishi I, Ueno K, Ohta T, Kiyama T, Kanno M, Kayahara M, and Miyazaki I. The results and problems of extensive radical surgery for carcinoma of the head of the pancreas. Jap J Surg 1991; *21:*262–267.

41. Nagakawa T. Pancreaticoduodenectomy. Geka Shinryo 1996; *38:*437–444 (in Japanese).

42. Manabe T, Baba N, Nonaka A, Asano N, Yamaki K, Shibamoto Y, et al. Combined treatment using radiotherapy for carcinoma of the pancreas involving the adjacent vessels. Int Surg 1988; *73:*153–156.

43. Manabe T, Ohshio G, Baba N, Miyashita T, Asano N, Tamura K, et al. Radical pancreatectomy for ductal cell carcinoma of the head of the pancreas. Cancer 1989; *64:*1132–1137.

44. Matsuno S and Sato T. Surgical treatment for carcinoma of the pancreas. Am. J. Surg 1988; *152:*499–504.

45. Tsuchiya R, Tsunoda T, and Yamaguchi T. Operation of choice for resectable carcinoma of the head of the pancreas. Int J Pancreatol 1990; *6:*295–306.

46. Hanyu F, Imaizumi T, Nakasako T, Harada N, Hatori T, Ozawa F, Suzuki T, and Tenma N. Pancreatic cancer. Gastroenterol Surg 1995; *18:*323–330 (in Japanese).

47. Nakao A, Harada K, Nonami T, Kaneko T, Inoue S, Takeuchi A, et al. Radical surgery and adjuvant therapy for carcinoma of the pancreatic head region. Jpn J Gastroenterol Surg 1994; 2341–2346 (in Japanese).
48. Nitecki SS, Sarr MG, Colby TV, and van Heerden JA. Long-term survival after resection of ductal carcinoma of the pancreas. Is it really improving? Ann Surg 1995; *221:*59–61.
49. Griffin JF, Smallery SR, Jewell W, Paradelo JC, Reymond RD, Hassanein RES, and Evans RG. Patterns of failure after curative resection of pancreatic carcinoma. Cancer 1990; *66:*56–61.
50. Wade TP, Radford DM, Virgo KS, and Jonson FE. Complications and outcomes in the treatment of pancreatic adenocarcinoma in the United States veteran. J Am Coll Surg 1994; *179:*38–48.
51. Gall FP, Kessler H, and Hermanek P. Surgical treatment of ductal pancreatic carcinoma. Eur J Surg Oncol 1991; *17:*173–181.
52. Gudjonsson B. Carcinoma of the pancreas: critical analysis of costs, results of resections, and the need for standardized reporting. J Am Coll Surg 1995; *181:*483–503.
53. Warren KW, Choe DS, Plaza J, and Relihan M. Results of radical resection for periampullary cancer. Ann Surg 1975; *181:*534–540.
54. Hannoun L, Christophe M, Ribeiro J, Nordlinger B, Elrinwini M, Tiret E, and Parc R. A report of forty-four instances of pancreaticoduodenal resection in patients more than seventy years of age. Surg Gynecol Obstet 1993; *177:*556–560.
55. Baumel H, Huguier M, Mandersheid JC, Fabre JM, Houry S, and Fagot H. Results of resection for cancer of the exocrine pancreas: a study from the French Association of Surgery. Br J Surg 1994; *81:*102–107.
56. Tannapfel A, Wittekind C, and Hunefeld G. Ductal adenocaricinoma of the pancreas. Histopathological features and prognosis. Int J Pancreatol 1992; *12:*145–152.
57. Kümmerele F and Ruckert K. Surgical treatment of pancreatic cancer. World J Surg 1984; *8:*889–894.
58. Tsuchiya R, Harada N, Tsunoda T, Miyamoto T, and Ura K. Long-term survivors after operation on carcinoma of the pancreas. Int J Pancreatol 1988; 3:491–496.
59. Beger HG, Link KH, Poch B, and Gansauge F. Pancreatic cancer-rencent progress in diagnosis and treatment. pancreas. In: Neoptolemos JP, (eds), Pancreatic cancer, et al., Blackwell, London 1996; pp. 227–235 In: Go VLN, (eds), The pancreas: biology, pathobiology, and disease, 2nd ed., Raven, New York 1993; pp. 913–929.
60. Kawarada Y, Naganuma T, Vaidya P, et al. Extended resection for cancer of the pancreas and prognostic factors. Asian J Surg (in print).
61. Böttger TC, Strokel S, Wellek S, Stockle M, and Junginger T. Factors influencing survival after resection of pancreatic cancer. Cancer 1994; *73:*63–73.
62. Fortner JS, Kimustra DS, Senie RT, and Maclean BJ. Tumor size is the primary prognosticator for pancreatic cancer after regional pancreatectomy. Ann Surg 1996; *223:*147–153.
63. Cubilla AC, Fortner J, and Fitzgerald PJ. Lymph node involvement in carcinoma of the head of the pancreas. Cancer 1978; *41:*880–887.
64. Vaidya P, Isaji S, Kato K, Tanigawa K, Okamura Y, Ogura Y, et al. Adjuvant therapy following resection of pancreatic head carcinoma according to the histopathological and biological features. In: Recent advances in management of digestive cancers, Springer-Verlag/Tokyo Press, Hong Kong, 1993; pp. 779–781.
65. Saito Y. The annual report of pancreatic cancer. Pancreatic Cancer Register Committee, Japan Pancreas Society 1993. Suizo 1994; *9:*499–527 (in Japanese).
66. Cangemi V, Volpino P, Mingazini P, Fiori E, Gentili S, Ansali A, and Piat G. Role of surgery in ductal carcinoma of the pancreas. Int Surg 1992; *77:*158–163.
67. Martin FM, Rossi RL, Dorrucci V, Silverman L, and Braasch JW. Clinical and pathologic correlations in patients with periampullary tumors. Arch Surg 1990; *125:*723–726.

68. Funovics JM, Karner J, Pratschner Th, and Fritsch A. Current trends in the management of carcinoma of the pancreatic head. Hepat-gastroenterology 1989; *36:*450–455.
69. Conlon K, Kimstra DS, and Brennan MF. Long-term survival after curative resection for pancreatic ductal adenocarcinoma: clinicopathologic analysis of 5-year survivors. Ann Surg 1996; *223:*273–279.
70. Lillemoe Kd, Cameron JL, Yeo CJ, Sohn TA, Nakeeb A, Sauter PK, et al. Pancreatico-duodenectomy. Does it have a role in the palliation of pancreatic cancer? Ann Surg 1996; *223:*718–728.

13

Endoscopic Stents for Palliation in Patients with Pancreatic Cancer

Richard C. K. Wong and David L. Carr-Locke

INTRODUCTION

Pancreatic carcinoma is a common, biologically aggressive malignancy that has a very poor prognosis. Management requires a multidisciplinary approach, with input from the subspecialties of surgery, gastrointestinal endoscopy, oncology, radiology, and radiation oncology. The only potentially curative form of treatment is surgical resection, although most patients present late in the course, with unresectable disease. Approximately 20% of patients presenting with malignant obstructive jaundice undergo some form of surgery (either resection or palliative bypass). The remaining 80% are managed nonsurgically. For this group of patients, who either have unresectable disease, refuse surgery, or are medically unfit for surgery, endoscopic palliation of symptoms should be strongly considered. Indeed, over the last decade, endoscopic palliation of malignant biliary obstruction has become an acceptable, and preferred, alternative to surgical bilioenteric bypass; this is achieved by the endoscopic placement of either plastic or metallic endoprostheses (stents).

Symptoms may be caused by at least five different effects of pancreatic cancer, the first three of which are amenable to endoscopic stent therapy: biliary obstruction, local-regional invasion, pancreatic/obstructive-type pain, metastatic disease, and paraneoplastic manifestations. Biliary obstruction is a common occurrence and may result in pruritis, malaise, anorexia, jaundice, cholangitis, malabsorption, progressive hepatic failure, coagulopathy, and renal dysfunction. Local-regional invasion may result in duodenal or gastric outlet obstruction, and intermittent pancreatic pain may be caused by obstruction of pancreatic ductal drainage.

The aims of treatment in patients with unresectable disease, or in those who are unfit for surgery, are to provide prompt and effective relief of symptoms with minimum disturbance, so that the patient should be able to enjoy as good a quality of life as possible for the remaining weeks or months. The morbidity associated with endoscopic stent insertion varies from 0 to 36% (1–12), but major morbidity is probably well under 10%.

Mortality within 1 mo of the procedure is 10–18%, and median survival is about 6 mo *(1–3)*. Another option for biliary obstruction, apart from surgical bypass, would include percutaneous drainage. However, an endoscopic approach has been shown to be superior to both surgical and percutaneous methods of drainage *(4,5,7,8,13)*.

THE ENDOSCOPIC APPROACH

Patient Selection

The first decision that must be made in evaluating the patient with jaundice is to distinguish between hepatocellular (e.g., from intrahepatic metastases) and obstructive or cholestatic jaundice. Usually, these can be easily differentiated by the clinical presentation of the patient, the profile of the liver function tests, and hepatobiliary imaging by ultrasound, CT, or MRI. Ultrasound is usually the initial test, because it is readily available and relatively inexpensive. However, a CT scan may be preferred over ultrasound because it provides additional information about surrounding structures (e.g., involvement of the porta hepatis, the duodenum, vasculature, and so on), and its interpretation is less operator-dependent.

Once the diagnosis of malignant biliary obstruction is made and the patient is deemed nonresectable, the subsequent management focuses on deciding the optimal form of palliation. In patients who are in the terminal stages of their disease, an aggressive approach may be inappropriate, and this decision should be made early. Nevertheless, in most instances, the best approach is endoscopic. There are circumstances, however, in which consideration should be given to other forms of palliative treatment. For example, in a patient presenting with both malignant biliary and duodenal obstruction, a double surgical bypass procedure, such as a gastrojejunostomy and bilioenteric anastomosis, should be considered. In addition, the optimal treatment for patients with a complex obstructing lesion in the hilum of the liver has not been determined. In this situation, the endoscopic, as well as the percutaneous transhepatic, approach needs to be considered. The optimal treatment would greatly depend on available expertise. Nevertheless, in most circumstances endoscopic cholangiography is the preferred method, because it is less invasive and carries fewer complications than the transhepatic route. Furthermore, endoscopic retrograde cholangiopancreatography (ERCP) provides information about the duodenum, the major papilla, and the pancreatic ductal system, as well as the biliary tree, and offers a wide spectrum of therapy, with a high technical success rate in biliary stent placement (80–90%), and relief of jaundice in the overwhelming majority of cases *(2,4,6,11,14)*. In expert centers, a technical success rate of at least 95% should be expected *(1–11)*. Furthermore, endoscopic transpapillary brush cytology *(15–17)*, forceps biopsy *(18)*, or needle aspiration *(19)* can be used alone or in combination to obtain diagnostic tissue from biliary or pancreatic duct strictures during ERCP.

Plastic Endoprostheses

The methodology and range of plastic endoprosthesis equipment currently available has been well standardized *(1–9,20*; Fig. 1). Hydrophilic guidewires may speed the process, and often permit access across strictures resistant to standard guidewires. Steerable and torque-stable wires have made some difference to selective intrahepatic cannulation. A sphincterotome can also be used as a deflecting device *(21)*. Two wires can

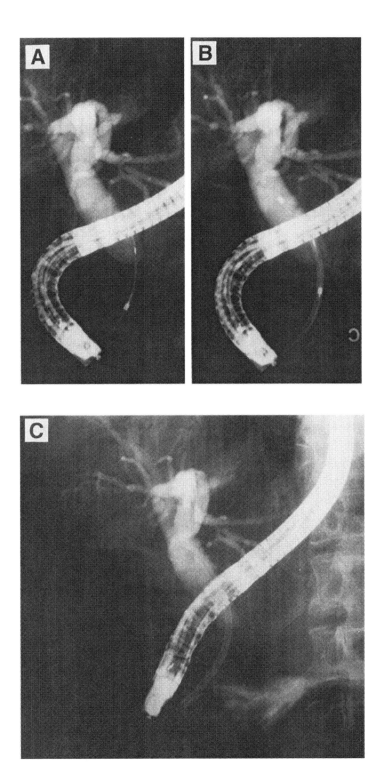

Fig. 1. ERCP sequence showing (**A**) cytology sample being taken through guide catheter of stent insertion system; (**B**) 10-Fr diameter polyethylene stent being placed over guide catheter–cytology brush combination; (**C**) final appearance of stent immediately after placement.

be placed through the channel of an endoscope into both hepatic ducts in hilar lesions. Many experts do not routinely perform sphincterotomy for stent insertion unless the placement of more than one stent is planned.

Stent occlusion may occur from 1 wk to over 15 mo after placement, with a mean of about 5 mo. Patients may present with malaise, low-grade fever, liver function test abnormalities, or frank cholangitis *(22–32)*. Several variables may be involved in the occlusion process: bile flow, bile composition, bacterial contamination, and endoprosthesis characteristics such as stent diameter, length, shape, design, position, number, and material. Attempts at manipulating all of these have been made in vitro *(22–28)*, with little impact on clinical practice, although a recently developed Teflon stent shows promise *(29)*. The maximum outside diameter of such stents is limited by the diameter of the instrument channel in the duodenoscope and 10–11.5-French stents are now standard and perform better than smaller diameter endoprostheses *(33)*. Endoscopic replacement of a clogged stent is usually technically simple, and is associated with prompt resolution of symptoms. Small diameter, 7-French plastic stents can be easily removed with a snare and pulled up the accessory channel, while maintaining a short endoscope position. The removal of larger stents (10 or 11.5 French) depends on the diameter of the endoscope channel. If the diameter of the channel is larger than the stent, then it is possible to remove it in a fashion similar to the 7-French stent. However, in order for this to be successful, the snare must be positioned tightly around the distal few millimeters of the stent. Other alternatives are to remove the snare, stent, and endoscope together from the patient (thus necessitating repeat introduction of the endoscope), or to remove the stent with the snare, or to place the stent in the stomach (retrieving it at the end of the procedure). In addition, other techniques have been used particularly for complex or difficult strictures. In these cases, the lumen of the occluded stent is cannulated with a guidewire, and then is retrieved using a snare ("snare over-the-wire" technique; Fig. 2) or, with a cork-screw type stent extractor, a guidewire is placed alongside the stent ("snare beside-a-wire" technique) *(34)*. These latter techniques maintain guidewire access across the bile duct stricture, while retrieving the stent via the channel of the endoscope.

Macroscopically, the material in a blocked stent resembles biliary sludge or brown pigment stones, consisting mostly of calcium bilirubinate, with some calcium palmitate and unidentified organic material, together with bacteria *(22–25)*. Bacteria form biofilms by polysaccharide production, which cements the bacterial cell to the surface and mediates adhesion to sister cells. The polysaccharide matrix protects the bacteria from the host defense mechanisms and from toxic substances, such as antibiotics, biocides, and surfactants. It is probable that this layer is the first step in the clogging process *(22–24)*. Crystals of calcium bilirubinate, calcium palmitate, and cholesterol are embedded within the matrix, and the bacteria are attached to the stent surface by a fibrillar matrix. In most instances, the use of antibiotic- or bacteriostatic-impregnated stents have not prevented this clogging phenomenon from occurring, nor have the use of gallstone dissolution agents, mucolytics, or choleretics been of use *(26–28)*.

The predictability of occlusion, with its serious and potentially life-threatening complication of sepsis, mitigates in favor of planned removal and replacement at approx 4-mo intervals *(1–3)*. The variability of stent survival, however, would, in the appropri-

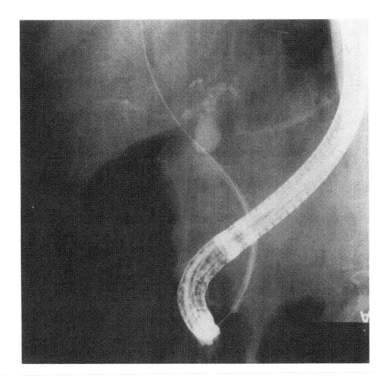

Fig. 2. ERC showing hydrophilic guidewire placed through stent lumen prior to snare extraction through the endoscope.

ate patient, support the alternative approach of close clinical follow-up to anticipate early symptoms of biliary obstruction or cholangitis.

Metallic Expandable Endoprostheses

In search of a solution to the problem of plastic stent occlusion, larger diameter expandable metallic stents were developed, and initial experience was with the percutaneous transhepatic route *(33,35–39)*.

There is limited experience with the endoscopic Gianturco Z stent (Wilson-Cook, Winston-Salem, NC), available as single 8 × 30 mm units when fully expanded *(37,39,40)*, which can be linked end-to-end to cover the necessary stricture length. The Strecker stent (Microvasive, Boston Scientific, Natick, MA) has a single tantalum thread, interlocking woven meshwork construction, attains a maximum diameter of 8 mm, and is available in lengths of 4, 6, and 8 cm. It requires balloon expansion at the time of placement, there are technical failures in up to 18%, and there is no subsequent self-expansion in its original form *(44)*. One randomized trial *(33)* compared the use of plastic (polyethylene) stents with those made of metal for the treatment of malignant obstruction of the common bile duct. It was found that the early results (<1 mo) were similar in the two groups. However, the long-term results (median of 5 mo) revealed that, compared to metallic stents, the plastic ones had significantly worse outcome. That is, the cholangitis rate was higher with plastic stents, as was the total

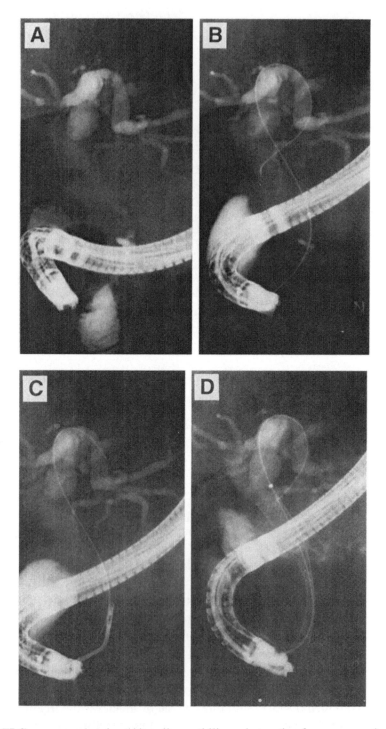

Fig. 3. ERC sequence showing (**A**) malignant biliary obstruction from pancreatic cancer invasion; (**B**) placement of hydrophilic guidewire across stricture into obstructed bile duct; (**C**) forceps biopsy alongside guidewire; (**D**) placement of 10 × 68 mm Wallstent with guidewire still in place; (**E**) appearances immediately after stent deployment and endoscope withdrawal, showing some constriction of the stent at the stricture site.

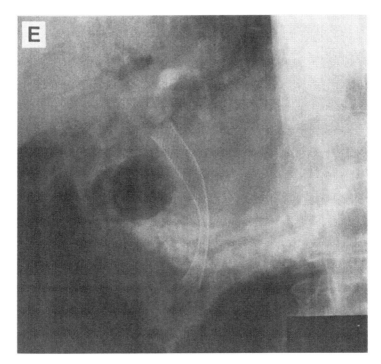

Fig. 3. (Continued)

duration of hospital stay. The plastic stents were also not cost-effective when retreatment costs for stent malfunction and stent exchange were considered.

Most experience has been gained with the self-expanding metallic Wallstent (Schneider Stent, Minneapolis, MN), which is delivered on a 7.5 or 8-French-gage system, but expands to 30-French gage in its fully expanded form of 42, 68, or 80 mm in length *(32,33,35–50)* (Fig. 3). Initial open studies were conducted in Europe *(33,36–38,50)* in a total of 293 patients with malignant biliary obstruction. Early morbidity was very low, but late occlusion by tumor ingrowth or overgrowth appeared in 10%. However, occlusion by sludge was only reported in 2%. Three randomized controlled trials have now been reported *(33,47,48)* from the United States and Europe comparing Wallstents with plastic in 380 patients. Prolonged stent patency, lower stent occlusions, and a reduction in subsequent interventions for Wallstents were demonstrated, with significant impact on cost-effectiveness. The problem of tumor ingrowth through the meshwork may be overcome by the development of a silicone covering *(51)* or the emergence of newer metallic stents, which do not have an open framework *(52)* (Fig. 4).

It is important to remember that the placement of a metallic stent is permanent, because, once fully deployed, the metallic stent cannot easily be removed. Indeed, a recent article clearly demonstrated that the struts of uncovered Wallstents become incorporated either into tumor tissue or into the wall of the normal organ (above and below the tumor) *(53)*. Therefore, if there is any doubt about the nature of a biliary stricture, then a plastic endoprosthesis should be placed first, until malignancy is proven.

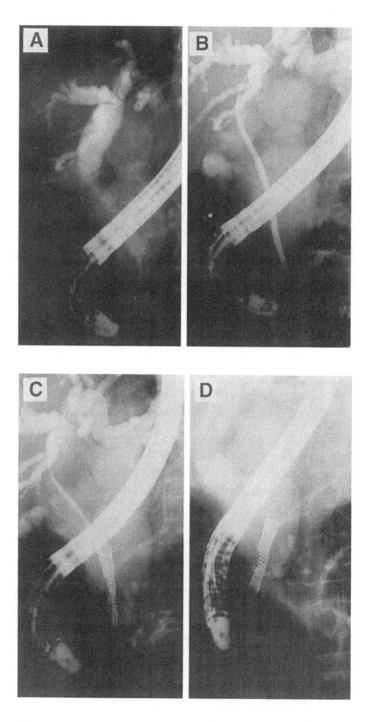

Fig. 4. ERCP sequence showing **(A)** distal bile duct stricture caused by pancreatic cancer involvement; **(B)** insertion of Endocoil (Instent-Medtronic, Minneapolis, MN) delivery system over guidewire, with stent fully compressed; **(C)** appearance as Endocoil is released from delivery catheter; **(D)** appearance of Endocoil immediately after removal of delivery catheter and guidewire; **(E)** position of Endocoil after removal of endoscope, showing-almost complete expansion and coil closure.

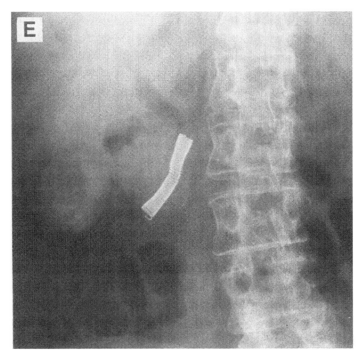

Fig. 4. (Continued)

Complications of Endoprosthesis Placement

These can be divided into acute and delayed. The acute complications are related to the performance of the ERCP and stent insertion, and may include acute pancreatitis, cholangitis, acute cholecystitis, and bile duct and duodenal perforation. Delayed complications may also include acute cholecystitis and duodenal perforation, in addition to stent migration, fracture, and occlusion *(54–58)*.

Biliary sepsis is an acute and serious complication of ERCP with stent insertion. Current recommendations from the American Society for Gastrointestinal Endoscopy (ASGE) are for the administration of prophylactic antibiotics before ERCP is attempted in all patients with biliary obstruction *(59)*. However, other authorities argue for the selective use of antibiotics following ERCP procedures in which adequate biliary drainage has not been achieved *(60)*. A prospective, randomized controlled study has not been done comparing these two strategies. However, it is crucial to remember that contrast should not be injected into an obstructed duct that is subsequently left undrained because there is a very high risk of cholangitis occurring in this segment. Hence, the endoscopist performing the procedure must be capable of both diagnostic and therapeutic ERCP. If cholangitis does develop following stent insertion, then the obstructed ductal system must be drained in a prompt and efficacious manner. In most cases, this will require a repeat ERCP, both for diagnostic localization of the undrained segment(s) and for therapeutic drainage. Occasionally, biliary drainage may need to be provided by the percutaneous transhepatic route or the combined percutaneous–endoscopic route (so-called "rendez-vous" technique) *(61)*.

Plastic stent migration is a complication that is encountered with an incidence of approx 5%. In particular, it should be thought of if jaundice recurs soon after stent placement. Migration can occur either proximally or distally. Factors that appear to favor stent migration include larger diameter stents, proximal bile duct strictures, and whether a sphincterotomy was performed for stent placement *(56)*. Various endoscopic techniques have been used to retrieve proximally migrated stents, with a success rate in the range of 86% *(62)*.

Stent occlusion is a delayed complication that can occur with both plastic and metallic endoprostheses. In general, the expandable metallic endoprostheses occlude less readily, and, consequently, there is less need for endoscopic intervention *(33,47,48)*. Occlusion also occurs by different mechanisms: plastic stents tend to occlude with biliary sludge; metallic stents tend to occlude by either tumor ingrowth or overgrowth. The management of stent occlusion depends on whether the stent is plastic or metal. In general, occluded plastic stents can be easily dealt with endoscopically by repeat ERCP and stent replacement. The occluded stent can be removed with a snare or basket, or by using guidewire-assisted techniques (as above). The latter method is particularly useful when a tight, complex stricture is anticipated, based on the prior ERCP, because it allows maintenance of biliary access via the guidewire *(34,63–65)*. It is important to measure the length of the stricture again, because a longer stent may be needed. On the other hand, the currently available metallic stents should be considered permanent, and, as such, cannot be removed when occluded. Different methods can be used to treat occluded metallic stents, depending on the nature of the occlusion *(66)*. If the occlusion is from tumor ingrowth or overgrowth, then another stent (either plastic or metal) can be placed inside the lumen of the first (Fig. 5). If the occlusion is from sludge (uncommon), then a balloon can be used to clean the lumen of the stent.

ENDOSCOPIC VS SURGICAL PALLIATION OF MALIGNANT OBSTRUCTIVE JAUNDICE

Surgical resection with or without adjuvant therapy is the only treatment with the potential for cure in the patient who presents with obstructive jaundice secondary to pancreatic malignancy. Thus, all patients should be initially considered for surgery, but most will either have advanced disease, or be medically unfit for major surgery. Occasionally, the pancreatic malignancy is found early, i.e., a 2-cm diameter tumor localized to the head of the pancreas. In the latter scenario, surgical resection should be the treatment of choice, unless the patient has serious co-morbid disease, refuses surgery, or is otherwise medically unfit for surgery.

In the majority of patients in whom palliation is the focus, endoscopic, percutaneous transhepatic, and surgical options should be considered. The decision process should involve a multidisciplinary team approach, and include the gastroenterologist, surgeon, interventional radiologist, and oncologist. In addition to the available expertise, other factors important to consider include: the biological age of the patient and co-morbid diseases, the site of biliary obstruction, coexisting duodenal obstruction, and the preference of the informed patient. In a young patient, a trial of surgery is often undertaken, in the absence of unfavorable features in preoperative imaging, because sur-

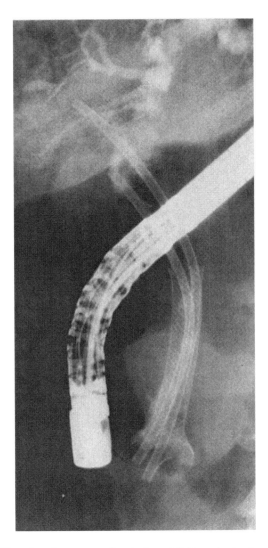

Fig. 5. Post-ERC film showing two polyethylene 10-French stents placed through an occluded Wallstent previously placed endoscopically.

gical resection gives the only potential for cure. In metastatic lesions involving the hilum of the liver, it is still unclear whether endoscopic or percutaneous transhepatic drainage is the optimal mode of treatment. Surgical bypass is usually technically difficult in this situation. In general, if there is combined biliary and duodenal obstruction and the patient is an operative candidate, surgical palliation should be recommended. The technique of placement of expandable metallic stents in both the bile duct and duodenum (endoscopic double-bypass), however, is being developed.

Two randomized trials have compared endoscopic plastic stent placement vs surgical palliation in the management of malignant obstructive jaundice mainly caused by pancreatic cancer *(5,8)*. The success rate in relieving jaundice was similar in both

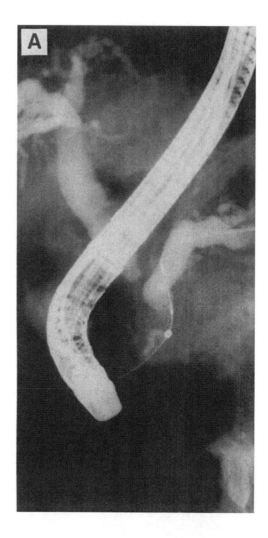

Fig. 6. ERCP sequence showing **(A)** Brush cytology obstructing main pancreatic duct stricture in the head; **(B)** guidewire placement across stricture, and insertion of 7-French polyethylene pancreatic duct stent; **(C)** final position of stent across malignant stricture (cytology positive.)

groups (approx 90%). However, there was a significantly higher morbidity procedure-related mortality, 30-d mortality, and longer initial hospital stay in the group treated by surgical bypass. Nevertheless, the endoscopy group had a higher rate of subsequent duodenal obstruction (but under 10%), and needed more frequent admissions for stent exchange because of occlusion. Overall, the length of survival was similar in both groups. Although patient and physician preference is important, cost analysis would appear to favor the endoscopic approach *(4)*. With the development of expandable metallic endoprostheses, the endoscopic double-bypass procedure, and advances in laparoscopic techniques for bilioenteric bypass, the management algorithm will need to be re-examined in appropriate designed, prospective trials.

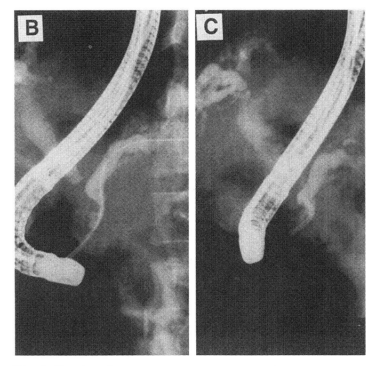

Fig. 6. (Continued)

PALLIATION OF OBSTRUCTIVE-TYPE PANCREATIC PAIN

Abdominal pain is a common symptom in pancreatic malignancy. Its cause is multifactorial; possible mechanisms are neural tumor infiltration, increased parenchymal pressure secondary to pancreatic duct obstruction, superimposed pancreatic inflammation, and biliary-type pain secondary to biliary obstruction.

The authors and others *(67)* have attempted to identify those patients with obstructive symptoms not responding to analgesia, who might benefit from pancreatic ductal drainage. Placement of 5 or 7-French-gage pancreatic stents across the malignant stricture in such patients has produced impressive alleviation of pain *(67)*, with prolonged benefit in 75% of patients. In a series of seven patients in whom the authors placed either plastic or expandable metallic stents across the malignant pancreatic duct stricture (Fig. 6), they have similarly demonstrated successful relief of pain in this patient group. Patients should be selected based either on a clinical history of obstructive pancreatic pain, that is, intermittent pain, or overt pancreatitis following the ingestion of food. However, greater experience is needed before the role of pancreatic duct stenting for this indication is established.

METALLIC STENTS FOR GASTRIC OUTLET OBSTRUCTION

The traditional method for treating gastric outlet obstruction caused by duodenal invasion with pancreatic cancer has been by surgical gastroenterostomy. However, this carries with it a morbidity of up to 30% *(68)*. Moreover, one retrospective study concluded that, in patients with pancreatic cancer presenting with luminal obstructive

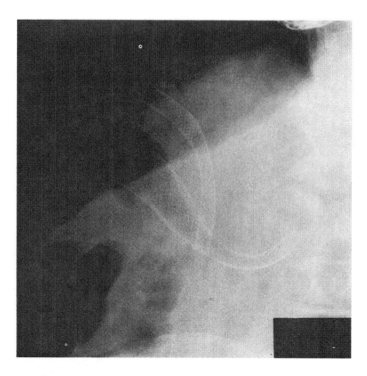

Fig. 7. Post-ERCP radiograph showing 10 × 80 biliary Wallstent placed across a malignant biliary stricture from pancreatic cancer involvement, with the distal end of the stent across the papilla and two 22-mm enteral Wallstents overlapped to bridge a long malignant stenosis of the first, second, and third parts of the duodenum, with the proximal end (fully expanded) within the gastric antrum.

symptoms such as nausea and vomiting, only 10% of such patients had a "good" outcome *(69)*. Hence, less invasive approaches have been sought for this group of patients with advanced disease. One promising option is the placement of expandable metallic endoprostheses across the area of duodenal obstruction *(70)*. Initially, this was accomplished by inserting a biliary metallic stent via a percutaneous endoscopic gastrostomy, because the stent delivery system was not long enough to use endoscopically *(71)*. The authors have had early experience using specially designed Wallstents of 16-mm diameter and 60–90 mm in length (Fig. 7). Thus far, good results have been obtained in 11 of 13 patients. In the two patients in which the stent failed, both had their stricture length underestimated by measurement under fluoroscopy. In the authors' experience, the most difficult aspects of stent deployment are accurate measurement of the length of the malignant stricture and the correct positioning of the stent across the stricture. The latter is particularly important, because the Wallstent is designed to shorten by 30% upon deployment. Improved methods need to be developed for placement of these types of stents. For instance, one recent study used a plastic overtube to stabilize the stent as it tranversed the gastric cavity *(72)*. Although the preliminary results are encouraging with duodenal metal stents, more experience and long-term assessment are required before it can be recommended.

CONCLUSION

The minimally invasive approach of endoscopic stenting has revolutionized the palliative management of malignant biliary obstruction caused by pancreatic carcinoma. It has enabled patients to experience a shorter index hospital stay, a lower 30-d mortality rate, and is cost-effective when compared to traditional surgical palliation. The advent of expandable metallic endoprostheses has tipped the equation even more in favor of endoscopic management. In addition, the possibilities of a double-bypass procedure, and of ameliorating refractory obstructive-type pancreatic pain, holds great promise. Nevertheless, corresponding advances are being made in hepatobiliary surgery and in percutaneous transhepatic intervention. Thus, there is a great need for prospective randomized trials comparing these innovative developments, in order to define the optimal palliative management of pancreatic carcinoma.

REFERENCES

1. Cotton PB. Endoscopic methods for relief of malignant obstructive jaundice. World J Surg 1984; *8:*854–861.
2. Huibregtse K, Katon RM, Coene PP, and Tytgat GNJ. Endoscopic palliative treatment in pancreatic cancer. Gastrointest Endosc 1986; *32:*334–338.
3. Siegel JH and Snady H. The significance of endoscopically placed prostheses in the management of biliary obstruction due to carcinoma of the pancreas: results of nonoperative decompression in 277 patients. Am J Gastroenterol 1986; *81:*634–641.
4. Brandabur JJ, Kozarek RA, Ball TJ, Hofer BO, Ryan JA, Traverso LW, Freeny PC, and Lewis GP. Nonoperative versus operative treatment of obstructive jaundice in pancreatic cancer: cost and survival analysis. Am J Gastroenterol 1988; *83:*1132–1139.
5. Sheperd HA, Royle G, Ross APR, Diba A, Arthur M, and Colin-Jones D. Endoscopic biliary endoprosthesis in the palliation of malignant obstruction of the distal common bile duct—a randomized trial. Br J Surg 1988; *75:*1166–1168.
6. Deviere J, Baize M, DeToeuf J, and Cremer M. Long-term follow-up of patients with hilar malignant stricture treated by endoscopic internal biliary drainage. Gastrointest Endosc 1988; *34:*95–101.
7. Andersen JR, Sorensen SM, Kruse A, Rokkjaer M, and Matzen P. Randomized trial of endoscopic endoprosthesis versus operative bypass in malignant obstructive jaundice. Gut 1989; *30:*1132–1135.
8. Dowsett JF, Russell RCG, Hatfield ARW, Cotton PB, Speer AG, Houghton J, et al. Malignant obstructive jaundice: What is the best management? A prospective randomized trial of surgery vs endoscopic stenting. Gut 1989; *30:*128.
9. Cullingford GL, Srinivasan R, and Carr-Locke DL. Endoscopic endoprosthesis for malignant biliary obstruction. Gut 1989; *30:*A1458.
10. Mizuma Y, Ikeda E, Mukai H, Yasuda K, and Nakajima M. ERBD vs PTBD in the management of inoperable malignant obstructive jaundice. Gastroenterol 1992; *102:*A323.
11. Boender J, Nix GA, Schutte HE, Lameris JS, van Blankenstein M, and Dees J. Malignant common bile duct obstruction: factors influencing the success rate of endoscopic drainage. Endoscopy 1992; *22:*259–262.
12. Marsh WH and Cunningham JT. Endoscopic stent placement for obstructive jaundice secondary to metastatic malignancy. Am J Gastroenterol 1992; *87:*985–990.
13. Motte S, Deviere J, Dumonceau J-M, Serruys E, Thys J-P, and Cremer M. Risk factors for septicemia following endoscopic biliary stenting. Gastroenterology 1991; *101:*1374–1381.
14. Frakes JT, Johanson JF, and Stake JJ. Optimal timing for stent replacement in malignant biliary tract obstruction. Gastrointest Endosc 1993; *39:*164–167.

15. Ferrari AP, Lichtenstein DR, Slivka A, Chang C, and Carr-Locke DL. Brush cytology during ERCP for the diagnosis of biliary and pancreatic malignancies. Gastrointest Endosc 1994; *40:*140–145.

16. Foutch PG, Kerr DM, Harlan JR, Manne RK, Kummet TD, and Sanowski RA. Endoscopic retrograde wire-guided brush cytology for diagnosis of patients with malignant obstruction of the bile duct. Am J Gastroenterol 1990; *85:*791–795.

17. Venu RP, Geenen JE, Kini M, Hogan WJ, Payne M, Johnson GK, and Schmalz MJ. Endoscopic retrograde brush cytology: a new technique. Gastroenterology 1990; *99:*475–479.

18. Kubota Y, Takaoka M, and Tani K. Endoscopic transpapillary biopsy for diagnosis of patients with pancreaticobiliary ductal strictures. Am J Gastroenterol 1993; *88:*1700–1704.

19. Howell DA, Beveridge RP, Bosco J, and Jones M. Endoscopic needle aspiration biopsy at ERCP in the diagnosis of biliary strictures. Gastrointest Endosc 1992; *38:*531–535.

20. Kadakia SC and Starnes E. Comparison of 10 French gauge stent with 11.5 French gauge stent in patients with biliary tract diseases. Gastrointest Endosc 1992; *38:*454–459.

21. Slivka A. Directed guide wire placement during ERCP using a papillotome. Gastrointest Endosc 1996; *44:*187–189.

22. Leung JWC, Ling TKW, Kung JLS, and Vallance-Owen J. The role of bacteria in the blockage of biliary stents. Gastrointest Endosc 1988; *34:*19–22.

23. Huibregtse K. Endoscopic biliary and pancreatic drainage, Georg Thieme Veriag, Stuttgart, 1988.

24. Speer AG, Cotton PB, Rhode J, Seddon AM, Neal CR, Holton J, and Costerton JW. Biliary stent blockage with bacterial biofilm. Ann Intern Med 1988; *108:*546–553.

25. Speer AG, Cotton PB, and MacRae KD. Endoscopic management of malignant biliary obstruction: stents of 10 French gauge are preferable to stents of 8 French gauge. Gastrointest Endosc 1988; *34:*412–417.

26. Coene PPLO. Endoscopic biliary stenting: Mechanisms and possible solutions of the clogging phenomenon. MD Thesis. CIP-DATA Koninklijke Bibliotheek den Haag, 1990.

27. Sung JY, Shaffer EA, Lam K, and Costerton JW. Inhibition of *E. coli* adhesion on biliary stents by bile salts with different hydrobicites. Gastrointest Endosc 1992; *38:*263.

28. Hurwich DB, Poterucha JJ, Nixon DE, Cockerill FR, Moyer TP, and Thistle JL. Preventing biliary stent occlusion. Gastrointest Endosc 1992; *38:*268.

29. Seitz U, Vadeyar H, and Soehendra N. Prolonged patency with a new-design Teflon biliary prosthesis. Endoscopy 1994; *26:*478–482.

30. Johanson JF and Frakes JT. Optimal timing for stent replacement in malignant biliary strictures. Gastrointest Endosc 1992; *38:*254.

31. Cessot F, Sauterau D, Le Sidaner A, Moesch C, Berry P, Florence J, Deviois B, and Pillegand B. Obstruction delay of biliary endoprostheses. Gastroenterol 1992; *102:*A304.

32. Soehendra N. A new method for exchanging biliary stents. Endoscopy 1990; *22:*271–272.

33. Knyrim K, Wagner HJ, Pausch J, and Vakil N. A prospective, randomized, controlled trial of metal stents for malignant obstruction of the common bile duct. Endoscopy 1993; *25:*207–212.

34. Tarnasky PR, Morris J, Hawes RH, Hoffman BJ, Cotton PB, and Cunningham JT. Snare beside-a-wire biliary stent exchange: a method that maintains access across biliary strictures. Gastrointest Endosc 1996; *44:*185–187.

35. Yoshioka T, Sakaguchi H, Yoshimura H, Tamada T, Ohishi H, Uchida H, and Wallace S. Expandable metallic biliary endoprostheses: preliminary clinical evaluation. Radiology 1990; *177:*253–257.

36. Lammer J. Biliary endoprothesis, plastic versus metal stents. Radiol Clin North Am 1990; *28:*1211–1222.

37. Kozarek RA, Ball TJ, and Patterson DJ. Metallic self-expanding stent application in the upper gastrointestinal tract: caveats and concerns. Gastrointest Endosc 1992; *38:*1–6.

38. Salomonowitz EK, Antonucci F, Heer M, Stuckmann G, Egloff B, and Zollikofer CL. Biliary obstruction: treatment with self-expanding metal prostheses. J Vasc Interv Radiol 1992; *3:*365–370.
39. Jackson JE, Roddie ME, Chetty N, Benjamin IS, and Adam A. The management of occluded metallic self-expandable biliary endoprostheses. Am J Roentgenol 1991; *157:*291–292.
40. Shim CS, Lee MS, Kim JH, and Cho SW. Endoscopic application of Gianturco-Rosch biliary Z-stent. Endoscopy 1992; *24:*436–439.
41. Neuhaus H, Hagenmuller F, and Classen M. Self-expanding biliary stents, preliminary clinical experience. Endoscopy 1989; *21:*225–228.
42. Nicholson DA, Chetty N, Jackson JE, Roddie ME, and Adam A. Patency of side branches after peripheral placement of metallic biliary endoprostheses. J Vasc Interv Radiol 1992; *3:*127–130.
43. Kawase Y, Takemura T, and Hashimoto T. Endoscopic implantation of expandable metal Z stents for malignant biliary strictures. Gastrointest Endosc 1993; *39:*65–67.
44. Bethge N, Wagner HJ, Knyrim K, Zimmerman HB, Starck E, Pausch J, and Vakil N. Technical failure of biliary metal stent deployment in a series of 116 applications. Endoscopy 1992; *24:*395–400.
45. Huibregtse K, Carr-Locke DL, Cremer M, Domschke W, Fockens P, Foerster E, et al. Biliary stent occlusion: a problem solved with self-expanding metal stents? Endoscopy 1992; *24:*391–394.
46. Cotton PB. Metallic mesh stents: Is the expanse worth the expense? Endoscopy 1992; *24:*421–423.
47. Carr-Locke DL, Ball TJ, Connors PJ, Cotton PB, Geenen JE, Hawes RH, et al. Multicenter randomized trial of Wallstent biliary endoprosthesis versus plastic stents. Gastrointest Endosc 1993; *39:*A310.
48. Davids PHP, Groen AK, Rauws EAJ, Tytgat GNJ, and Huibregtse K. Randomized trial of self-expanding metal stents versus polyethylene stents for distal malignant biliary obstruction. Lancet 1992; *340:*1488–1492.
49. Cremer M, Deviere J, Sugai B, and Baize M. Expandable biliary metal stents for malignancies: endoscopic insertion and diathermic cleaning for tumor ingrowth. Gastrointest Endosc 1990; *36:*451–457.
50. Dertinger S, Ell C, Fleig WE, Hóchberger J, Karn M, Gurza L, and Hahn EG. Long-term results using self-expanding metal stents for malignant biliary obstruction. Gastroenterol 1992; *102:*A310.
51. Sievert CE, Silvis SE, Vennes JA, Abeyta B, and Brennecke LH. Comparison of covered vs uncovered wire stents in the canine biliary tract. Gastrointest Endosc 1992; *38:*A262.
52. Goldin E, Wengrower D, Fich A, Safra T, Verstandig A, Globerman O, and Beyar M. A new self-expandable and removable metal stent for biliary obstruction. Gastrointest Endosc 1992; *38:*A251.
53. Bethge N, Sommer A, Gross U, von Kleist D, and Vakil N. Human tissue responses to metal stents implanted in vivo for the palliation of malignant stenoses. Gastrointest Endosc 1996; *43:*596–602.
54. Leung JWC, Chung SCS, Sung JY, and Li MKW. Acute cholecystitis after stenting of the common bile duct for obstruction secondary to pancreatic cancer. Gastrointest Endosc 1989; *35:*109–110.
55. Gould J, Train JS, Dan SJ, and Mitty HA. Duodenal perforation as a delayed complication of placement of a biliary endoprosthesis. Radiology 1988; *167:*467–469.
56. Johanson JF, Schmaltz MJ, and Geenen JE. Incidence and risk factors for biliary and pancreatic stent migration. Gastrointest Endosc 1992; *38:*341–346.
57. Matsuda Y, Shimakura K, and Akamatsu T. Factors affecting the patency of stents in malignant biliary obstructive disease: univariate and multivariate analysis. Am J Gastroenterol 1991; *86:*843–849.

58. Mallat A, Saint-Marc Girardin MF, Meduri B, Liguory C, and Dhumeaux D. Fracture of biliary endoprosthesis after endoscopic drainage for malignant biliary obstruction. Report of two cases. Endoscopy 1986; *18:*243–244.

59. ASGE Report. Antibiotic prophylaxis for gastrointestinal endoscopy. Gastrointest Endosc 1995; *42:*630–635.

60. Vandervoort J, Tham TCK, Wong RCK, Lichtenstein DR, Van Dam J, Ruymann F, Hughes M, and Carr-Locke DL. Is there a need for prophylactic antibiotics prior to ERCP for suspected bile duct obstruction? Gastrointest Endosc 1996; *43:*323.

61. Hall RI, Denyer ME, and Chapman AH. Palliation of obstructive jaundice with a biliary endoprosthesis. Comparison of insertion by the percutaneous–transhepatic and the combined percutaneous–endoscopic routes. Interv Radiol 1989; *40:*186–189.

62. Tarnasky PR, Cotton PB, Baillie J, Branch MS, Affronti J, Jowell P, et al. Proximal migration of biliary stents: attempted endoscopic retrieval in forty-one patients. Gastrointest Endosc 1995; *42:*513–519.

63. Martin DF. Wire guided balloon assisted endoscopic biliary stent exchange. Gut 1991; *32:*1562–1564.

64. Sherman S, Hawes RH, Uzer MF, Smith MT, and Lehman GA. Endoscopic stent exchange using a guide wire and mini-snare. Gastrointest Endosc 1993; *39:*794–799.

65. Soehendra N, Maydeo A, Eckmann B, Bruckner M, Nam VC, and Grimm H. A new technique for replacing an obstructed biliary endoprosthesis. Endoscopy 1990; 22:271–272.

66. Tham TCK, Vandervoort J, Wong RCK, Carr-Locke DL, Chow S, Bosco JJ, et al. Management of occluded biliary Wallstents. Gastrointest Endosc 1996; *43:*400.

67. Costamagna G, Gabbrielle A, Mutignani M, Perri V, and Crucitti F. Treatment of obstructive pain by endoscopic drainage in patients with pancreatic head carcinoma. Gastrointest Endosc 1993; *39:*774–777.

68. Sarr MG, Gladen HE, Beart RW, Jr., and van Heerden JA. Role of gastroenterostomy in patients with unresectable carcinoma of the pancreas. Surg Gyn Obstet 1981; *152:*597–600.

69. Weaver DW, Wiencek RG, Bouwman DL, and Walt AJ. Gastrojejunostomy: Is it helpful for patients with pancreatic cancer? Surgery 1987; *102:*608–613.

70. Kozarek RA, Ball TJ, and Patterson DJ. Metallic self-expanding stent application in the upper gastrointestinal tract: caveats and concerns. Gastrointest Endosc 1992; *38:*1–6.

71. Keymling M, Wagner H-J, Vakil N, and Knyrim K. Relief of malignant duodenal obstruction by percutaneous insertion of a metal stent. Gastrointest Endosc 1993; *39:*439–441.

72. Feretis C, Benakis P, Dimopoulos C, Georgopoulos K, Milas F, Manouras A, and Apostolidis N. Palliation of malignant gastric outlet obstruction with self-expanding metal stents. Endoscopy 1996; *28:*225–228.

14

Laparoscopic Biliary and Gastric Bypass

Kevin C. Conlon and Stanley W. Ashley

INTRODUCTION

In the United States, pancreatic cancer is the fourth leading cause of cancer death in men and the fifth in women *(1)*. It is estimated that, in 1998, 27,600 new cases will be diagnosed, with the majority dying of their disease *(2)*. In spite of some recent progress in diagnosis and treatment, the outlook for the majority of patients remains bleak.

Adenocarcinoma accounts for more than 90% of pancreatic tumors, and is a particularly aggressive lesion; at the time of diagnosis, the tumor is confined to the pancreas in fewer than 10% of patients, 40% have locally advanced disease, and over 50% have distant spread *(3,4)*. More than 95% of patients eventually die of their disease, most within the first year *(5)*. Radiation and chemotherapy have been shown to be of only marginal benefit *(6,7)*; the primary mode of therapy continues to be surgical resection *(8)*. However, only 20–25% of patients actually prove to have resectable disease at the time of exploration.

Resectability is determined based on the presence or absence of distant metastases and local invasion of the major retroperitoneal vascular structures, particularly the portal and superior mesenteric veins and the superior mesenteric artery. It has been reported that resectability can be determined with an accuracy of 90% using the combination of abdominal computerized tomography (CT), angiography, and laparoscopy *(9)*.

In fact, it has been suggested that, even with a negative CT scan, 40% of patients have small hepatic or omental metastases that can be visualized laparoscopically, although this study was reported before the advent of the most recent generation spiral CT scanners or endoscopic ultrasound *(9)*. However, a recent prospective study from Memorial Sloan-Kettering Cancer Center likewise demonstrated that the combination of a contrast-enhanced CT scan and laparoscopy could accurately predict resectability in over 90% of patients, thus sparing a significant proportion of patients unnecessary surgery, while not precluding potentially curative surgery to those who would benefit *(10)*. Recently refined techniques of endoscopic biliary stenting have made preoperative determinations of resectability more desirable; however, there continue to be prob-

253

lems with gastric outlet obstruction, requiring rehospitalization, and, sometimes, operation *(11)*.

Obstructive jaundice develops in about 70% of patients with pancreatic cancer at some time in their course, and there are several reasons to relieve it *(4)*. Biliary obstruction impairs liver function and may lead to frank hepatic failure. Ten percent of patients develop cholangitis. Anorexia and malabsorption may also ensue. Approximately 25% of patients develop pruritus, which is often impossible to relieve medically. There are a number of surgical options for drainage of the biliary tree *(4)*. A T-tube placed in the common duct effectively relieves the obstruction, but fluid and electrolyte losses are difficult to manage, and patients are seldom satisfied with an external biliary fistula. Despite extensive controversy in the literature *(11)*, both cholecysto- and choledochoenteric bypasses, if selected appropriately, have comparable results regarding reducing serum bilirubin. In a recent analysis of the Memorial Sloan-Kettering experience *(12)*, the authors were unable to demonstrate any differences between these two methods. Cholecystojejunostomy is simpler if the cystic duct is patent and enters the bile duct away from the tumor. This is usually the case, and can be confirmed by cholangiography at the time of operation. Roux-en-Y jejunostomy is theoretically better than a simple loop, because it prevents reflux of intestinal contents into the biliary tree. However, this has never been clearly demonstrated to be of any consequence, and, since most of these patients die within 8 mo, a simpler loop reconstruction is usually performed. Jaundice is effectively relieved in 85–90% of patients *(4)*.

Duodenal obstruction develops in 30–40% of patients with pancreatic cancer at sometime in their course, and is effectively relieved by a gastrojejunostomy in most patients *(5)*. The value of gastrojejunostomy as a prophylactic measure in the patient who has not yet developed clinical evidence of such obstruction continues to be debated; however, there is no evidence to suggest that the morbidity or mortality rates of the biliary bypass alone are increased when gastrojejunostomy is performed as either a therapeutic or prophylactic measure.

Rationale for Laparoscopic Bypass

Although these palliative procedures are relatively minor operations, because of the debilitated state of the patients, there is major morbidity in 30–40% and mortality in 15–20% *(4,5,10,11)*. It is the authors' clinical impression that, particularly after a complicated postoperative course, some patients never regain their preoperative performance status, and commence a slow inexorable slide in their quality of life (QOL) until death. Minimal access surgery offers a new approach to this problem, in theory, at least, associated with decreased surgical morbidity, reduced hospital stay, shorter recovery, and potentially improved QOL. Laparoscopy as an initial step permits the identification of patients with small metastases precluding curative resection, who are not identified by abdominal CT, and who then are candidates for laparoscopic bypass. If metastases are identified, the patency of the cystic duct may be assessed by laparoscope-directed cholangiography through the gallbladder wall, or by laparoscopic ultrasonography, and then bypass may be performed. Patients who are not candidates for laparoscopic bypass could be converted to open laparotomy, at which time a choledochojejunostomy would be performed.

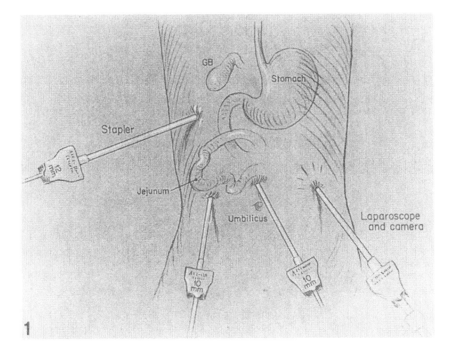

Fig. 1. Schematic diagram showing the sites for placement of the trocars, laparoscope, and stapler. GB, gallbladder. (Used, with permission from ref. *14.*)

ANIMAL EXPERIENCE

Nathanson and coworkers *(13)* reported the first series of animal experiments designed to test the feasibility of laparoscopic bypass in an animal model. They utilized a sutured cholecytojejunostomy in six pigs, five of whom subsequently underwent ligation of their common bile ducts. In all cases, at 4 wk following the procedure, the bilioenteric anastomosis was noted to be patent and the bilirubin was <5 mol/L.

The authors recently examined the combined operation in the porcine model *(14)*. The purpose of the study was to determine the feasibility of laparoscopic double bypass regarding safety and operating time. We also compared stapled and sutured anastomoses.

Methods

Animals were fasted preoperatively and liver function tests were obtained. After induction of anesthesia, the pigs were placed in Trendelburg position, a Veress needle was inserted, and the abdomen insufflated to a pressure of 12–14 mmHg with CO_2. After removal of the needle, an 11-mm trocar was introduced in the left linea semilunaris at the level of the infracostal margin (Fig. 1). The laparoscope was inserted and a complete inspection of the abdomen was performed. The animals were then placed in reverse Trendelenburg position and two more trocars (10-mm) were placed, under direct vision, in the right linea semilunaris and in the midline at the level of the infracostal margin. A fourth trocar (12-mm) was inserted just below the junction of the right costal margin for insertion of the ENDOGIA stapler (Autosuture).

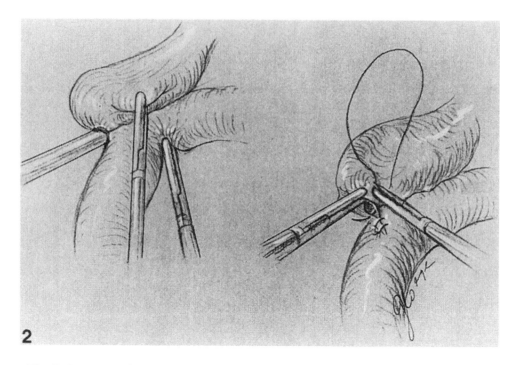

Fig. 2. Laparoscopic cholecystojejunsotomy. The stapled anastomosis was created by passing the stapler through the right lateral port. The anastomosis was created with jejunum distal to the gastrojejunostomy. (Used with permission from ref. *14*.)

An initial laparoscopic examination was performed to assess the liver, gallbladder, pancreas, and peritoneal cavity. To simulate the demonstration of cystic duct patency, the gallbladder was grasped and elevated. Using the laparoscopic aspirator needle, the fundus was punctured and the bile suctioned. Approximately 25 cc of half-strength Hypaque was injected and a cholangiogram was obtained using the fluoroscopic C arm.

Johann atraumatic forceps (Micro-France) were introduced, and the entire small bowel was examined, beginning at the ileocecal valve. This procedure was necessary in order to choose the most appropriate position for the cholecystojejustomy. The fundus of the gallbladder was grasped and elevated, and a loop of jejunum, approx 40 cm distal to the ligament of Treitz, was brought up and approximated to the gallbladder with two stay sutures of 2–0 silk on either side of the projected line of anastomosis. The intention was that the anastomosis be approx 3 cm in diameter. For the hand-sutured anastomoses, enterotomies were made in both the jejunum and gallbladder, parallel to the projected line of anastomosis. The cholecytojejunostomy was created using a continuous 3–0 absorbable suture. For the stapled anastomoses, enterotomies were made at the medial end of the projected line of anastomosis in both the jejunum and gallbladder. The 3-cm ENDOGIA stapler was introduced into the enterotomies and the anastomosis was created with single cartridge. The stapler was then removed and the resulting defect was closed with a continuous 3–0 absorbable suture tied intracorporeally (Fig. 2).

Attention was then directed to the gastrojejunostomy (Fig. 3). A dependent position on the anterior surface of the stomach near the greater curvature was identified and a

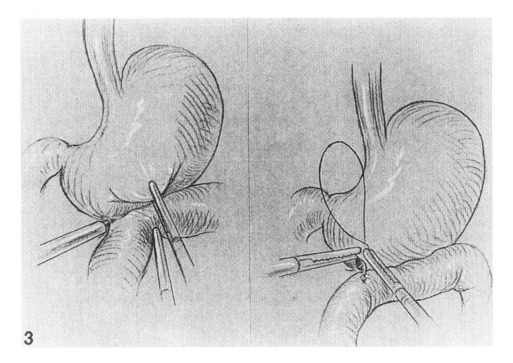

Fig. 3. Laparoscopic gastrojejunsotomy. The stapled anastomosis was created by passing the stapler again through the right lateral port. The enterotomy was then closed using a continuous suture. (Used with permission from ref. *14.*)

loop of jejunum, 10 cm long, located 20 cm distal to the ligament of Trietz, was brought up in an antecolic, isoperistaltic fashion, so that there was no tension on the biliary anastomosis. Again, after placement of two stay sutures on either end of the projected line of anastomosis, enterotomies were made in both the jejunum and stomach, and an approx 3-cm diameter anastomosis was created. Side-to-side gastrojejunostomy was performed, using either a handsewn, continuous 3-0 suture or a combination of stapling with suture, to close the enterotomies. In the latter technique, the 3-cm ENDOGIA stapler was introduced and used to create the anastomosis, using a single cartridge. The stapler was then removed and the resulting defect was closed with a continuous absorbable suture, tied intracorporeally.

Following completion of the anastomoses, a No. 10 Jackson-Pratt closed suction drain was placed through the medial trocar site and positioned in close proximity to the biliary and gastric anastomoses. The abdomen was irrigated with heparinized saline and partially desufflated. The trocar sites were then examined for evidence of bleeding and the remainder of the gas was removed. After the trocars were taken out, the fascia at the larger sites was approximated with figure-of-eight sutures, and the skin was closed in a subcuticular fashion. Total operating time was noted at the end of each case.

Results

Animals were allowed free access to water immediately and were given a regular diet beginning on the second postoperative day. The drains were removed when the quantity was <25 cc/d. At 1 mo postoperatively, all animals were sedated, weighed,

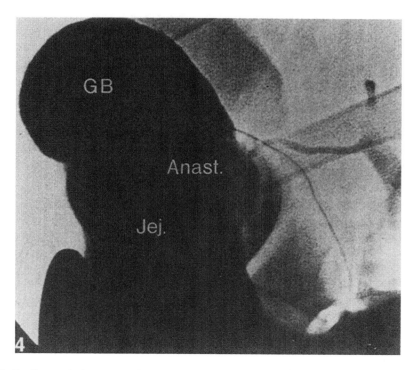

Fig. 4. Radiograph demonstrating patency of the cholecystojejunostomy 1 mo postoperatively. Contrast was injected through a catheter in the efferent limb. Anast., anastomosis; Jej., jejunum; GB, gallbladder. (Used with permission from ref. *14*.)

and blood was drawn for liver function tests. The animals were then sacrificed, and, after laparotomy, a catheter was placed in the efferent limb, the afferent limb was occluded, and contrast was injected to demonstrate the patency of the anastomoses.

Mean operating time was 199 ± 18 min, and was significantly less for the stapled vs handsewn technique (150 ± 21 vs 230 ± 13 min, $p < 0.05$). A closed suction drain was placed near the anastomosis and drained a total of 26 ± 7 cc; in four, this was bilious, but all cleared by postoperative d 5. All pigs recovered completely and were given free access to water 2 h after the operative procedure. Animals resumed a regular diet on postoperative d 2. They did not require any postoperative analgesia.

At 1 mo postoperatively, there was no significant change in the animals' weight as a result of the procedure (63 ± 3 preop vs 66 ± 4 kg at sacrifice). Likewise, there was no significant difference in liver function tests pre- and postoperatively (bilirubin, 0.2 ± 0.2 vs 0.3 ± 0.3 mg/dL; alkaline phosphatase, 39 ± 3 vs 41 ± 9 IU/L; SGOT, 35 ± 5 vs 39 ± 8 IU/L). At necropsy, all anastomoses appeared to be grossly and radiographically patent (Figs. 4 and 5), although three of the gastrojejunostomies (two stapled, one handsewn anastomosis) were significantly narrowed (arbitrarily defined as <1 cm in diameter); the authors believe that a 6-cm diameter anastomosis would prevent significant narrowing. This is supported by animal studies performed by Rhodes and colleagues *(15)*, who showed that there is a 0% anastomostic stricture formation at 12 wk if a 6-cm anastomosis is created. Two of the cholecytojejunostomies (one stapled, one handsewn anastomosis) were also <1 cm in these unobstructed animals; we

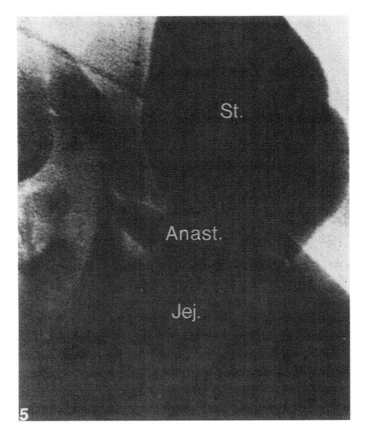

Fig. 5. Radiograph demonstrating patency of the gastrojejunostomy at 1 mo postoperatively. Contrast was injected through a catheter in the efferent limb. St., stomach. (Used, with permission, from ref. *14.*)

do not consider this to be significant, in view of the patency demonstrated both macroscopically and radiographically.

CLINICAL EXPERIENCE

In contrast to the voluminous literature concerned with open surgical approaches to biliary or gastric bypass in patients with unresectable pancreatic cancer, little has been written regarding the results of a laparoscopic approach. Most reports are anecdotal or contain limited numbers of patients.

Shimi and colleagues *(16)* from Dundee University, in 1992, were the first to report a series of biliary bypass procedures performed laparoscopically. They performed a cholecystojejunostomy in five patients with advanced cancer of the pancreas, using a similar technique developed in the animal model. Four patients had an excellent result, recovering from the procedure with minimal morbidity, and complete relief of their biliary obstruction. The remaining patient required further surgical intervention to clear an obstructed anastomosis. Nonetheless, the authors felt that this procedure had merit in selected patients and may avoid the hazards of endoscopic stenting, such as recur-

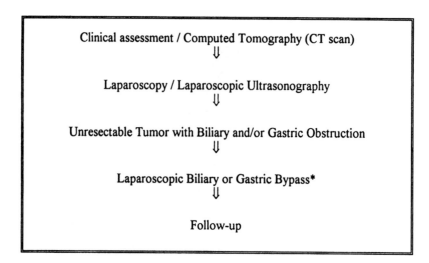

Clinical assessment / Computed Tomography (CT scan)
⇓

Laparoscopy / Laparoscopic Ultrasonography
⇓

Unresectable Tumor with Biliary and/or Gastric Obstruction
⇓

Laparoscopic Biliary or Gastric Bypass*
⇓

Follow-up

Fig. 6. Diagnostic and therapeutic algorithm for patients with unresectable pancreatic adenocarcinoma.

rent biliary obstruction or cholangitis. Fletcher and Jones, also in 1992, reported a case in which they had used the endoscopic linear stapler to construct the complete anastomosis *(17)*. At follow-up 1 mo after the procedure, the patient was neither icteric or symptomatic. Hawasli *(18)* described a similar technique in two patients, both of whom were discharged within 4 d following their procedure.

The first report of laparoscopic gastroenterostomy for malignant duodenal obstruction was by Wilson and Verma *(19)*. They reported on two cases in which duodenal obstruction was successfully relieved by means of an antecolic gastrojejunostomy. The nasogastric tube was removed on the first postoperative day and a regular diet was achieved by the fourth day. Rangraj and coworkers *(20)* reported a similar technique in 1994. In their case, they used the laparoscopic stapler to complete the entire anastomosis, rather than suturing the initial enterotomy/gastrotomy.

Memorial Sloan-Kettering Cancer Center Experience

At Memorial Hospital, laparoscopy is routinely performed prior to open exploration, for patients with potentially resectable tumors *(10,21)*. Under general anesthesia, a multiport technique, which mimics open exploration, is used. Patients with unresectable disease who have biliary or gastric obstruction are candidates for a laparoscopic bypass. Figure 6 illustrates the staging and therapeutic sequence.

Controversy exists concerning the utility of cholecystojejunostomy for biliary drainage. Based on a study by DiRooij and colleagues published from Memorial Sloan-Kettering Cancer Center in 1992 *(12)*, it is the authors' practice to perform a cholecystojejunostomy in selected patients. Patients with a patent cystic duct and at least 1-cm clearance from the upper extent of the tumor are candidates for this procedure. However, if at laparoscopy it is determined that a cholecystojejunostomy would not be appropriate (i.e., prior cholecystectomy, diseased gallbladder, blocked cystic duct, low insertion of cystic duct, or tumor encroachment on cystic duct or gallbladder), conversion to an open procedure will take place and a standard surgical bypass performed.

Surgical Technique

The patient is placed in 10° of reverse Trendelenberg position with 10° of left lateral tilt. The trocars used in the staging laparoscopy can be utilized. In order to accommodate a linear stapler, the right upper quadrant 10-mm trocar is converted into a 12-mm trocar.

A loop of jejunum approx 30 cm distal to the ligament of Treitz is selected and brought in an antecolic position to the gallbladder. Using an intracorporeal suturing technique, the jejunum is approximated to the gallbladder by two 3-0 coated, braided lactomer 9-1 sutures (Polysorb, U.S. Surgical, Norwalk, CT). Small incisions (0.5 mm) are made in the gallbladder and jejunum. Hemostasis is secured by electrocautery. Because of the increased intra-abdominal pressure, enteric leakage is minimal; however, any spillage can be dealt with by a suction device placed through the left upper quadrant port. An ENDOGIA 30-mm stapler (U.S. Surgical) is inserted through the 12-mm RUQ port, and manipulated into the gallbladder and jejunum. Often, this is difficult because of the proximity of the port site to the gallbladder. The stapler heads are approximated and the instrument fired. After removing the stapler, the anastomosis is inspected, hemostasis is confirmed, and the gallbladder interior aspirated and irrigated with saline.

The resultant enterotomy can be closed by using either a completely intracorporeal or laparoscopically assisted approach. Using an intracorporial technique, the defect is closed with a continuous seromuscular 3-0 coated, braided lactomer 9-1 suture, with knots tied using an intracorporeal technique. The laparoscopically assisted method is suitable in the thin patient. Two stay sutures are placed on either side of the anastomotic defect. These sutures are cut long. The 12-mm trocar is removed and the incision enlarged to 20 mm. Using retraction on the stay sutures, the newly created biliary–enteric anastomosis can be exteriorized and the enterotomy closed in a standard fashion. When this is completed, the bowel is returned to the abdominal cavity and the wound closed. The abdomen is reinsufflated and the anastomosis inspected. This technique allows for the construction of a 2.5-cm cholecystojejunal anastomosis without any bowel narrowing (Fig. 7). No intra-abdominal drains are used.

The technique for fashioning a gastrojejunostomy is similar. A proximal loop of jejunum is brought in an antecolic position to the stomach. The left upper quadrant 5-mm laparoscopic trocar is converted to a 12-mm trocar. Two 3-0 coated, braided lactomer 9-1 sutures (Polysorb; U.S. Surgical) are used to approximate the jejunum to the stomach. Enterotomies are made in both stomach and jejunum, an EndoGIA 30-mm stapler (U.S. Surgical) is inserted through the 12-mm LUQ port, and manipulated into both enterotomies. The instrument is positioned and fired. The stapler is removed and reloaded, being returned into the anastomosis and refired. This creates an anastomosis approx 5-cm in length. The anterior defect then can be closed in a fashion similar to the cholecystojejunostomy. Any defects in the anastomosis can be repaired with individual 3-0 sutures.

The authors have used the techniques described above in 12 patients with unresectable pancreatic cancer. There were six male and six female patients. The mean age was 60.8 yr (range, 35–80 yr). Five patients underwent a cholecystojejunostomy, two a gastrojejunostomy, and two received both a biliary and gastric bypass. Eleven patients

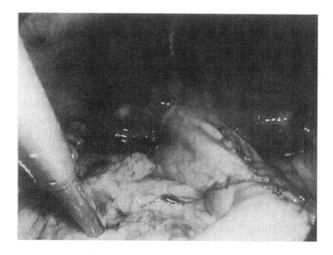

Fig. 7. Completed laparoscopic cholecystojejunostomy.

had a satisfactory result. In one patient with obstructive jaundice, who underwent a cholecystojejunostomy, bilirubin levels did not decrease postoperatively. An endoscopic stent was subsequently placed. The ERCP demonstrated a long biliary stricture with an occluded cystic duct. At the time of the original procedure, the cystic duct and common bile duct junction was not identified and laparoscopic ultrasonography was not available. None of the other patients required further intervention regarding biliary or gastric obstruction during their illness. The median survival for these patients was 8 mo.

CONCLUSION

The ideal palliative procedure for biliary or gastric obstruction should be effective in relieving jaundice or gastric outlet obstruction, have minimal morbidity, be associated with a short hospital stay, have a low symptomatic recurrence, and maintain quality of life. Animal experiments and preliminary clinical data suggest that laparoscopic procedures have the potential to achieve these goals. However, their true utility is currently undetermined and awaits the results of future clinical trials.

REFERENCES

1. Raijman I and Levin B. Exocrine tumors of the pancreas. In: Go VLW (eds). The pancreas: biology, pathobiology, and disease, 2-nd ed., Raven, New York, 1993; pp. 899–912.
2. Cancer facts and figures—1997. American Cancer Society, Atlanta, GA.
3. Singh SM and Reber HA. Surgical palliation for pancreatic cancer. Surg Clin N Am 1989; *69*:599–611.
4. Singh SM, Longmire WP, Jr., and Reber HA. Surgical palliation for pancreatic cancer. The UCLA experience. Ann Surg 1990; *212*:132–139.
5. Warshaw AL and Swanson RS. Pancreatic cancer in 1988. Possibilities and probabilities. Ann Surg 1988; *208*:541–553.
6. Gastrointestinal Tumor Study Group. Further evidence of effective adjuvant combined radiation and chemotherapy following curative resection of advanced pancreatic cancer. Cancer 1987; *59*:2006–2010.

7. Gastrointestinal Tumor Study Group. Treatment of locally unresectable carcinoma of the pancreas. Comparison of combined-modality therapy (chemotherapy plus radiotherapy) to chemotherapy alone. J Natl Cancer Inst 1988; *80:*751–755.

8. Warshaw AL, Gu GY, Wittenberg J, and Waxman AC. Preoperative staging and assessment of resectability of pancreatic cancer. Arch Surg 1990; *125:*230–233.

9. Warshaw AL, Tepper JE, and Shipley WU. Laparoscopy in the staging and planning of therapy for pancreatic cancer. Am J Surg 1986; *158:*76–80.

10. Conlon KC, Dougherty E, Klimstra DS, Coit DG, Turnbull ADM, and Brennan MF. The value of minimal access surgery in the staging of potentially resectable peri-pancreatic malignancy. Ann Surg 1996; *223:*134–140.

11. Watanapa P and Williamson RCN. Surgical palliation for pancreatic cancer: Developments during the past two decades. Br J Surg 1992; *79:*8–20.

12. DeRooij PD, Rogatko A, and Brennan MF. Evaluation of palliative surgical procedures in unresectable pancreatic cancer. Br J Surg 1991; *78:*1053–1058.

13. Nathanson LK, Shimi S, and Cuschieri A. Sutured laparoscopic cholecystojejunostomy evolved in a animal model. J R Coll Surg Edinburgh 1993; *37:*215–220.

14. Patel AG, McFadden DW, Hines OJ, Reber HA, and Ashley SW. Palliation for pancreatic cancer. Feasibility of laparoscopic cholecytojejunostomy and gastrojejunostomy in a porcine model. Surg Endosc 1996; *10:*639–643.

15. Rhodes M, Nathanson L, and Fielding G. Laparoscopic biliary and gastric bypass: a useful adjunct in the treatment of carcinoma of the pancreas. Gut 1990; *36:*778–780.

16. Shimi S., Banting S., and Cuschieri A. Laparoscopy in the management of pancreatic cancer: endoscopic cholecytojejunostomy for advanced disease. Br J Surg 1992; *79:*317–319.

17. Fletcher DR and Jones RM. Laparoscopic cholecystjejeunostomy as palliation for obstructive jaundice in inoperable carcinoma of the pancreas. Surg Endosc 1992; *6:*147–149.

18. Haswasli A. Laparoscopic cholecysto-jejunostomy for obstructing pancreatic cancer: technique and report of two cases. J Laparoendosc Surg 1992; 2:351–355.

19. Wilson RG and Varma JS. Laparoscopic gastroenterostomy for malignant duodenal obstruction. Br J Surg 1992; *79:*1348.

20. Rangraj MS, Mehta M, Zale G, Maffucci L, and Herz B. Laparoscopic gastrojejunostomy: a case presentation. J Laparoendosc Surg 1994; *4:*81–87.

21. Conlon KC and Minnard EA. The value of laparoscopic staging in upper gastrointestinal malignancy. Oncologist 1997; *2:*10–17.

15

Chemotherapy of Pancreatic Cancer

Margaret Tempero

INTRODUCTION

In contrast to the improvements in overall survival for most other gastrointestinal tract cancers, the 5-yr survival of patients with pancreatic cancer sits at a dismal 4% *(1)*, suggesting that there has been no significant improvement in early diagnosis or therapy. In 1998, an estimated 27,600 new cases will be diagnosed *(1)*. This disease is the fourth leading cause of cancer death in men and the fifth cause of cancer death in women.

In spite of these grim statistics, there has been notable progress in the overall care of patients with pancreatic adenocarcinoma. Three-dimensional imaging techniques, such as computed tomography, magnetic resonance imaging, and endoscopic ultrasound have provided more accurate staging, with minimally invasive procedures *(2,3)*. The widespread availability of fine-needle aspiration to diagnose this malignancy has resulted in fewer laparotomies. The availability of improved biliary stents (especially expandable metal stents) *(4)* placed endoscopically or transhepatically, can provide good palliation for biliary obstruction and can sometimes obviate the need for surgical bypass procedures. Finally, improvements in our understanding of appropriate therapy for cancer pain, including celiac plexus block *(5)*, and for cancer related depression *(6)*, has improved the supportive care of patients with pancreatic adenocarcinoma. For those patients who present with resectable disease (approx 15%), advances in surgical care have resulted in a steep drop in perioperative mortality. It is now clear that, in centers with extensive experience, a perioperative mortality rate of less than 1% can be achieved *(7)*.

Approximately 85% of patients who present with pancreatic cancer have metastatic or locally advanced and unresectable disease. Patients with locally unresectable disease may be candidates for radiation therapy, which is usually given with radiation-sensitizing chemotherapy. Patients with metastatic disease are often offered chemotherapy. In most centers, investigational approaches are encouraged. The purpose of this chapter is to review the role of chemotherapy in the treatment of pancreatic adenocarcinoma. Recent advances in drug development provide cautious optimism that the chemoresistant barrier, which has prevented us from making more progress against this malignancy, may be broken.

END POINTS FOR EFFICACY

Traditional end points in determining efficacy of therapy have included objective response rate, survival, and, less commonly, quality of life. Objective response is generally accepted as a 50% or greater reduction in the sum of the products of all bidimensional measurable lesions (7a). These criteria were actually developed prior to the advent of three-dimensional imaging, and were generally applied to nodules on chest X-ray or palpable masses and skin lesions; however, in contemporary trials, the criteria have often been extended to lesions seen on computed tomography scans or magnetic resonance images. Although this approach appears to be a valid one for many malignancies, such as breast or colorectal cancer, applying this to pancreatic cancer is fraught with pitfalls. One of the histologic hallmarks of pancreatic adenocarcinoma is an associated desmoplastic reaction. It is not uncommon for a biopsy of a pancreatic adenocarcinoma to reveal that the majority of the mass represents tumor-associated desmoplasia. In addition, the presence of a malignancy in the pancreas can create other anatomic abnormalities that may be radiographically difficult to distinguish from the margin of the malignancy, (8) including pseudocysts and varying degrees of acute and chronic pancreatitis from pancreatic duct obstruction. Furthermore, the location of the pancreas in the retroperitoneum, with its proximity to un- or poorly opacified small bowel, can make accurate measurements of masses in the pancreas difficult to obtain. Thus, determining the initial dimensions of a primary pancreatic adenocarcinoma can be challenging, and, if the lesion is predominantly composed of desmoplastic tissue, successful therapy can result in minimal change in measurement. For these reasons, there is growing interest in identifying alternative end points with which to gage effective therapy.

Although improved survival remains a very powerful end point for the success of any treatment, improved quality of life or diminished tumor-associated symptoms are also laudable goals. More than 95% of patients with pancreatic adenocarcinoma present with some or all of the following symptoms: pain, weight loss and/or fatigue, and depression, which can interfere with the ability to carry out activities of daily living. Thus, patients with pancreatic carcinoma are appropriate candidates for studies using symptom assessment as an end point for efficacy. Unfortunately, these studies are more difficult to conduct, and require a randomized trial design to discriminate between symptom relief produced by a new therapy from a placebo effect that can occur with any treatment. In practice, the use of symptom assessment or quality of life parameters to monitor pancreatic cancer therapy has been uncommon; historically, most single-agent or combination chemotherapy regimens have been accepted or dismissed, based on objective response criteria.

RECENT DEVELOPMENTS IN CHEMOTHERAPY

Discussions of chemotherapy in pancreatic adenocarcinoma often begin with a historical overview. A somewhat different approach will be used here because recent developments suggest that results of chemotherapy in pancreatic adenocarcinoma need to be re-examined.

As mentioned, pancreatic adenocarcinoma has been considered to be a chemoresistant disease. The effectiveness of virtually all forms of chemotherapy treatment have been challenged, and some authors have concluded simply that there is no effective chemotherapy. Recent studies with a new agent, gemcitabine (2′, 2′-difluorodeoxycytidine) have forced investigators to re-examine this issue. The initial phase II experience with gemcitabine was performed at Memorial Sloan-Kettering Cancer Center *(9)*. The objective response rate was modest (11%), but those who responded appeared to have more durable benefit (up to 20+ mo), and 32% of the patients had stable disease for >4 mo. Although the median survival was only 5.6 mo, 23% of the patients were alive at 1 yr. The authors noted that many of the patients reported improvement in symptoms that seemed out of proportion to objective responses achieved. A similar European study also reported a marginal response rate of 6.3%, but up to 28% of patients had some improvement in symptoms *(10)*.

Based on these results, a phase III randomized trial *(11)* was conducted, in which patients were randomized to gemcitabine treatment (1000 mg/m^2 weekly for up to 7 wk, followed by a week of rest, and then 3 times weekly every 4 wk thereafter), or to 5-fluorouracil (5-FU) (600 mg/m^2 weekly). End points in this study were unique: In addition to objective response and survival, patients were observed for a clinical benefit response. This end point incorporated elements of pain intensity, analgesic consumption, performance status, and weight. Again, the objective response rate in this study was low. Only 5.4% of the patients treated with gemcitabine experienced an objective response, compared to 0.0% of the patients treated with 5-FU. There was a small improvement in survival for gemcitabine-treated patients (5.65 vs 4.41 mo); however, this was statistically significant. One year survival with gemcitabine treatment was 18%, compared to 2% for 5-FU treatment. More importantly, 23.8% of the gemcitabine-treated patients experienced clinical benefit, compared with 4.8% of the 5-FU-treated patients. This clinical benefit was confirmed in a crossover study in which 5-FU refractory patients were treated with gemcitabine; symptom improvement occurred in 27% *(12)*.

The results of these studies with gemcitabine raise important issues. It must be acknowledged that the clinical benefit response is a new tool for evaluating treatment efficacy. Because this tool measures only certain symptoms, it is dissimilar from more global quality of life assessment tools. Nonetheless, it was applied rigorously in a randomized trial design, which clearly showed that both symptoms and survival can be significantly improved in spite of a very low objective response rate. This important observation strengthens the argument that objective response cannot adequately be measured in this disease, using standard criteria. The following discussion of single- and multiple-agent chemotherapy will emphasize available survival data.

SINGLE AGENT THERAPY

Table 1 depicts the results of single-agent chemotherapy with a variety of approved and unapproved drugs. Some of the older studies employed nonstandardized response criteria, which may have overstated the response rate. Although median survival is not always reported (particularly in older literature), it is clear from reviewing Table 1 that the median survival of patients treated with single-agent chemotherapy ranges from 2 to 8.3 mo. Among the cited trials, a median survival of greater than 5 mo was achieved only with actinomycin-D*(13)*, amsacrine *(14)*, carmofur *(15)*, epirubicin *(16)*, gemcitabine *(9,11)*, groserelin *(17)*, ifosfamide *(18)*, mitoguazone *(19)*, octreotide *(20)*, 5-

Table 1
Single Agents

Agent(s)	No. of patients	% Response	Median survival (mos) (range)	% >1 yr survival (no.)	Ref.
Aclacinomycin	16	0	3	0	53
Actinomycin-D	28	2	6 (.25–15+)	ns	13
Amonafide	14	0	2.7 (1.5–5+)	ns	54
Amonafide	36	0	2.5	ns	55
Amsacrine	31	0	8.5	ns	14
Amsacrine	27	0	ns	ns	23
Azinidinylbenzoquinone (AZQ)	21	0	2	ns	19
Baker's Antifol	31	0	2.9	19	25
BCNU	31	0	ns	ns	56
β-2′-deoxythioguanosine	32	6	2.4	ns	57
Brequinar sodium	17	0	ns	ns	58
Carmofur	31	3.2	8.3 (1.3–20.3)	ns	15
CCNU	19	16	ns	ns	59
Chlorozotocin (Low dose)	27	0	2.65	ns	60
Chlorozotocin (High dose)	30	10	2	ns	60
Cyproterone acetate	32	ns	4.25	15	22
Diaziquone	21	0	2	ns	25
Diaziquone	21	0	4.5	ns	61
Dihydroxyanthracenedione (DHAD)	29	0	2.7	ns	19
Dihydraxyanthracenedione (DHAD)	23	0	2.5	0	53
Dihydroxyanthracenedione (DHAD)	10	0	ns	ns	62
Dianhydrogalactitol	40	2.5	2.3	ns	57
Doxorubicin	25	8	3 (.25–14.5)	ns	13
Edatrexate	40	2	3.5	ns	63
Edatrexate	17	0	2.5	ns	64
Epirubicin	34	24	5 (2–18+)	10	16
Epirubicin	16	5	2	12	24
Epirubicin	34	5	2.5	12	25
Esorubicin	47	6	4	18	65
Esorubicin	18	0	4.2	ns	66
Etoposide	21	0	3	ns	52
Etoposide	26	0	ns	ns	67
Fazarabine	14	0	ns	ns	68
5-FU (Bolus) (11 trials)	169	15	ns	ns	21
Fludarabine	20	0	3 (1–8)	0	69
Gemcitabine	44	11.4	5.6 (ns–20+)	23 (ns)	9
Goserelin	18	0	5 (0.5–15)	22 (4)	17
Goserelin	7	0	7	28 (2)	28
Hexamethylmelamine	55	7	2.7	ns	57
Idarubicin	32	7	ns	ns	70
Ifosfamide	27	22	6 (1–15+)	ns	18
Ifosfamide	30	6	3 (1–26+)	ns	26
Ifosfamide	30	10	3	ns	27
Iproplatin	32	10	ns	ns	71
1-Asparaginase	10	0	ns	ns	72
m-AMSA	24	0	3	ns	73
Maytansine	48	0	2.3	ns	60
Melphalan	39	2	2	ns	74
Melphalan	15	13	4 (.5–36+)	ns	75

Table 1 (continued)
Single Agents

Agent(s)	No. of patients	% Response	Median survival (mos) (range)	% >1 yr survival (no.)	Ref.
Menogaril	38	5.2	3.1	ns	76
Menogarol	15	0	ns	ns	77
Merbarone	29	6.9	ns	ns	78
Merbarone	17	0	2.8 (1.2–14.1)	ns	79
Methotrexate	25	4	2 (.25–25 +)	ns	13
Methyl-CCNU	15	13	ns	ns	56
Methyl-CCNU	68	6	2	ns	80
Metoprine	24	0	ns	ns	81
Mitogauzone (MGBG)	32	6.3	7.6	ns	19
Mitoguazone	33	6	ns	ns	82
Mitomycin-C (4 trials)	44	27[a]	ns	ns	59
Mitoxantrone	30	0	ns	ns	83
MK-329	18	0	ns	ns	84
MoAb 17-1A (Panorex)	18	5.6	2.5 (ns–36 +)	ns	85
Octreotide	22	0	5 (1–17)	9 (2)	20
Paclitaxel	39	8	5	ns	86
Pibenzimol	23	0	ns	ns	87
Pibenzimol	26	0	ns	ns	88
Piroxantrone	35	0	3	ns	89
Razoxane	29	7	2.4	ns	56
Somatuline (BIM 23014)	18	5.6	3 (2–14)	ns	90
Spirogermanium	20	0	3	ns	53
Streptozotocin	27	11[a]	ns	ns	59
Tamoxifen	37	ns	5.25	20	22
Tamoxifen	26	0	4.4	ns	91
Tamoxifen	24	ns	7	25	29
6-thioguanine	30	3.3	ns	ns	92
Tumor Necrosis Factor	22	0	2.9	ns	93

ns = not stated.
[a] Response rate may be overstated because of nonstandardized response criteria.

fluorouracil (5-FU) *(21)*, and tamoxifen *(22)*. Confirmatory trials of amsacrine *(23)*, epirubicin *(24,25)*, and ifosfamide *(26,27)* did not reproduce these findings. In some instances, confirmatory studies have suggested that a median survival of 5 or more months can be sustained; however, some of the data must be interpreted with caution, because of low numbers of patients studied. Agents for which more than one trial has suggested that a median survival of 5 mo or greater can be achieved include 5-FU *(21)*, goserelin *(28)*, tamoxifen *(29)*, and gemcitabine *(11)*. The results with gemcitabine have already been discussed. 5-FU, goserelin, and tamoxifen are discussed below.

Historically, 5-FU has been considered to be a modestly active, but leading single agent in the treatment of pancreatic adenocarcinoma. An analysis by Ahlgren *(21)*, re-

Table 2
5-FU Modulation

Agents	No. of patients	% Response	Median survival (mos.) (range)	% >1 yr survival (no.)	Ref.
5-FU + α-interferon	46	4	5.5	ns	*94*
5-FU + α-interferon + leucovorin	32	12	5.5 (2–17)	ns	*33*
5-FU + leucovorin (GITSG)	42	7	6.2 (0.2–33)	17 (7)	*31*
5-FU + leucovorin (5-day)	20	0	2.5 (.5–25+)	ns	*32*
5-FU + PALA	35	35	5.1 (1–19)	5	*95*
5-FU + PALA	20	20	2 (1.5–13)	5	*96*
24HR IV 5-FU ± PALA (I)	17	17.6	ns	ns	*97*

ns, Not stated.

viewing 11 published trials, concluded that the objective response rate was approx 15%. Median survival information is not available in all the studies analyzed; however, a contemporary trial conducted by the North Central Cancer Treatment Group (NCCTG), comparing 5-FU to other combination regimens, reported a median survival of 5.1 mo, with a 1 yr survival of 12% *(30)*. Surprisingly, there has been very little effort to study protracted infusion schedules of 5-FU. This schedule may have a different mechanism of action; higher antitumor activity with protracted infusion of 5-FU has been suggested in other gastrointestinal tract cancers. 5-FU can be biochemically modulated with a number of agents, such as leucovorin, α interferon, and *N*-(phosphonacetyl)-L-aspartate (PALA). These results are outlined in Table 2. Although most of the authors had little enthusiasm for biochemical modulation therapy, it should be noted that DeCaprio et al. *(31)* reported a median survival of 6.2 mo, and a 1 yr survival of 17% using 5-FU and leucovorin. A similar study by Crown et al. *(32)* reported a median survival of only 2.5 mo, and the percent of patients surviving greater than 1 yr was not stated; however, the latter trial included previously treated patients with a less likely chance of improved outcome. A third trial conducted by Scheithauer et al. *(33)*, using 5-FU, α interferon, and leucovorin, reported a median survival of 5.5 mo; the 1 yr survival was not stated. Although randomized trials have not been conducted with biochemical modulation of 5-FU, the reported results do not point to superiority over monotherapy using single-agent 5-FU.

Among the agents with an encouraging median survival in single-arm trials are hormonal therapy with goserelin and tamoxifen. Goserelin, an LHRH agonist, was tested following the identification of low- and high-affinity LHRH receptors on pancreatic tumor cells. Initial trial of goserelin reported by Philip et al. *(17)* evaluated 18 patients, and reported no objective remissions. However, a median duration of survival of 5 mo, and a 1 yr survival of 22%, was noted. A follow-up study reported by Allegretti et al. *(28)* evaluated only seven patients, and accrual was stopped because no objective responses were reported. Only three patients had measurable metastatic disease, but two patients survived longer than 12 mo. Quality of life or symptom assessment was not conducted in these trials. A randomized trial comparing goserelin to supportive care or other treatment modalities has not been conducted.

Analogous to the experience with goserelin, the finding of estrogen receptors in pancreatic cancer has prompted the evaluation of tamoxifen. As with the LHRH receptors, it is not clear whether these receptors are functional. Early reports suggested prolonged survival with tamoxifen, and at least three studies have shown median survivals of 5.25, 7, and 8.5 mo (22,29,34). It is also worth noting that these studies reported a 1 yr survival of greater than, or equal to, 20%. Wong et al. (29) suggested that the best survival was observed in postmenopausal women. A randomized trial conducted by Keating et al. (22) compared tamoxifen to cyproterone acetate (an antiandrogen) or no therapy. Treatment with tamoxifen produced the longest median survival (5.25 mo), compared to a 3.0-mo median survival for patients who received no treatment. However, according to the analyses used, this did not represent a significant difference.

COMBINATION THERAPY

Table 3 lists published combination chemotherapy trials in patients with pancreatic cancer. An early study by Smith et al.(35) evaluated combination therapy using 5-FU, adriamycin, and mitomycin-C, and reported a median survival of 6 mo and a 1-yr survival of 20%. Unfortunately, a subsequent randomized trial by the NCCTG (30) failed to show superiority of this regimen over monotherapy with 5-FU, and the median survival in that study fell short, at 4.7 mo, with a 1-yr survival of 12%. A modification of this regimen, with addition of streptozotocin, was reported by Bukowski et al. (36) to produce a median survival of 6.7 mo and a 1-yr survival of 28%. Although this median survival fell somewhat short at 4.8 mo, in a subsequent Southwest Oncology Group study (19), the survival did appear to be superior, compared to the survival of patients treated with other single agents undergoing phase II testing. A further modification of this regimen, with deletion of the adriamycin (leaving a triplet of 5-FU, mitomycin-C, and streptozocin [SMF]), has been studied by a number of groups. Both the Gastrointestinal Study Group (GITSG) (37) and the Cancer and Leukemia Group B (CALGB) (38) were unable to show superiority over treatment with FAM. The Southwest Oncology Group (39) was unable to identify superiority over 5-FU and mitomycin. Initially, promising results were reported using cisplatin, cytosine, and arabinoside and caffeine (39% partial response, median survival 6.1 mo) (40). A subsequent phase III trial comparing SMF to this regimen demonstrated a significantly prolonged median survival (10 vs 5 mo) for SMF (41). Despite this encouraging median survival, the authors concluded that, because of the low observed objective response rates, neither regimen constituted effective treatment for advanced pancreatic cancer.

With the possible exception of SMF, there are no published studies demonstrating a consistent improved median survival for any combination regimen when compared to other combinations to monotherapy. The 1-yr survival of all of the randomized trials of combination chemotherapy has either not been reported or has been reported to be <20%. Given the large sample size and improved statistical design in many of the more contemporary trials evaluating combination chemotherapy in pancreatic cancer, it is difficult to cull out any advantage for combination chemotherapy, compared to monotherapy. However, a randomized trial comparing SMF to 5-FU monotherapy has not been conducted.

Table 3
Combined Modalities

Agents	No. of patients	% Response	Median survival (mos) (range)	% >1 yr survival (no.)	Ref.
Cisplatin + ARA-C + caffiene	40	5	5 (.5–16)	ns	*41*
vs					
5-FU + mitomycin-C + streptozotocin	42	10	10 (.3–23)	ns	*41*
Epirubicin + ifosfamide	32	12.5	5	ns	*98*
5-FU + adriamycin + mitomycin-C	39	37	6 (1–17)	20 (8)	*35*
5-FU + adriamycin + mitomycin-C + streptozotocin	25	48	6.7 (1–25)	28 (7)	*36*
5-FU + CCNU	65	0	3	ns	*44*
vs					
Best supportive care	87	0	3.9	ns	*44*
5-FU + methyl CCNU	41	10	3.3	ns	*74*
vs					
5-FU + methyl CCNU + streptozocin	43	7	2.9	ns	*74*
vs					
Melphalan	43	2	1.8	ns	*74*
CALGB:					
5-FU + doxorubicin + mitomycin-C	63	14	6.1	ns	*38*
vs					
5-FU + streptozotocin + mitomycin-C	66	4	4.2	ns	*38*
GITSG:					
5-FU + doxorubicin + mitomycin-C	29	14	2.7	5%	*37*
vs					
5-FU + streptozotocin + mitomycin-C (1)	28	14	4	12%	*37*
vs					
5-FU + streptozotocin + mitomycin-C (II)	27	15	3.1	12%	*37*
NCCTG:					
5-FU	64	7	4.5	6	*43*
vs					
5-FU + doxorubicin + cisplatin	59	15	3.5	8	*43*
vs					
5-FU + mitomycin-C + methotrexate + vincristine + cyclophosphamide	61	21	4.5	8	*43*
SWOG:					

(continued)

Table 3
Combined Modalities

Agents	No. of patients	% Response	Median survival (mos) (range)	% >1 yr survival (no.)	Ref.
5-FU + doxorubicin + mitomycin-C + streptozotocin	71	11	4.8	ns	*19*
SWOG: 5-FU + mitomycin-C	41	10	4 (1–27)	10	*39*
vs 5-FU + mitomycin-C + streptozotocin	43	7	5 (1–32)	12	*39*

↓SS = insufficient sample size.
ns = not stated.

This section cannot be concluded without acknowledgment of some studies that have compared combination chemotherapy to best supportive care. Perhaps the most encouraging results were reported with the Mallinson regimen using a five-drug program with 5-FU, mitomycin-C, methotrexate, vincristine, and cyclophosphamide *(42)*. A subsequent NCCTG trial could not demonstrate an advantage of this regimen compared to monotherapy with 5-FU*(43)*. A large study of 5-FU and CCNU conducted by as a Veteran's Administration Cooperative Group Study also showed no improvement in median survival compared to best supportive care *(44)*. Similarly, Glimelius et al. *(45)* initially evaluated the cost-effectiveness of palliative chemotherapy in advanced gastrointestinal cancer, and could not identify a survival advantage for chemotherapy treatment in patients with pancreatic and biliary tract cancer. A subsequent analysis by the same group, using a much larger sample size, did demonstrate prolonged survival and improved quality of life in treated patients *(46)*. Finally, a recent study by Palmer et al. *(47)* also using a randomized trial design, suggested that treatment with FAM prolongs the median survival (33 wk) compared to supportive care (15 wk). It should be noted that the median survival with FAM treatment in this study is somewhat better than has been previously reported, and the median survival of the control group was somewhat worse than previous reports, raising concern about balance between the groups.

CHEMOTHERAPY IN COMBINATION WITH RADIATION

A detailed review of chemoradiation is beyond the scope of this chapter. However, it is important to note the role of chemotherapy as a radiation sensitizer in patients with pancreatic cancer. This has been studied in the adjuvant setting and as therapy for locoregional, but unresectable, disease.

A pivotal randomized study of adjuvant therapy in pancreatic cancer was performed by the GITSG *(48)*. In this study, patients were randomized, following resection, to observation or radiation therapy combined with bolus 5-FU. Radiation therapy was given using a split course and a total dose of 4000 cGy. 5-FU was given as a bolus treatment in a dose of 500 mg/m^2 daily for 3 d at the beginning of each 2-wk radiation cycle. 5-FU was then continued weekly after completion of radiation for a full 2 yr. The 2-yr actuarial survival was 43% in the treatment group, compared to 18% in the control group. A follow-up study, in which patients were simply randomized to the treatment confirmed a high survival rate in the treated groups *(49)*. These reports have led to wide acceptance of this form of therapy after resection from pancreatic adenocarcinoma. A contemporary study by the European Organization for Research and Treatment of Cancer (EORTC) is being conducted, in the hope of confirming these results. New approaches to adjuvant therapy have included the use of neoadjuvant therapy (preoperative therapy), primarily with various schedules of 5-FU *(50,51)*, but trials employing gemcitabine (also a radiosensitizing agent) are in progress. These studies suggest that an improvement in the resection rate may be achieved, but the overall impact of neoadjuvant therapy on long-term survival is not clear.

Only 22% of patients who present with pancreatic adenocarcinoma have potentially resectable disease. The standard oncologic management of such patients often includes therapy with combination of radiation and 5-FU. The selection of radiation dose and 5-FU regimen is usually based on an older study performed by the GITSG *(52)*. In this trial, combination of 5-FU and split-course radiation (total dose 4000 cGy) was compared to a radiation dose of 6000 cGy alone, or 6000 cGy combined with 5-FU. The regimen containing 5-FU and 4000 cGy radiation resulted in a near twofold increase in median survival (22.9–42.2 wk), compared to radiation alone. Although this approach has been studied extensively with various schedules of 5-FU, and with alternate radiotherapy techniques, including brachytherapy, new approaches are incorporating study of new chemotherapy agents, including paclitaxel and gemcitabine, which appear to have important radiation-sensitizing attributes.

SUMMARY

Pancreatic adenocarcinoma remains a relatively chemoresistant disease. However, improvements in the development of more appropriate clinical end points for efficacy in pancreatic cancer will permit higher discrimination between marginally and modestly effective treatment regimens. The recent introduction of new drugs, such as gemcitabine, with some efficacy in this disease, raises hope for improved agents with greater efficacy for the future.

REFERENCES

1. Parker SL, Tong T, Bolden S, and Wingo PA. Cancer Statistics, 1997. CA Can J Physicians 1997; *47:*5–27.
2. Brand R and Matamoros A. Imaging techniques in the evaluation of adenocarcinoma of the pancreas. Dig Dis 1997; in press.
3. Muller ME, Meyenberger C, Bertschinger P, Schaer R, and Marincek B. Pancreatic tumors: evaluation of endoscopic US, CT, and MR imaging. Radiology 1994; *190:*745–751.
4. Carr-Locke DL, Ball TJ, Connors PJ, Cotton PB, Geenen JE, Hawes RH, et al. Multicenter randomized trial of wallstent biliary endoprosthesis versus plastic stents. Gastrointest Endosc 1993; *3:*310.
5. Lillemoe KD, Cameron JL, Kaufman HS, Yeo CJ, Pitt HA, and Sauter PK. Chemical splanchnicectomy in patients with unresectable pancreatic cancer. A prospective randomized trial. Ann Surg 1993; *217:*447–455.
6. Passik SD and Breithart WS. Depression in patients with pancreatic carcinoma: Diagnostic and treatment issues. Cancer 1996; *78:*615–626.

7. Crist DW and Cameron JL. The current status of the Whipple operation for periampullary carcinoma. Adv Surg 1994; *25:*21–49.

7a. Green S and Weiss GR. Southwest Oncology Group standard response criteria, endpoint definitions and toxicity criteria. Invest New Drugs 1992; *10:*239–253.

8. Freeny PC. Radiologic diagnosis and staging of pancreatic ductal adenocarcinoma. Radiol Clin North Am 1989; *27:*121–128.

9. Casper ES, Green MR, Kelsen DP, Heelan RT, Brown TD, Flombaum CD, Trochanowski B, and Tarassoff PG. Phase II trial of gemcitabine (2,2′-difluorodeoxycytidine) in patients with adenocarcinoma of the pancreas. Invest New Drugs 1994; *12:*29–34.

10. Carmichael J, Fink U, Russell RCG, Spittle MF, Harris A, Spiessl G, et al. Phase II study of gemcitabine in patients with advanced pancreatic cancer. Br J Cancer 1995; *73:*101–105.

11. Burris HA, Moore MJ, Andersen J, Green MR, Rothenberg ML, Modiano MR, et al. Improvements in survival and clinical benefit with gemcitabine as first-line therapy for patients with advanced pancreatic cancer: a randomized trial. J Clin Oncol 1997; *15:*2403–2413.

12. Rothenberg ML, Moore MJ, Cripps MC, Andersen JS, Portenoy RK, Burris HA, et al. A phase II trial of gemcitabine in patients with 5-FU refractory pancreas cancer. Ann Oncol 1996; *7:*347–353.

13. Schein PS, Lavin PT, Moertel CG, Frytak S, Hahn RG, O'Connell MJ, et al. Randomized phase II clinical trial of adriamycin, methotrexate, and actinomycin-D in advanced measurable pancreatic carcinoma: a Gastrointestinal Tumor Study Group report. Cancer 1978; *42:*19–22.

14. Inamasu M, Oishi N, Chen T, Legha S, McCracken J, Balcerzak S, et al. Phase II trial of amsacrine in pancreatic carcinoma: a Southwest Oncology Group study. Cancer Treatment Rep 1984; *68:*1411–1412.

15. Kajanti MJ and Pyrhönen SO. Phase II trial of oral carmofur in advanced carcinoma. Ann Oncol 1991; *2:*765–766.

16. Wils J, Bleiberg H, Blijham G, Dalesio O, Duez N, Lacave A, and Splinter T. Phase II study of epirubicin in advanced adenocarcinoma of the pancreas. Eur J Cancer Clin Oncol 1985; *21:*191–194.

17. Philip PA, Carmichael J, Tonkin K, Buamah PK, Britton J, Dowsett M, and Harris AL. Hormonal treatment of pancreatic carcinoma: a phase II study of LHRH agonist goserelin plus hydrocortisone. Br J Cancer 1993; *67:*379–382.

18. Loehrer PJ, Williams SD, Einhorn LH, and Ansari R. Ifosfamide: an active drug in the treatment of adenocarcinoma of the pancreas. J Clin Oncol 1985; *3:*367–372.

19. Bukowski RM, Fleming TR, Macdonald JS, Oishi N, Taylor SA, and Baker LH. Evaluation of combination chemotherapy and phase II agents in pancreatic adenocarcinoma. A Southwest Oncology Group study. Cancer 1993; *71:*322–325.

20. Friess H, Büchler M, Beglinger C, Weber A, Kunz J, Fritsch K, Dennler HJ, and Beger HG. Low-dose octreotide treatment is not effective in patients with advanced pancreatic cancer. Pancreas 1993; *8:*540–545.

21. Ahlgren JD. Pancreatic cancer: chemotherapy of advanced disease. In: Ahlgren JD and Macdonald JS (eds), Gastrointestinal Oncology, JB Lippincott, Philadelphia, 1992; pp. 227–235.

22. Keating JJ, Johnson PJ, Cochrane AMG, Gazzard BG, Krasner N, Smith PM, et al. A prospective randomised trial of tamoxifen and cyproterone acetate in pancreatic carcinoma. Br J Cancer 1989; *60:*789–792.

23. Omura GA, Bartolucci AA, Lessner HE, and Hill GJ. Phase II evaluation of amsacrine in colorectal, gastric, and pancreatic carcinomas: a Southeastern Cancer Study Group trial. Cancer Treatment Rep 1984; *68:*929–930.

24. Hochster H, Green MD, Speyer JL, Wernz JC, Blum RH, and Muggia FM. Activity of epirubicin in pancreatic carcinoma. Cancer Treatment Rep 1986; *70:*299–300.

25. Gastrointestinal Tumor Study Group. Phase II trials of single agents Baker's antifol, diaziquone, and epirubicin in advanced pancreatic cancer. Cancer Treatment Rep 1987; *71:*865–867.

26. Ajani JA, Abbruzzese JL, Goudeau P, Faintuch JS, Yeomans AC, Boman BM, Nicaise C, and Levin B. Ifosfamide and mesna: marginally active in patients with advanced carcinoma of the pancreas. J Clin Oncol 1988; *6:*1703–1707.

27. Gastrointestinal Tumor Study Group. Ifosfamide is an inactive substance in the treatment of pancreatic carcinoma. Cancer 1989; *64:*2010–2013.

28. Allegretti A, Lionetto R, Saccomanno S, Paganuzzi M, Onetto M, Martinoli C, et al. LH-RH analogue treatment in adenocarcinoma of the pancreas: a phase II study. Oncology 1993; *50:*77–80.

29. Wong A, Chan A, and Arthur K. Tamoxifen therapy in unresectable adenocarcinoma of the pancreas. Cancer Treatment Rep 1987; *71:*749–750.

30. Cullinan SA, Moertel CG, Fleming TR, Rubin JR, Krook JE, Everson LK, et al. A comparison of three chemotherapeutic regimens in the treatment of advanced pancreatic and gastric carcinoma. JAMA 1985; *253:*2061–2067.

31. DeCaprio JA, Mayer RJ, Gonin R, and Arbuck SG. Fluorouracil and high-dose leucovorin in previously untreated patients with advanced adenocarcinoma of the pancreas: results of a phase II trial. J Clin Oncol 1991; *9:*2128–2133.

32. Crown J, Casper ES, Botet J, Murray P, and Kelsen DP. Lack of efficacy of high-dose leucovorin and fluorouracil in patients with advanced pancreatic adenocarcinoma. J Clin Oncol 1991; *9:*1682–1686.

33. Scheithauer W, Pfeffel F, Kornek G, Marczell A, Wiltschke C, and Funovics J. A phase II trial of 5-fluorouracil, leucovorin, and recombinant alpha-2b-interferon in advanced adenocarcinoma of the pancreas. Cancer 1992; *70:*1864–1866.

34. Thieve NO, Pousette A, and Carlstrom K. Adenocarcinoma of the pancreas: a hormone sensitive tumour? A preliminary report on Nolvadex treatment. Clin Oncol 1983; *9:*193–197.

35. Smith FP, Hoth DF, Levin B, Karlin DA, Macdonald JS, Woolley PV, and Schien PS. 5-fluorouracil, adriamycin and mitomycin-C(FAM) chemotherapy for advanced adenocarcinoma of the pancreas. Cancer 1980; *46:*2014–2018.

36. Bukowski RM, Schacter LP, Groppe CW, Hewlett JS, Weick JK, and Livingston RB. Phase II trial of 5-fluorouracil, adriamycin, mitomycin-C, and streptozotocin (FAM-S) in pancreatic carcinoma. Cancer 1982; *50:*197–200.

37. Gastrointestinal Tumor Study Group. Phase II studies of drug combinations in advanced pancreatic carcinoma: fluorouracil plus doxorubicin plus mitomycin C and two regimens of streptozotocin plus mitomycin C plus fluorouracil. J Clin Oncol 1986; *4:*1794–1798.

38. Oster MW, Gray R, Panasci L, and Perry MC. Chemotherapy for advanced pancreatic cancer: a comparison of 5-fluorouracil, adriamycin, and mitomycin (FAM) with 5-fluorouracil, streptozotocin, and mitomycin (FSM). Cancer 1986; *57:*29–23.

39. Bukowski RM, Balcerzak SP, O'Bryan RM, Bonnet JD, and Chen TT. Randomized trial of 5-fluorouracil and mitomycin C with or without streptozotocin for advanced pancreatic cancer. Cancer 1983; *52:*1577–1582.

40. Dougherty J, Kelsen D, Kemeny N, et al. Advanced pancreatic cancer: a phase I-II trial of cisplatin, high dose cytarabine, and caffeine. J Natl Cancer Inst 1989; *81:*1735–1738.

41. Kelsen D, Hudis C, Niedzwiecki D, Dougherty J, Casper E, Botet J, Vinciguerra V, and Rosenbluth R. A phase III comparison trial of streptozotocin, mitomycin, and 5-fluorouracil with cisplatin, cytosine arabinoside, and caffeine in patients with advanced pancreatic carcinoma. Cancer 1991; *68:*965–969.

42. Mallinson CN, Rake MO, and Cocking JD. Chemotherapy in pancreatic cancer. Br Med J 1980; *281:*1589–1591.

43. Cullinan S, Moertel CG, Wieand HS, Schutt AJ, Krook JE, Foley JF, et al. A phase II trial on the therapy of advanced pancreatic carcinoma: evaluations of the Mallinson regimen and combined 5-fluorouracil, doxorubicin, and cisplatin. Cancer 1990; *65:*2207–2212.

44. Frey C, Twomey P, Keehn R, Elliott D, and Higgins G. Randomized study of 5-FU and CCNU in pancreatic cancer. Cancer 1981; *47:*27–31.

45. Glimelius B, Hoffman K, Graf W, et al. Cost-effectiveness of palliative chemotherapy in advanced gastrointestinal cancer. Ann Oncol 1995; *6:*267–274.

46. Glimelius B, Hoffman K, Sjödén PO, Jacobson G, Sellström H, Enander LK, Linné T, and Svensson C. Chemotherapy improves survival and quality of life in advanced pancreatic and biliary cancer. Ann Oncol 1996; *7:*593–600.

47. Palmer KR, Kerr M, Knowles G, Cull A, Carter DC, and Leonard RC. Chemotherapy prolongs survival in inoperable pancreatic carcinoma. Br J Surg 1994; *81:*882–885.

48. Gastrointestinal Tumor Study Group. Pancreatic cancer: Adjuvant combined radiation and chemotherapy following curative resection. Arch Surg 1985; *120:*899–903.

49. Gastrointestinal Study Group. Further evidence of effective adjuvant combined radiation and chemotherapy following curative resection of pancreatic cancer. Cancer 1987; *59:*2006–2010.

50. Hoffman JP, Weese JL, Solin LJ, Engstrom P, Agarwal P, Barber LW, et al. A pilot study of preoperative chemoradiation for patients with localized adenocarcinoma of the pancreas. Am J Surg 1995; *169:*71–77.

51. Evans EB, Rich TA, Byrd DR, Cleary KR, Connelly JH, Levin B, et al. Preoperative chemoradiation and pancreaticoduodenectomy for adenocarcinoma of the pancreas. Arch Surg 1992; *127:*1335–1339.

52. Moertel CC, Fryta KS, Hahn RG, O'Connell MJ, Reitemeier RJ, Rubin J, et al. Therapy of locally unresectable pancreatic carcinoma: a randomized comparison of high dose (6,000 rads) radiation alone, moderate dose radiation (4,000 rads + 5 fluorouracil), antidose radiation + 5 fluorouracil: the Gastrointestinal Tumor Study Group. Cancer 1981; *48:*1705–1710.

53. Ashbury RF, Cnaan A, Johnson L, Harris J, Zaentz SD, and Haller DG. An Eastern Cooperative Oncology Group phase II study of single agent DHAD, VP-16, Aclacinomycin, or spirogermanium in metastatic pancreatic cancer. Am J Clin Oncol 1994; *17:*166–169.

54. Linke K, Pazdur R, Abbruzzese JL, Agani JA, Winn R, Bradof JE, Daugherty K, and Levin B. Phase II study of amonafide in advanced pancreatic adenocarcinoma. Invest New Drugs 1991; *9:*353–356.

55. Leichman CG, Tangen C, Macdonald JS, Leimert T, and Fleming TR. Phase II trial of amonafide in advanced pancreas cancer: a Southwest Oncology Group study. Invest New Drugs 1993; *11:*219–221.

56. Moertel CG, Schutt AJ, Reitemeier RJ, and Hahn RG. Therapy for gastrointestinal cancer with the nitrosoureas alone and in drug combination. Cancer Treatment Rep 1976; *60:*729–732.

57. Gastrointestinal Tumor Study Group. Phase II trials of hexamethylmelamine, dianhydrogalactitol, razoxane, and β-2'-deoxythioguanosine as single agents against advanced measurable tumors of the pancreas. Cancer Treatment Rep 1985; *69:*713–716.

58. Moore M, Maroun J, Robert F, Natale R, Neidhart J, Dallaire B, Sisk R, and Gyves J. Multicenter phase II study of brequinar sodium in patients with advanced gastrointestinal cancer. Invest New Drugs 1993; *11:*61–65.

59. Carter SK and Comis RL. The integration of chemotherapy into a combined modality approach for cancer treatment. Cancer Treatment Rev 1975; *2:*193–214.

60. Gastrointestinal Tumor Study Group. Phase II trials of maytansine, low-dose chlorozotocin, and high-dose chlorozotocin as single agents against advanced measurable adenocarcinoma of the pancreas. Cancer Treatment Rep 1985; *69:*417–420.

61. Tilchen EJ, Fleming T, Mills G, Oishi N, Bonnett JD, Natale RB, Harker G, and Coltman CA. Phase II evaluation of diaziquone in pancreatic carcinoma: a Southwest Oncology Group study. Cancer Treatment Rep 1987; *71:*1309–1310.

62. Bedikian AY, Karlin D, Stroehlein J, Valdivieso M, Korinek J, and Bodey GP. Phase II evaluation of dihydroxyanthracenedione (DHAD, NSC 301739) in patients with upper gastrointestinal tumors. Am J Clin Oncol 1983; *6:*473–476.

63. Moore DF, Pazdur R, Abbruzzese JL, Ajani JA, Dubovsky DW, Wade JL, et al. Phase II trial of edatrexate in patients with advanced pancreatic adenocarcinoma. Ann Oncol 1994; *5:*286–287.

64. Casper E, Schwartz GK, Johnson B, and Kelsen DP. Phase II trial of edatrexate in patients with pancreatic adenocarcinoma. Invest New Drugs 1992; *10:*313–316.

65. Vaughn CB, Salmon SE, and Fleming TR. Phase II evaluation of esorubicin (4'deoxydoxorubicin) in pancreatic adenocarcinoma: a Southwest Oncology Group study. Invest New Drugs 1990; *8:*81–85.

66. Blayney DW, Goldberg DA, Leong LA, Carr BI, and Doroshow JH. Phase II trial of epirubicin in advanced pancreatic adenocarcinoma. Cancer Treatment Rep 1986; *70:*683–684.

67. Sternberg CN, Magill GB, Cheng EW, Applewhite A, and Sordillo PP. Etoposide (VP-16) in the treatment of advanced adenocarcinoma of the pancreas. Am J Clin Oncol 1988; *11:*172–173.

68. Casper ES, Schwartz GK, and Kelsen DP. Phase II trial of fazarabine (arabinofuranosyl-5-azacytidine) in patients with advanced pancreatic adenocarcinoma. Invest New Drugs 1992; *10:*205–209.

69. Kilton LJ, Benson AB, Greenberg A, Johnson P, Shapiro C, Blough R, French S, and Weidner L. Phase II trial of fludarabine phosphate for adenocarcinoma of the pancreas. An Illinois Cancer Center study. Invest New Drugs 1992; *10:*201–204.

70. Mittelman A, Magill GB, Raymond V, Sternberg CN, Cheng EW, Sordillo PB, and Young CW. Phase II trial of idarubicin in patients with pancreatic cancer. Cancer Treatment Rep 1987; *71:*657–658.

71. Hubbard KP, Pazdur R, Ajani JA, Braud E, Blaustein A, King M, Llenado-Lee M, Winn R, Levin B, and Abbruzzese JL. Phase II evaluation of iproplatin in patients with advanced gastric and pancreatic cancer. Am J Clin Oncol 1992; *15:*524–527.

72. Lessner HE, Valenstein S, Kaplan R, DeSimone P, and Yunis A. Phase II study of L-asparaginase in the treatment of pancreatic cancer. Cancer Treatment Rep 1980; *64:*1359–1361.

73. Sternberg CN, Magill GB, Sordillo PP, Cheng E, and Currie VE. Phase II evaluation of *m*-AMSA (4'-(9-acridinylamino)-methane-sulfon-*m*-anisidide) in patients with adenocarcinoma of the pancreas. Am J Clin Oncol 1983; *6:*459–462.

74. Horton J, Gelber RD, Engstrom P, Falkson G, Moertel C, Brodovsky H, and Douglass H. Trials of a single-agent and combination chemotherapy for advanced cancer of the pancreas. Cancer Treatment Rep 1981; *65:*65–68.

75. Smith DB, Kenny JB, Scarffe JH, and Maley WV. Phase II evaluation of melphalan in adenocarcinoma of the pancreas. Cancer Treat Rep 1985; *69:*917–918.

76. Brown TD, Goodman PJ, Fleming TR, Baker LH, and Macdonald JS. Phase II trial of menogaril in adenocarcinoma of the pancreas. A Southwest Oncology Group study. Invest New Drugs 1991; *9:*77–78.

77. Sternberg CN, Magill GB, Cheng EW, and Hollander P. Phase II trial of menogarol in the treatment of advanced adenocarcinoma of the pancreas. Am J Clin Oncol 1988; *11:*174–176.

78. Kraut EH, Fleming T, Macdonald JS, Spiridonidis CH, Bradof JE, and Baker LH. Phase II trial of merbarone in pancreatic cancer: a Southwest Oncology Group study. Am J Clin Oncol 1993; *16:*327–328.

79. Jones DV, Ajani JA, Winn RJ, Daugherty KR, Levin B, and Krakoff IH. A phase II study of merbarone in patients with adenocarcinoma of the pancreas. Cancer Invest 1993; *11*:667–669.

80. Moertel CG, Douglass HO, Hanley J, and Carbone PP. Phase II study of methyl-CCNU in the treatment of advanced pancreatic carcinoma. Cancer Treatment Rep 1976; *60*:1659–1661.

81. Sternberg CN, Magill GB, Sordillo PP, Cheng EW, and Kemeny N. Phase II evaluation of metoprine in advanced pancreatic adenocarcinoma. Cancer Treatment Rep 1984; *68*:1053–1054.

82. Inamasu MS, Oishi N, Chen TT, Kraut EH, Grozea PN, Costanzi JJ, and Bonnet JD. Phase II study of mitoguazone in pancreatic cancer: a Southwest Oncology Group study. Cancer Treatment Rep 1986; *70*:531–532.

83. DeSimone PA, Gams R, and Bartolucci A. Weekly mitoxantrone in the treatment of pancreatic carcinoma. A Southeastern Cancer Study Group Trial. Cancer Treatment Rep 1986; *70*:929–930.

84. Abbruzzese JL, Gholson CF, Daugherty K, Larson E, DuBrow R, Berlin R, and Levin B. A pilot clinical trial of cholecystokinin receptor antagonist MK-329 in patients with advanced pancreatic cancer. Pancreas 1992; *17*:165–171.

85. Weiner LM, Harvey E, Padavic-Shaller K, Willson JKV, Walsh C, LaCreta F, et al. Phase II multicenter evaluation of prolonged murine monoclonal antibody 17-1A therapy in pancreatic cancer. J Immunother 1993; *13*:110–116.

86. Whitehead RP, Jacobson J, Brown TD, Taylor SA, Weiss GR, and Macdonald JS. Phase II trial of paclitaxel and granulocyte colony-stimulating factor in patients with pancreatic carcinoma: a Southwest Oncology Group study. J Clin Oncol 1997; *15*:2414–2419.

87. Kraut EH, Fleming T, Segal M, Neidhart JA, Behrens BC, and MacDonald J. Phase II study of pibenzimol in pancreatic cancer. Invest New Drugs 1991; *9*:95–96.

88. Patel SR, Kvols LK, Rubin J, O'Connell MJ, Edmonson JH, Ames MM, and Kovach JS. Phase I-II study of pibenzimol hydrochloride (NSC 322921) in advanced pancreatic carcinoma. Invest New Drugs 1991; *9*:53–57.

89. Jenkins TR, Tangen C, Macdonald JS, Weiss G, Chapman R, and Hantel A. A phase II trial of piroxantrone in adenocarcinoma of the pancreas. A Southwest Oncology Group study. Invest New Drugs 1993; *11*:329–331.

90. Canobbio L, Boccardo F, Cannata D, Gallotti P, and Epis R. Treatment of advanced pancreatic carcinoma with somatostatin analogue BIM 23014. Cancer 1992; *69*:648–650.

91. Scheithauer W, Kornek G, Haider K, and Depisch D. Unresponsiveness of pancreatic adenocarcinoma to antioestrogen therapy. Eur J Cancer 1990; *26*:851–852.

92. Ajani JA, Pazdur R, Winn RJ, Abbruzzese JL, Levin B, Belt R, Young J, Patt YZ, and Krakoff IH. Phase II study of intravenous 6-thioguanine in patients with advanced carcinoma of the pancreas. Invest New Drugs 1991; *9*:369–371.

93. Brown TD, Goodman P, Fleming T, Macdonald JS, Hersh EM, and Braun TJ. A phase II trial of recombinant tumor necrosis factor in patients with adenocarcinoma of the pancreas: a Southwest Oncology Group study. J Immunother 1991; *10*:376–378.

94. Pazdur R, Ajani JJ, Abbruzzese JL, Belt RJ, Dakhil SR, Dubovsky D, et al. Phase II evaluation of fluorouracil and recombinant α-2a-interferon in previously untreated patients with pancreatic adenocarcinoma. Cancer 1992; *70*:2073–2076.

95. Rosvold E, Schilder R, Walczak J, DiFino SM, Flynn PJ, Banerjee TK, et al. Phase II trial of PALA in combination with 5-fluorouracil in advanced pancreatic cancer. Cancer Chemother Pharmacol 1992; *29*:305–308.

96. Morrell LM, Bach A, Richman SP, Goodman P, Fleming TR, and Macdonald JS. A phase II multi-institutional trial of low-dose N-(phosphonacetyl)-L-aspartate and high-dose 5-flu-

orouracil as a short-term infusion in the treatment of adenocarcinoma of the pancreas. Cancer 1991; *67:*363–366.

97. Ardalan B, Singh G, and Silberman H. A randomized phase I and II study of short-term infusion of high-dose fluorouracil with or without N-(phosphonacetyl)-L-aspartic acid in patients with advanced pancreatic and colorectal cancer. J Clin Oncol 1988; *6:*1053–1058.

98. Wils J, Bleiberg H, Buyse M, Wagener DT, Splinter T, Veenhoe C, Herben M, and Duez N. An EORTC Gastrointestinal Group Phase II evaluation of epirubicin combined with ifosfamide in advanced adenocarcinoma of the pancreas. Eur J Cancer Clin Oncol 1989; *25:*1119–1120.

16

Radiation Therapy for Pancreatic Cancer

Tyvin A. Rich

INTRODUCTION

Adenocarcinoma of the pancreas was diagnosed in about 28,000 persons in 1997 in the United States, and the prognosis for most remains poor. A minority of patients present with localized disease amenable to curative surgery and have a median survival of 18–24 mo. Better prognosis is found in those with resected periampullary cancers, or in those with pancreatic adenocarcinoma with negative lymph nodes, and in patients with islet cell cancers *(1)*. Survival appears to be helped slightly by adjuvant postoperative irradiation and chemotherapy (chemoradiation) *(2,3)*. For the majority of patients with locally advanced, unresected disease, however, chemoradiation results in a median survival of only 3–10 mo, and nearly all die within 24 mo of diagnosis. Recent advances in combinations of primary irradiation with newer chemotherapy, radiotherapy treatment planning, and new external irradiation treatment techniques offer some hope to control this cancer better.

ETIOLOGIC FACTORS AND RADIATION SENSITIVITY

Clinical research into the etiology of pancreatic cancer strongly implicates tobacco smoking; as public health awareness of the hazards of cigarette smoking increases, some leveling off of this diagnosis may occur. Currently, these epidemiologic observations are interesting, but provide little insight into radiation sensitivity.

Recent observations regarding the molecular biology of the mutated *ras* oncogene in pancreatic cancer may be of some interest to the radiation biologist. Since the K-*ras* mutation is common in pancreatic cancer *(4)*, this knowledge may eventually have some significance for radiation biology, since this is one of a class of oncogenes that regulates signal-transduction pathways, which are known to alter radiation sensitivity *(5)*. Increased radiosensitivity occurs when mutated *ras* is transfected into NIH/3T3 cells *(6)*. Transfection of mutated *ras* can significantly alter radiation sensitivity, when there is also a mutation in p53 or cotransfection of the *myc* gene. These observations await correlative studies to define their role in clinical management.

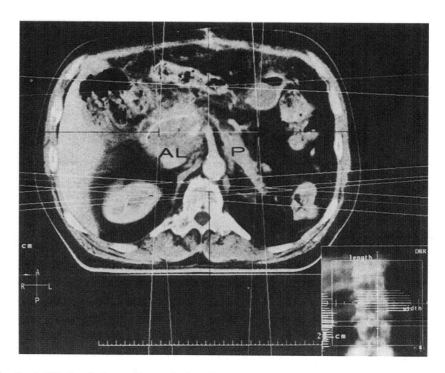

Fig. 1. A CT simulation radiograph showing the field placement around a resected pancreatic cancer. Shown in this figure are the pancreatic remnant (p) and the radiopaque stent that drains the pancreatic remnant into the afferent loop (al). Also shown are projections of the anterior/posterior and lateral irradiation beams. Note the posterior edge of the lateral beams, which are blocked to reduce the dose to the kidney.

EXTERNAL IRRADIATION

A mainstay of treatment for patients with advanced, localized pancreatic cancer has been external beam irradiation (ExBRT). One aspect of treatment that has made palliative radiotherapy better is the use of radiologic methods that accurately localize the cancer and thereby lessen irradiation of normal tissues. For patients with resected or unresected pancreatic cancers, computerized tomographic scanning (CT), with intravenous bolus contrast and 1.5-mm (thin) sections or spiral CT, facilitates precise demarcation of the treatment volume. CT with intravenous bolus contrast has been especially helpful in the initial diagnosis of hypodense lesions that have a high correlation with cancer *(7)*. With CT diagnosis, very few patients have been found to need surgical exploration for diagnosis or correction of jaundice, since determination of the extent of disease and the relief of obstruction can be corrected nonsurgically. For those with borderline resectable lesions, evaluation of response to ExBRT and the determination of resectability after preoperative infusional chemoradiation can also be made with CT *(8)*.

Simulation for ExBRT with CT and bolus contrast infusion is also helpful for patients treated postoperatively after pancreatic resection (Fig. 1) or for those with unresectable disease (Fig. 2). In the former, the location of the pancreatic anastomosis can sometimes be identified by the radiopaque stent at the pancreaticoenteric anastomosis,

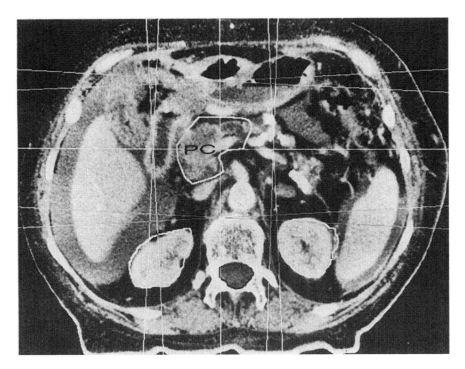

Fig. 2. A CT radiograph of a four-field treatment of an unresectable pancreatic cancer (pc).

but frequently this may not be present or easily visualized. The author has found that intravenous bolus contrast helps to demarcate the pancreatic remnant further, and can aid in field placement (Fig. 1). One treatment technique that further aids treatment accuracy is to place the patient in a comfortable supine position that allows the arms to rest above the head and out of the path of the lateral beams.

Modern treatment planning software allows the reconstruction of isodose curves, which allow an assessment of the dose delivered to the target volume and to the surrounding normal tissues. A typical CT treatment plan using multiple beams is shown in Fig. 3A,B, and the corresponding dosimetry is shown in Fig. 4. ExBRT doses of ~50 Gy are commonly used for palliation of local symptoms of pain, bleeding, and jaundice related to advanced malignancy. Higher doses to ≥60 Gy can be given by split-course techniques (over 10 wk), or in a continuous ExBRT, if the volume treated is very restricted *(9,10)*. ExBRT is given daily at a rate of 9 to 10 Gy/wk. The result of higher ExBRT doses is illustrated from a series that showed an improvement in median survival when ExBRT doses were increased from ~50 to >60 Gy, and with the addition of 5-FU *(9)*. Newer radiotherapeutic methods to improve treatment have included not only better target localization, but have also focused on higher doses given by intraoperative electron beam (EB-IORT), used to deliver ultra-high doses of radiotherapy directly to the pancreas, altered fractionation, hyperthermia, and high LET irradiation.

INTRAOPERATIVE RADIOTHERAPY

Intraoperative radiotherapy has been combined with external irradiation in order to increase the total radiation dose to the pancreas, and to provide for better local disease

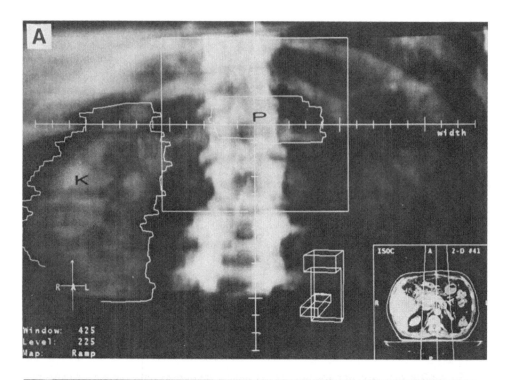

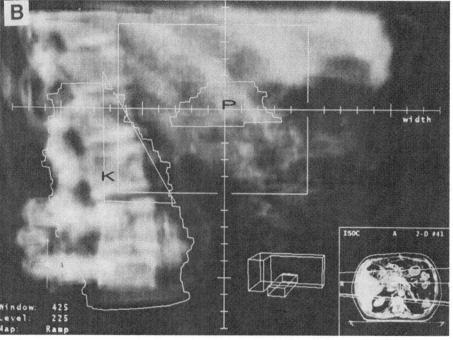

Fig. 3. (A) A CT digitally reconstructed radiograph showing the anterior treatment portal. The inset in the lower right shows the anterior beam projected onto the area surrounding the pancreatic remnant (p) and shows how the right kidney is just outside the beam edge (k). **(B)** A CT digitally reconstructed radiograph showing the lateral treatment portal. Note that the field edge is placed at the border of the kidney (k).

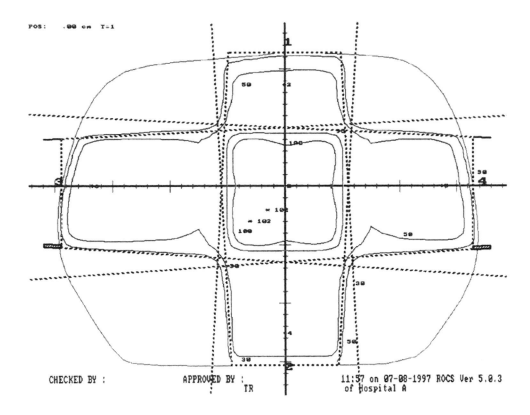

Fig. 4. An isodose treatment plan using the four fields shown in Fig. 3A,B. This plan is normalized to the isocenter and shows the 100, 95, and 50% isodose lines.

control and palliation *(11)*. This can be accomplished by the placement of radioactive seeds placed directly into the pancreas, usually at the time of surgical exploration. This technique allows an assessment of the abdominal contents and selection of the most favorable patients for this approach. In one report, the radioactive seeds are placed transcutaneously *(12)*. The results of this approach have failed to show a substantial benefit over that of ExBRT alone.

Another method used for delivery of higher radiation doses to the pancreas has been with EB-IORT, which has been shown to be associated with good palliation of symptoms for patients with advanced and metastatic disease. One of the attractions of this technique is the ability to deliver high doses quickly and safely, since there is no exposure to the operating room personnel with the use of single doses of 20–40 Gy *(11)*. Pain relief occurs in the majority of cases within 1 wk after doses of >20 Gy. Although this palliation alone may justify EB-IORT, this technique is more costly than conventionally fractionated ExBRT given for 2–6 wk postoperatively. EB-IORT with or without ExBRT for nonresectable pancreatic cancer in those without clinically evident distant metastasis or peritoneal seeding noted at laparotomy has been reported *(13–15)*. Those receiving both EB-IORT and ExBRT tend to have better survival, compared to those treated with surgical bypass or EB-IORT alone. Another benefit of EB-IORT and ExBRT is the potential reduction in acute complications with the combination, compared to single high doses of EB-IORT alone; the main complication of EB-IORT alone at these doses is a ~10% risk of hematochezia from radiation duodenitis.

In the United States, several institutions have used EB-IORT doses between 10 and 20 Gy in combination with pre- and postoperative ExBRT given at 45–50 Gy for 5–6 wk *(16)*. Pilot studies in the United States began in 1978 and used EB-IORT at the time of surgical exploration and postoperative ExBRT, if there was no evidence of metastatic disease. EB-IORT doses ranging from 15 to 30 Gy (16.5 Gy, average dose) were given with 15–29 MeV electrons. A median survival of 15 mo and individual survival times of 26–31 mo for some patients were reported *(13–16)*; 1-yr actuarial local control for unresectable pancreatic cancer as high as 82% has been reported *(15)*. These local control rates appear to be better than those of historic controls treated with ExBRT with or without 5-fluorouracil (5-FU). In spite of high local control rates at 1 yr, there is still an unacceptably high local failure rate and local symptom progression or growth of the pancreatic mass on CT scan within the high-dose volume. Other patterns of failure for unresectable pancreatic cancer patients include peritoneal failure occurring in ~30% and liver metastasis in >50% *(17)*.

OTHER RADIOTHERAPEUTIC APPROACHES
TO IMPROVE CONTROL OF UNRESECTED DISEASE

The use of hyperthermia has been tried for deep-seated cancers, because of the availability of equipment capable of delivering controlled heat to abdominal sites. One attractive approach for the treatment of pancreatic cancer is the use of intraoperative hyperthermia with either microwaves *(18)* or with intraoperative ultrasound *(19)*, when the normal tissues can be moved away from the site and thus spared radiation sensitization. Although these methods have been shown to be feasible, they must still be considered experimental, since there is no proof that local control or survival are benefited.

Another approach that has general applicability has been the use of altered fractionation schedules. This means that radiotherapy is administered in a schedule different than once per day in fraction sizes of ~2 Gy/d. One approach is hypofractionationated ExBRT, which has been found to be useful for the rapid palliation for selected patients who are not able to attend daily treatments; here a dose of 30 Gy in 6 fractions (two treatments/wk) are given over 3 wk, with or without chemotherapy. In a different approach, hyperfractionation or the administration of 1.2 Gy twice per day has been reported for the treatment of unresectable cancer. At present, there is no evidence that either of these approaches results in an improvement in either local control or distant failure, compared to conventional treatment schedules *(20)*.

Because of the apparent radioresistance of pancreatic cancer, some believe this is an ideal area to test high linear energy transfer (LET) beams, to determine if this approach can result in better tumor control. The preliminary studies showed no substantial improvement in local control, and that there were potentially more complications with this approach than with the use of conventional X-rays combined with chemotherapy *(21)*.

CHEMORADIATION

The rationale for chemoradiation is to exploit cytotoxic cooperation for local enhancement of the irradiation and for systemic effect *(22)*. In early clinical trials in patients with advanced gastrointestinal cancer, concomitant bolus (rapid injection) 5-FU 15 mg/kg/d, and modest doses of ExBRT (30–36 Gy), showed improved local tumor control; the dose limiting toxicities were leukopenia and stomatitis *(23)*. Later randomized controlled studies confirmed there was improved survival with the use of concomitant 5-FU plus 35–40 Gy *(24)*, or with 40–60 Gy *(10)* for patients with unresected pancreatic cancer. Combination chemotherapy, consisting of streptozocin, mitomycin, and 5-FU (SMF), showed some potential superiority over ExBRT alone or 5-FU chemoradiation in pilot studies *(25)*. However, SMF, compared to bolus 5-FU chemoradiation, showed a survival benefit in favor of the chemoradiation (41% vs 19% 1-yr survival) in a subsequent randomized trial *(26)*.

At M. D. Anderson Cancer Center, Houston, Tx investigators used chemoradiation in an administration schedule of prolonged, low-dose, continuous infusion (>30 d), 5-FU during ExBRT. Continuous infusion 5-FU in dosages of 250–300 mg/m^2/d for 5 or 7 d/wk has been given during ExBRT, employing total doses of 50–55 Gy in 5.5 wk given at 1.8 Gy/fraction *(16,22)*. This treatment is managed in the outpatient clinic, and 5-FU is given with a portable pump through a central venous catheter. Acute side effects include nausea, diarrhea and vomiting, weight loss, fatigue, and hand/foot syndrome, but rarely is leukopenia encountered. In employing this treatment for a variety of gastrointestinal cancer sites, the degree of acute toxicity is not related to treatment site, ExBRT dose, or 5-FU dose, but is associated with the weekly duration of 5-FU infusion. For example, the acute toxicity during 5-FU chemoradiation is well-tolerated by administration of 5-FU for 5 d/wk instead of 7 d/wk. The late-occurring treatment effects of combined modality therapy do not appear to be increased, compared to that seen with ExBRT alone.

As a further clinical innovation, wide-field irradiation to the liver and upper abdomen is now being investigated at M. D. Anderson for pancreatic cancers. This concept has been fostered by the apparent success of whole-abdomen irradiation for ovarian cancer, and the known pattern of tumor spread for pancreatic cancer, which includes regional lymph nodes and liver metastasis in a high percentage. In one pilot study using upper-abdomen chemoradiation and tumor/nodal treatment, 5-FU was administered by continuous infusion of 1000 mg/m^2/24 h for 3 d; there was an improvement in 2-yr survivorship when patients treated with wide-field XRT were compared with patients receiving local irradiation alone (20 vs 6.5%, respectively) *(27)*. Prophylactic hepatic 5-FU chemoradiation consisted of 23.4 Gy in 13 fractions over 2.5 wk, and high-dose chemoradiation to the pancreas (61.2 Gy/7 wk). The apparent reduction in hepatic metastasis by prophylactic treatment has been confirmed by the Radiation Therapy Oncology Group: The incidence of liver metastasis was reduced to 28%. In a single-institutional, pilot study with infusional 5-FU chemoradiation, there was unacceptable toxicity found when low-dose 5-FU was administered continuously (in a dosage of 300 mg/m^2), in conjunction with 23.4 Gy, to the whole liver. These data underscore the experimental nature of prophylactic hepatic irradiation and the need to study this approach only in prospective studies *(28)*.

A different chemoradiation study for localized, unresectable pancreatic cancer has investigated 5-FU in combination with streptozotocin and cisplatin plus ExBRT (RT-FSP). Recent results with RT-FSP show excellent palliation for patients with unresectable pancreatic cancer and should be explored further *(29)*.

Both acute and late treatment complications of upper gastrointestinal bleeding after chemoradiation with or without EB-IORT, in patients with unresected pancreatic tumors, can occur. Careful endoscopic evaluation is necessary whenever this symptom is encountered, to exclude the possibility of tumor regrowth, especially in patients with associated gastric outlet or biliary obstruction. These latter radiotherapeutic complications can be minimized by routine bypass of the distal bile duct. For patients having EB-IORT, the treatment of the second, third, and fourth portions of the duodenum can also be associated with bleeding. For the clinician using combined therapy, a cautionary note must be made regarding the need to control acute complications with this form of accelerated therapy. Accelerated radiotherapy treatment is defined as a treatment course that delivers the total radiotherapy dose in a shorter period that usual *(22)*. Chemoradiation is similar to accelerated radiotherapy, since simultaneous treatments are given daily, and the overall time of treatment for the two is thus shortened. These treatment approaches heighten the toxic effects in rapidly proliferating normal tissues, and, for pancreatic cancer patients, this usually means greater gastrointestinal toxicity. Acute tolerance is improved if the patient's nutritional status can be normalized prior to initiating treatment. A feeding tube for enteral feeding can be used at home for all patients who are unable to take in more than 1500 calories assessed at the beginning of irradiation.

Two of the newer agents that have become available for systemic use are the taxanes and gemcitabine. The use of paclitaxel has recently been shown to have a 31% response rate when weekly paclitaxel (up to 50 mg/kg/wk) was administered with 50 Gy *(30)*. The dose-limiting toxicities were acceptable levels of abdominal pain, nausea, and vomiting that were very well controlled with standard medications. A multicenter study to determine the feasibility of such an approach is underway in the RTOG. In another area of new radiation sensitizers, there is enthusiasm for the combination of gemcitabine and irradiation, since this drug has been shown to be a powerful radiation sensitizer in vitro *(31)* and in vivo *(32)*. There are no available data regarding the best schedule of gemcitabine and irradiation, but there have been reports of increased normal tissue toxicity with this combination, so that its use must still be considered experimental.

ADJUVANT TREATMENT

Postoperative Chemoradiation

Local-regional tumor recurrence after pancreatic resection occurs in 50–90% of cases *(33,34)*. This high local failure rate is related to the propensity for pancreatic cancer to invade adjacent nerves, blood vessels, and lymphatics. Moreover, the close proximity of large blood vessels constrains the basic oncologic principle of *en-bloc* removal. From an analysis of surgical specimens for the presence of positive margins or retroperitoneal tumor extension, there is clear evidence that poor local control and poor survival may occur as a result of positive margins *(35)*. Based on these patterns of failure, a rationale for more aggressive local treatment is justified, and the use of adjuvant radiotherapy with chemotherapy has been tested in numerous nonrandomized *(36)* and randomized *(37)* trials. In the prospective randomized study of surgery alone vs surgery plus adjuvant chemoradiotherapy for resected pancreatic cancer, conducted by the Gastrointestinal Tumor Study Group, 49 patients were randomized, 20 of whom received adjuvant therapy consisting of two courses of 20 Gy each, separated by an interval of

Radiation Therapy Oncology Group: A phase III study of pre- and post- chemoradiation: 5-FU vs. pre- and post- chemoradiation Gemcitabine (dFdC) for postoperative adjuvant treatment of resected pancreatic adenocarcinoma.

Schema:

S T R A T I F Y   nodal involvement / tumor diameter / tumor location / CA 19-9 / Surgical margins   R A N D O M O I Z E

Arm 1: 5-FU + chemoXRT* + 5-FU

Arm 2: dFdC + chemoXRT + dFdC

* ChemoXRT= 50.4 Gy + infusional 5-FU.

Fig. 5. Schema of the proposed RTOG/intergroup adjuvant postoperative chemoradiation protocol (to be opened 1998).

2 wk, for a total dose of 40 Gy *(37)*. 5-FU (iv bolus) was given concurrently during the first 3 d of each 2-wk course of irradiation, at a dosage of 500 mg/m². The results demonstrated a significant improvement in survival throughout the follow-up period ($p = .03$) for those patients receiving adjuvant therapy. Disease-free recurrence at 2 yr was 15% for the control group and 42% for the adjuvant chemoradiation group. An additional 30 patients were registered to this protocol after the preliminary report, and demonstrated a beneficial effect of adjuvant chemoradiation. The median survival time in the 30 patients was 18 mo and the 2-yr actual survival rate was 46%. Although these data are based on a small patient study, they support the concept that, by reducing the local recurrence rate, there can be a beneficial effect on overall survival. Additional studies are warranted, and the proposed schema for a new RTOG is shown in Fig. 5. This study builds on the knowledge gained in the adjuvant treatment of rectal cancer, and is designed to enroll patients with resected pancreatic cancer and offer them a course of chemotherapy and chemoradiation.

Preoperative Chemoradation

For patients with adenocarcinoma of the pancreas, pancreaticoduodenectomy (PD) requires complete reconstruction of the upper gastrointestinal tract, including reanastomoses of the pancreas, bile duct, and stomach. A lengthy postoperative recovery sometimes prevents the timely delivery of postoperative therapy, and has been responsible for the slow patient accrual in postoperative adjuvant therapy studies. For example, in a recent report on 78 consecutive patients treated with PD for adenocarcinoma of the pancreatic head, 22 of the 78 (28%) patients did not receive postoperative adjuvant therapy, despite having undergone surgery at an institution with very low perioperative mortality (<1%) and morbidity *(38)*. Perioperative complications increase significantly at institutions performing PD infrequently, as shown in the experience from New York State, where the mean perioperative hospital stay was greater than 1 mo, and the risk-adjusted perioperative mortality was 12–19% *(39)*. One way to reduce the risk of delaying adjuvant therapy is to deliver chemoradiation before PD for patients with potentially resectable or locally advanced adenocarcinoma of the pancreas. One important radiobiologic consideration for this approach is that irradiation can be more effective on well-oxygenated cells that have not been devascularized by surgery. Also, in practical terms, peritoneal tumor cell implantation caused by the manipulation of surgery may be prevented by preoperative chemoradiation, as well as a reduction of the high frequency of positive-margin resections. Also, patients with disseminated disease, evident on restaging studies after chemoradiation, will not be subjected to laparotomy, and will thereby be spared the associated morbidity and risk of treatment-related mortality. Finally, delayed postoperative recovery, which has been frequent in postoperative adjuvant therapy studies, will have no effect on the delivery of all components of the multimodality treatment.

At M. D. Anderson, a pilot trial of preoperative 5-FU chemoradiation, surgical resection, and EB-IORT boost indicates that this combination of treatment is safe, and that local control may be improved *(16)*. Preliminary results show that complications of EB-IORT plus ExBRT and radical surgery are not increased above those experienced with surgery alone. Evaluation of preoperative chemoradiation, resection, and EB-IORT from other series indicates that local failure is ~15%, and is lowest in those patients treated with both ExBRT and EB-IORT, which is also suggested by similar studies from European centers.

THE ROLE OF RADIOTHERAPY IN THE TREATMENT OF ISLET CELL CANCERS

Islet cell tumors of the pancreas are rare, slow-growing neuroendocrine neoplasms that occur at an estimated prevalence of 1/100,000 *(40)*. Characteristic tumor syndromes develop in two-thirds of patients with hormone-producing tumors (e.g., glucagon, insulin, somatostatin, gastrin); the remainder have nonfunctioning islet cell cancer *(41)*. Patients with nonfunctioning tumors present with an older age, presumably because of the lack of clinical symptoms that would otherwise bring them to medical attention *(42)*. Islet cell tumors are malignant tumors and frequently metastasize to regional lymph nodes and the liver. Complete surgical resection is only possible in a minority of patients. Nonsurgical treatment for those with unresected, residual, or metastatic disease has used mainly cytotoxic chemotherapy and cytostatic hormone therapy *(43)*. The role for radiotherapy is not defined, since most reported series have too few cases to draw general conclusions regarding the utility of ExBRT. Adjuvant irradiation and chemotherapeutics for patients with resected disease is also unproven.

The author reviewed the records of 13 patients with nonfunctioning islet cell tumors treated with radiotherapy at M. D. Anderson between 1960 and 1991. The medical, surgical, and radiotherapy reports were analyzed for presenting symptomatology, type of surgery, details of radiotherapy and chemotherapy, treatment complications, tumor recurrence patterns, and length of follow-up.

There were five women and eight men. Abdominal pain was the most common presenting symptom, followed by diarrhea, back pain, nausea and vomiting, and jaundice. Seven tumors occurred in the head of the pancreas, and the remainder were located in the body or the tail. Three patients were diagnosed and treated prior to the age of 35, but the majority were not diagnosed until after age 50, and the mean age at treatment was 48.5 yr. All patients referred with unresected disease had nonfunctioning tumors, and one patient with a VIP-syndrome was referred after surgery.

Five patients had surgical resection and eight had unresectable disease. One patient with initially staged unresectable tumor had surgical resection following chemotherapy.

ExBRT was given to doses of 45–50 Gy in 25–30 fractions; five patients received EB-IORT boost in combination with ExBRT. The sequence of therapy varied, and was individualized according to the differing clinical presentations. Two patients received concurrent continuous infusion of 5-FU during ExBRT. Acute complications from ExBRT were limited to nausea, vomiting, and diarrhea, and were well controlled with medications. Long-term complications of pancreatic insufficiency requiring insulin replacement occurred in three patients; one patient developed esophageal varices secondary to portal vein hypertension from periportal fibrosis secondary to irradiation.

Follow-up ranged from 7 to 81 mo, with a median of 46 mo. The actuarial survival at 5 yr after ExBRT is 60%. There are five resected and one unresected patients alive. The longest survivor is alive without tumor progression 71 mo after irradiation for an unresected tumor. The overall status of these patients is seven of 13 are dead and the remaining six patients are alive without evidence of disease.

These data indicate that radiotherapy can be useful in the treatment of both unresected islet cell tumors and as postoperative adjuvant. ExBRT appears to extend the interval of local tumor control for patients with even large, unresected cancers. Acute and long-term side effects of ExBRT have been minimal. Since radiotherapy has not traditionally been used in the management of these tumors, it deserves further investigation. It is not possible to evaluate fully the value of chemoradiation or EB-IORT boost in the treatment of these tumors. However, the poor prognosis of those with unresected disease treated with ExBRT alone, and the possibility that better local control can be obtained with chemoradiation, without a great increase in toxicity, warrants the use of more aggressive local therapy.

SUMMARY

New treatment strategies for pancreatic cancer patients are emerging in the 1990s with the use of combined modality therapy. The use of preoperative chemoradiation with 5-FU infusion, plus ExBRT, is an exciting area to pursue, based on preliminary reports. Improved local control gained by these approaches may also influence overall survival, as has been demonstrated by the results of adjuvant chemoradiation with 5-FU infusion for operable rectal cancer. Newer combinations of chemotherapy and ExBRT will need to be tested. The use of combined modality therapy causes increased normal tissue reactions, and caution must be exercised during treatment, especially in the areas of nutrition and fluid balance. Selection of patients who may benefit the most for these treatment approaches are those with localized disease. The use of newer diagnostic measures like thin-slice CT scanning may help by more accurately diagnosing occult metastatic disease.

New radiotherapy techniques, such as EB-IORT boost, offer a potential to surely deliver higher total radiotherapy doses to the unresected tumor or to the resected tumor bed. Prospective trials are needed to establish the utility of EB-IORT boost. Prophylactic hepatic and whole-abdominal chemoradiation for occult liver disease is also being tested in clinical trials, since the liver is the single most frequent site of failure outside of the primary site.

The use of radiotherapy for islet cell cancers is a controversial area, since there are only a few small series reported. Our data indicate 100% local control for patients treated with adjuvant local therapy after resection of islet cell cancer. For patients with bulky unresected disease, longterm palliation can be achieved with ExBRT alone. The use of chemoradiation for these latter patients is indicated in order to obtain the best and most durable palliation.

REFERENCES

1. Crist DW and Cameron JL. Current status of pancreaticoduodenectomy for periampulary carcinoma. Hepato-Gastroenterology 1989; *36:*478–485.
2. Cancer of Pancreas Task Force. Staging of cancer of the pancreas. Cancer 1981; *47:*1631–1637.
3. Cancer facts and figures. American Cancer Society, 1992.
4. Lumadue JA, Griffin CA, Osman M, and Hruban RH. Familial pancreatic cancer and the genetics of pancreatic cancer. Surg Clin N Am 1995; *75:*845–855.
5. Hallahan DE, Virudachalam S, Schwartz JL, Panje N, Mustafi R, and Weichselbaum RR. Inhibition of protein kinases sensitizes human tumor cells to ionizing radiation. Rad Res 1995; *129:*345–350.
6. Maity A, Kao GD, Muschel RJ, and McKenna WG. Potential molecular targets for manipulating the radiation response. Int J Radiat Oncol, Biol, Phys 1997; *37:*639–653.
7. Fuhrman GM, Charnsangavej C, Abbruzzese JL, et al. Thin-section contrast-enhanced computed tomography accurately predicts the resectability of malignant pancreatic neoplasms. Am J Surg 1994; *167:*104–113.
8. Evans DB, Staley CA, Lee JE, et al: Adenocarcinoma of the pancreas: recent controversies, current management, and future therapies. GI Cancer 1996; *1:*149–161.
9. Whittington R, Solin L, Mohiuddin M, Canto RI, Rasato FE, Biermann WA, Weiss SM, and Pajak TF. Multimodality therapy of localized unresectable pancreatic adenocarcinoma. Cancer 1984; *54:*1991–1998.
10. Gastrointestinal Tumor Study Group. Further evidence of effective adjuvant combined radiation and chemotherapy following curative resection of pancreatic cancer. Cancer 1987; *59:*2006–2010.
11. Rich TA. Intraoperative radiotherapy. In: Mauch P and Loeffler J (eds), Radiation oncology: technology and biology, Saunders, Philadelphia, 1993, pp. 152–166.
12. Morrow M, Hilaris B, and Brennan M. Comparison of conventional surgical resection, radioactive implantation, and bypass procedures for exocrine carcinoma of the pancreas 1975–1980. Ann Surg 1984; *199:*1–5.
13. Gunderson LL, Martin JK, Martinez A, Kvols LK, Nagorney DM, Fieck JM, Earle JD, and O'Connell MJ. Intraoperative and external beam irradiation for locally advanced pancreatic cancer. Int J Radiat Oncol Biol Phys 1985; *11:*115.
14. Nishimura A, Sakata S, Iida K, et al. Evaluation of intraoperative radiotherapy for carcinoma of the pancreas: prognostic factors and survival analyses. Radiat Med 1988; *6:*85.

15. Roldan GE, Gunderson LL, Nagorney DM, et al. External beam versus intraoperative and external beam irradiation for locally advanced pancreatic carcinoma. Cancer 1989; *61:*1110.

16. Spitz FR, Abbruzzese JL, Lee JE, Pisters PW, Lowy AM, Fenoglio CJ, et al. Preoperative and postoperative chemoradiation strategies in patients treated with pancreaticoduodenectomy for adenocarcinoma of the pancreas. J Clin Oncol 1997; *15:*928–937.

17. Nagakawa T, Konishi I, and Ueno K. The results and problems of extensive surgery for carcinoma of the head of the pancreas. Jap J Surg 1991; *21:*262–267.

18. Ashayeri E, Bonney G, DeWitty RL, Goldson AL, Leffall LD, and Thomas JN. Preliminary survivorship report on combined intraoperative radiation and hyperthermia treatments for unresectable pancreatic adenocarcinoma. J Nat Med Ass 1993; *85:*36–40.

19. Colacchio TA, Coughlin C, Taylor J, Douple E, Ryan T, and Crichlow RW. Intraoperative radiation therapy and hyperthermia. Morbidity and mortality from this combined treatment modality for unresectable intra-abdominal carcinomas. Arch Surg 1990; *125:*370–375.

20. Seydel HG, Stablein BM, Leichman LP, Kinzie JJ, and Thomas TRM. Hyperfractionated radiation and chemotherapy for unresectable localized adenocarcinoma of the pancreas. Cancer 1990; *65:*1478–1482.

21. Thomas FJ, Krall J, Hendrickson F, Griffin TW, Saxton JP, Parker RG, and Davis LW. Evaluation of neutron irradiation of pancreatic cancer. Results of a randomized radiation therapy oncology group clinical trial. Am J Clin Oncol 1989; *12:*283–239.

22. Rich TA. Chemoradiation or accelerated fractionation: basic considerations. J Infusional Chemother 1992; *1:*2–8.

23. Moertel CG, Reitemeier RJ, Childs DS, et al. Advanced gastrointestinal cancer. Mayo Clin Proc 1964; *39:*767–771.

24. Moertel C, Childs D, Reiemeir R, Colby MY, and Holbrook MA. Combined 5-fluorouracil and supervoltage radiation therapy of locally unresectable gastrointestinal cancer. Lancet 1969; *2L:*865–867.

25. Smith FP, Stablein D, Korsmeyer S, et al. Combination chemotherapy for locally advanced pancreatic cancer: equivalence to external beam irradiation and implication for future management. J Clin Oncol 1983; *1:*413–415.

26. Douglass HO, Stablein DM, and Thomas PRM. An organized multi-institutional interdisciplinary evaluation of the role of radiation therapy alone or combined with chemotherapy in treatment of adenocarcinoma of the gastrointestinal tract. NCI Monogr 1988; *6:*253–257.

27. Komaki R, Hansen R, Cox JD, et al. Phase I–II study of prophylactic hepatic irradiation with local irradiation and systemic chemotherapy for adenocarcinoma of the pancreas. Int J Radiat Oncol Biol Phys 1988; *15:*1447–1452.

28. Komaki R, Wadler S, Peters T, et al. High dose localirradiation plus prophylactic hepatic irradiation and chemotherapy for inoperable carcinoma of the pancreas. A preliminary report of a multi-institutional trial (RTOG protocol 88-01). Cancer 1992; *69:*2807.

29. Bruckner HW, Kalnicki S, Dalton J, et al. Combined modality therapy increasing local control of pancreatic cancer. Cancer Investigation 1993; *11:*2⁺1–246.

30. Safran H, King TP, Choy H, Hesketh PJ, Wolf B, Altenhein E, et al. Paclitaxel and concurrent radiation for locally advanced pancreatic and gastric cancer: a phase I study. J Clin Oncol 1997; *15:*901–907.

31. Shewach DS and Lawrence TS. Gemcitabine and radiosensitization in human tumor cells. Invest New Drugs 1996; *14:*257–263.

32. Fujii T, Hunter N, Elshaikh M, Hittleman W, Plunchett W, Ang K, and Milas L. Gemcitabine improves the therapeutic ratio of radiotherapy in mouse tumors after single dose irradiation. Proc Radiation Research 45th annual meeting. p. 229.

33. Tepper J, Nardi G, and Suit H. Carcinoma of the pancreas. Review of MGH experience from 1963 to 1973: analysis of surgical failure and implications for radiation therapy. Cancer 1976; *37:*1519–1524.

34. Griffin JF, Smalley SR, Jewell W, et al. Patterns of failure after curative resection of pancreatic carcinoma. Cancer 1990; *66:*56–61.
35. Willet CG, Lewandrowski K, Warshaw AL, et al. Resection margins in carcinoma of the head of the pancreas: implications for radiation therapy. Ann Surg 1993; *217:*144–148.
36. Rich TA. Radiation therapy for pancreatic cancer: eleven year experience at the JCRT. Int J Radiat Oncol Biol Phys 1985; *11:*759–763.
37. Kalser MH and Ellenberg SS. Pancreatic cancer. Adjuvant combined radiation and chemotherapy following curative resection. Arch Surg 1985; *120:*899–903.
38. Yeo C, Cameron Th, Lillemore KD, et al. Pancreaticoduodenectomy for cancer of the head of the pancreas: 201 patients. Ann Surg 1995; *221:*721–733.
39. Lieberman MD, Kilburn H, Lindsey M, et al. Relation of perioperative deaths to hospital volume among patients undergoing pancreatic resection for malignancy. Ann Surg 1995; *222:*638.
40. Torrisi JR, Treat J, Zeman R, and Dritschilo A. Radiotherapy in the management of pancreatic islet cell tumors. Cancer 1987; *60:*1226–1231.
41. Eriksson B, Öberg K, and Skogseid B. Neuroendocrine pancreatic tumors: clinical findings in a prospective study of 84 patients. Acta Oncol 1989; *28:*373–377.
42. Venkatesh S, Ordenez NG, Ajani J, Schultz PN, Hickey RC, Johnston DA, and Samaan NA. Islet cell carcinoma of the pancreas: a study of 98 patients. Cancer 1990; *65:*354–357.
43. Moertel CG. An odyssey in the land of small tumors. J Clin Oncol 1987; *5:*1503–1522.

Gene Therapy for Pancreatic Cancer

Nicholas R. Lemoine

INTRODUCTION

There are a number of compelling reasons why cancer of the pancreas may be a particularly good model for the development of gene therapy strategies. First, the genetic basis of pancreatic cancer is becoming very well characterized because of intense activity in laboratories around the world (reviewed in refs. *1* and *2*), and each oncogene and tumor-suppressor gene identified represents a novel target for genetic therapy *(3)*. Second, the recognition that there may be familial inherited predisposition to pancreatic cancer, either alone *(4)* or in association with other malignancies such as melanoma *(5–7)*, offers the possibility of prevention by genetic intervention. Third, because of the poor response to conventional treatment and dismal prognosis of the disease, patients and clinicians are willing to explore such new therapies. This chapter reviews the latest possibilities for exploiting genetic technology in the treatment and prevention of pancreatic cancer, and highlights the most promising areas for clinical application.

SOMATIC AND GERM-LINE THERAPY

In principle, gene therapy could be applied either to somatic cells of an individual, or to a germ cell (ovum or, theoretically, even spermatozoon), in order to alter the genetic constitution of the individual produced on subsequent fertilization, as well as all their succeeding generations. At present, the permanent correction of an inherited genetic condition by gene transfer to germ cells has not been approved, but the possibility will remain the subject of continuing debate. Hence, somatic tissue is presently the arena for genetic intervention, which may be performed either ex vivo or in vivo, depending on the requirements of the strategy applied. However, before reviewing the technologies and strategies for gene transfer therapy, the author will first consider the potential of more familiar and conventional approaches to genetic intervention at the stage of embryonic or fetal development.

PREVENTION OF HEREDITARY PREDISPOSITION SYNDROMES

At present, prevention of cancer relies on epidemiological studies to identify factors involved in the etiology of the disease and the subsequent modification of behavioral patterns of the population at risk. However, these studies require extensive research and the implementation of new health education measures, both of which can take decades to come to fruition.

In recent years, it has become evident that some individuals are predisposed to neoplasia at predictable sites because of inherited genetic mutation. Unfortunately, until preventative measures or effective cures are developed, such individuals will live with the prospect of developing cancer in midlife or even childhood. At present, there are few methods for the prevention of cancer, and those that do exist are often unacceptable; for instance, carriers of *BRCA1* gene are offered prophylactic mastectomy and oophorectomy, even though it is still difficult to quantify the actual risk of disease *(8)*. It is difficult to envisage how an analogous organ removal approach could be operated for pancreatic cancer predisposition, although advances in transplantation technology may in future improve the prospects for individuals undergoing pancreatectomy.

With the progress reported for the prediction of inherited genetic diseases, such as cystic fibrosis and muscular dystrophy, it has been suggested that such prenatal techniques could be offered to couples with genetic traits predisposing to cancer, thereby preventing transmission of the gene to any offspring *(9)*. However, termination of a pregnancy after chorionic villus sampling (CVS) may prove unacceptable to many couples, when the baby would be otherwise normal. A more acceptable alternative may be in vitro fertilization coupled with preimplantation diagnosis. However, a prerequisite for the success of such an approach is the identification and characterization of the genes involved. There are essentially three categories of genetic cancer predisposition: Those in which mutation of an identified gene locus affecting the families is known, e.g., *CDKN2* in familial atypical mole and melanoma syndrome, in some cases associated with pancreatic cancer *(6,7)*, or the cationic trypsinogen gene in hereditary pancreatitis *(10)* (individuals in some families with this phenotype have a higher relative risk for pancreatic cancer) *(11)*; those in which a defined chromosomal linkage is known, but the gene has yet to be identified; and those in which there is familial site-specific cancer phenotype without definite linkage to a chromosomal locus (most kindreds with an excess incidence of pancreatic cancer presently fall into this category) *(4)*.

The diagnosis of genetic mutations after IVF involves the removal of one or two cells from the embryo, and the subsequent analysis of their DNA by polymerase chain reaction (PCR) amplification techniques. Such methods could be applied to mutations resulting in cancer predispositions, in which the mutation is well characterized and efforts are now directed to develop multiplex PCR systems to allow analysis of several exons or several genes simultaneously.

Important factors in implementing interventional strategies are the sheer scale of the problem of screening large genes with diverse mutation sites, and the realization that any one gene may be just one of many that can contribute to susceptibility to a given tumor type *(12)*. In addition, the involvement in pancreatic cancer of predisposition genes with only partial penetrance, such as *BRCA2*, seriously complicates interpretation of germline mutations *(13)*.

TECHNOLOGY FOR SOMATIC GENETIC INTERVENTION

Somatic gene therapy involves the insertion of genes into the diploid cells of an individual in whom the genetic material is not passed on to the subject's progeny. The transfer is achieved by physical means, or by using virus-mediated delivery, and is conventionally envisaged for application in patients with established cancer *(3)*. Gene transfer can be achieved ex vivo or in vivo, each of which has applications for particular therapeutic strategies.

Gene transfer ex vivo requires that the target cells are removed from the patient, and can be applied to the tumor cells for immunomodulation strategies, or to samples of normal host tissue, such as bone marrow, for the introduction of drug resistance genes. Gene transfer ex vivo has the great advantage that conditions can be optimized to achieve the highest efficiency, and the transfected cells can be selected and expanded before reimplantation.

Gene transfer in vivo is technically more difficult to achieve because of the relatively primitive vectors presently available, and because of problems of accessing target tissues. Most experimental protocols use viral vectors to introduce the therapeutic gene, but the realization that naked DNA can be taken up and expressed by somatic cells after simple injection *(14)* has led to an increased enthusiasm for this approach for clinical studies.

A variety of vector systems have been proposed for gene therapy, composed of biological systems (viruses and viral components), synthetic agents (liposomes and lipopolyamines) and physical systems (particle bombardment and electroporation).

Viral Vectors

Retroviral vectors were the first system to be engineered for gene transfer in clinical trial and have been the most widely used system since (reviewed in ref. *15)*. Although a variety of retroviruses (including murine mammary tumor virus [MMTV], human immunodeficiency virus type 1 [HIV-1], simian immunodeficiency virus [SIV] and human foamy viruses) could theoretically be utilized for the purpose, the vectors in clinical trials so far are exclusively based on Moloney murine leukemia virus (MMLV). Retroviruses were first used successfully ex vivo for marking human tumor-infiltrating lymphocytes (TIL) with an antibiotic resistance gene that could be used to track the reintroduced cells in biopsy samples *(16)*; currently most human clinical trials using retroviral gene transfer involve ex vivo transduction of target cells. The use of murine retroviruses in vivo is complicated by their sensitivity to destruction by human complement, but local administration of virus has been attempted, particularly for brain tumors *(17–19)*. Since complement resistance is a property of the viral surface proteins, hybrid vectors with envelope components from other viruses have been developed *(20,21)* and it may also be possible to block specific components of the complement pathway *(22,23)*.

Adenoviral vectors *(24)* can be prepared to much higher titers than retroviral vectors, and, because they do not possess an envelope, they are much more stable than retroviruses, with little sensitivity to human complement. They are able to mediate gene transfer into cells regardless of their proliferative state, which could be an advantage when targeting human tumors with a relatively low growth fraction, such as pancreatic cancer. However, adenoviruses do have some disadvantages, which limit their application. Since the majority of the viral genome is retained in most vector systems, there is a problem with unwanted expression of viral genes, which can result in toxicity and immune reactions that may be dose-limiting in clinical trial *(25–28)*; this may be overcome by the recent development of a vector in which all the viral coding regions are replaced by recombinant sequence *(29)*.

The adeno-associated virus (AAV) is a unique member of the parvovirus family, with some special features useful for gene therapy application *(30)*. The virus mediates stable and efficient integration of therapeutic gene sequence into the host genome, it is able to infect a variety of cell types, even when they are growth-arrested, and it is not associated with any known pathology. The disadvantages include difficulty in achieving high viral titers and potential for contamination with wild-type virus in large-scale production.

Vaccina virus has applications for immunization strategies against tumor antigens and has been used for the construction of recombinant vectors to express a variety of potential epitopes. Since the original virus is very large, with a number of nonessential regions, there is a possibility of inserting multiple therapeutic genes for simultaneous expression.

Nonviral Vectors

Naked DNA may be injected directly in vivo, either intravascularly or into tissues such as skeletal muscle or skin. The efficiency of this apparently primitive approach is surprisingly high, with transfection levels reported to be similar to those of transfecting fibroblasts in vitro by conventional co-precipitation technology, and expression persists for months, even in the absence of chromosomal integration *(31)*. Transfection rates can be increased by manipulations such as injection of hypertonic sucrose or bupivacaine into the tissue before exposure to DNA *(32,33)*. When injected intravenously, naked DNA is rapidly taken up by the liver, with 60% being cleared within 1.5 min of administration *(34,35)*, and there are powerful nucleases in serum that degrade the surviving plasmid. Naked DNA injection does not appear to result in formation of anti-DNA antibodies even in primates *(36)*, and so the technique may be particularly exploited for developing vaccines against the expressed product.

Liposomes are stable microscopic vesicles formed by phospholipids and such amphipathic lipids, which can be combined with other components, such as virosomes (empty viral particles) or polyamines, to improve gene delivery *(37)*. Cationic lipids form a complex with DNA, which binds to the negatively charged surface of cells and allows internalization for gene transfer. In vivo administration of cationic lipid–plasmid DNA complexes produces no antibody or cell-mediated immune reponse, which is a significant advantage over viral systems when considering repeated injection. However, the efficiency of present-generation liposomes is around 100–1000 times less than an adenoviral vector system, so large doses of complexed DNA are required to achieve a given biological end point. Several clinical trials have been performed using cationic lipid–DNA complexes, and these have shown that there can be therapeutic effect, with only low levels of toxicity after intranasal administration in cystic fibrosis patients *(38,39)* and intratumoral injection in melanoma patients *(40,41)*. Attempts have been made to target liposome complexes and increase delivery efficiency by, for instance, incorporating an antibody conjugate *(42,43)* or modifying the lipid moiety to interact with the asialoglycoprotein receptors on hepatocytes *(44)*, but these approaches have not yet been tested in vivo. Co-administration of adenovirus, given simultaneously, can significantly enhance the efficacy of gene transfer by cationic lipid and lipopolyamine complexes *(45–49)*. This appears to be a result of the ability of adenovirus to mediate escape of the conjugate from the endosomal–lysosomal pathway after internalization.

Particle bombardment is a technique that is particularly suited to gene delivery to superficial tissues, but could be applied to deeper organs intraoperatively. Particles (typically of gold) coated with DNA are accelerated to high velocity either by electrical charge or helium pulse, so that they can penetrate up to 50 cell layers deep into an organ *(50–52)*. Larger beads can be used to bombard a tissue to produce multiple microscopic channels that enhance penetration of viral or other vectors administered subsequently. Although transgene expression is only temporary and there may be problems with damage to bombarded tissues, the relative simplicity and speed of the technique make it attractive for applications such as DNA vaccination or cytokine gene expression *(53,54)*.

Antisense Technology

Naturally occurring antisense interactions are known to modulate gene expression in prokaryotes, and similar mechanisms are thought to occur also in eukaryotes *(55)*. As a consequence, there has been an explosion in the development of antisense technology to target specifically cellular transcription and translation. Initial attempts to downregulate genes in vitro, using antisense oligonucleotides, have been extended as a result of increasing interest in their potential therapeutic application in vivo *(56,57)*.

There are four strategies for the use of antisense agents, which are all based on complementary base pairing. Antisense sequences can be administered exogenously as synthetic oligonucleotides, or produced endogenously from an antisense-expression vector *(56)*. The most widely documented involves the exogenous introduction of short complementary single-stranded oligonucleotides (normally DNA molecules 15–20 nucleotides in length), which are thought to act by binding specifically to their corresponding cellular mRNA partner, blocking translation *(56)*. These antisense oligonucleotides may target several different stages of the translation pathway. Cleavage by RNase H specifically degrades the RNA subunit in the DNA–RNA hybrid. Antisense oligonucleotides, which target the 5′ untranslated region, may sterically hinder the binding of the 40S ribosomal subunit. Similarly, those binding close to the initiation codon (AUG) could prevent assembly of the translation initiation complex. In some instances, it has been suggested that antisense oligonucleotides that bind to the more restricted pool of cytoplasmic hrRNA may provide a better target because less antisense agent would be required to downregulate gene expression. It has also been suggested that targeting hrRNA intron/exon junctions may afford a higher degree of specificity *(56)*.

The second approach involves specific binding of oligonucleotides to gene targets prior to transcription, by forming a triple helix. This can be manipulated to produce irreversible binding at a genetic locus, or even selective cleavage, resulting in loss of gene expression and cell death.

The third approach targets the transcription machinery. Certain proteins, including transcription factors, DNA polymerases, and RNA polymerases, have the ability to recognize nucleic acid motifs. These factors, which are essential for transcription initiation, can be sequestered away from the genetic site by providing the cell with double-stranded oligodeoxynucleotides, which act as traps or decoys *(58–60)*.

The fourth approach uses ribozymes, which are small oligoribonucleotides with a specific base sequence, resulting in a self-splicing activity. Although their mode of action is significantly different from the other three antisense technologies described above, their targets and the outcome of their activity is similar. The ribozyme activity can be directed against various RNAs by the incorporation of flanking antisense regions around the ribozyme, although some targets are better cleaved than others (the sequences GUC, GUA, GUU, CUC, and UUC are most favored).

REPLACEMENT OF TUMOR-SUPPRESSOR GENE FUNCTION

Experimental models suggest that introduction of a single tumor-suppressor gene can produce dramatic antitumor effects, but there are a number of problems associated with gene augmentation/replacement as a clinical strategy, not least being heterogeneity of molecular profile. It also appears that individual tumor-suppressor genes may be important only at particular points in tumor evolution, so that there may be a limited window of opportunity for therapeutic intervention. Introduction of the normal gene could be envisaged either in the tumor cells of an established cancer, or in the stem cells of the pancreas in an individual with an inherited defect predisposing to cancer of this organ.

For the preventive strategy, the ideal scenario would be to replace a defective tumor-suppressor gene directly in its normal genomic position by the process of homologous recombination *(61)*. Such gene targeting can already be used to repair genetic defects in cultured cells, but the process is very inefficient in mammalian cells: Even in highly favorable conditions created in vitro, the proportion of transfected cells that become targeted is of the order of $10^{-6}–10^{-8}$. It is inconceivable that this approach could work for an established tumor cell population in vivo, but it might one day be adapted for correcting a defect in, for instance, the preneoplastic ductal cells of an individual with pancreatic cancer predisposition. The first challenge for this to be possible is the identification of stem cells in pancreatic tissue; even in the most experimentally tractable models, such as skin *(62)*, these are very rare, difficult to assay, and expand in culture without losing their pluripotentiality. Given the present efficiency of gene targeting, one would need to transfect around 10^{10} stem cells to obtain a single targeted result. The second challenge would be to reintroduce the genetically corrected stem cell(s) and induce them to repopulate the ductal system, which would require some form of positive advantage over the existing population. Since introduction of a tumor-suppressor gene is usually associated with inhibition of proliferation, compared to the mutant parent cells, this may be difficult to achieve.

The majority of protocols for tumor-suppressor gene therapy for established cancer have concentrated on the tumor-suppressor gene *TP53*. The protein product of this gene plays a pivotal role in arresting cell growth in response to DNA damage, so that repair or apoptosis can occur. More than 50% of pancreatic tumors have some type of gene alteration, and up to 80% show allelic loss (deletion of one copy of the gene) at the *p53* locus 17p13 *(63–69)*. The p53 protein forms a tetramer in solution, and the consensus DNA binding site has a symmetry that corresponds with an interaction with tetrameric protein. Mutated forms of *p53* lose their transactivating function and inhibit the activity of any wild-type protein co-expressed, but multiple studies have now demonstrated that ex vivo introduction of a wild-type *p53* gene into tumor cells expressing mutant *p53* can suppress malignant growth both in vitro and in vivo *(70–72)*. Replication-in-competent adenoviruses have been used to deliver the *p53* gene into a variety of tumor cell types, including ovarian cancer, lung cancer, head and neck cancer, prostate cancer, hepatocellular cancer, bladder cancer, and cervical cancer *(73–85)* and this approach is being applied to pancreatic cancer in this laboratory (unpublished data). Multiple daily dosing of an adenoviral construct expressing wild-type *p53* via hepatic artery infusion in a rat model of hepatocellular carcinoma showed suppression of tumor growth without effect on normal hepatocyte metabolism and regenerative capacity *(83,86)*. An exciting possibility is that genetic intervention may potentiate the effects of conventional anticancer therapies. Recent studies have shown that induction of apoptosis by chemotherapeutic drugs and radiotherapy is dependent on the *p53* status of tumor cells. Direct injection of an adenoviral construct expressing *p53* into lung cancer cells growing as subcutaneous xenografts in nude mice, followed by intraperitoneal administration of cisplatin, produced massive tumor cell death by apoptosis, with little evidence of systemic toxicity *(87)*.

A related tumor-suppressor gene of interest is the *p53*-inducible *WAF1* which encodes *p21*[Waf]. This binds to and inhibits cyclin-dependent kinases (cdk) by forming a quaternary structure with cdks, cyclins, and proliferative cellular nuclear antigen (PCNA)*(88)*. In the vast majority of tumors, the activity of cdks is uncontrolled because of loss of *p21*[Waf] expression. It has been demonstrated that overexpression of *p21*[Waf] in *p53*-deficient cells suppressed tumor growth *(89)*. Only the N-terminal domain of this protein is required to act as a suppressor, and, indeed, two tructated subunits of *p21*[Waf] (amino acids 1-80 and 1-89) showed an increased activity against tumor cell proliferation, compared to the wild-type *p21*[Waf]. These studies look promising for the development of high-efficiency synthetic suppressor genes for replacement therapies.

CDKN2 (also known as *p16*) is another candidate suppressor gene that could be exploited in augmentation therapies. This gene encodes *p16*, which inhibits cyclin-dependent kinase-4 in complex with cyclin D1. Deletions in exons 1 and 2 of *CDKN2* have been found in a high proportion of pancreatic cancers *(90–93)*. Ectopic expression of *p16* blocks entry into S phase of the cell cycle if the cells express functional retinoblastoma protein, and, since this condition is satisfied in the majority of pancreatic cancers, a *CDKN2* replacement strategy might be feasible for this disease.

BLOCKADE OF DOMINANT GENE EXPRESSION BY ANTISENSE TECHNOLOGY

An in vitro study of H460 human lung cancer cells showed that protein expression of a mutant K-ras oncogene could be suppressed by 95% using an antisense construct, and this was accompanied by a threefold reduction in cell growth relative to controls *(94)*. In vivo studies of xenografts in nude mice treated with the construct demonstrated substantial reductions in both K-ras expression and tumor growth; treatment of an orthotopic human lung cancer model by intratracheal instillation in nude mice gave similar results *(95)*. Liposome-mediated in vivo gene transfer of an antisense K-ras construct was used to treat human pancreatic cancer (AsPC-1) cells inoculated intraperitoneally in nude mice *(96,97)*. Not only was there significant suppression of tumor progression (only two of 12 mice treated with the construct showed evidence of tumor, compared to nine of 10 control mice), but there was no evidence of systemic toxicity, even though gene transfer had evidently occurred in most organs except the brain.

Because mutated *p53* can act as a transforming oncogene in some conformations, it has been targeted for antisense suppression, using both synthetic oligonucleotides delivered exogenously and antisense constructs expressed endogenously. Synthetic agents have even been used in clinical trial for patients with acute myeloid leukemia, and although there was no evidence of clinical benefit, neither was there evidence of systemic side effects *(98,99)*. This is particularly surprising in view of the evidence from experiments in pancreatic cancer cells that agents targeted to this gene sequence have serious toxic side effects *(57)*. It has been reported that a retroviral construct delivering an anti-*p53* ribozyme able to cleave *p53* pre-mRNA at the intron 5–exon 6 boundary dramatically reduced the level of mutant p53 protein and suppressed the growth of tumor cells in vitro *(100)*. Another ribozyme targeted to the intron 7–exons 8 boundary did not suppress tumor cell growth, even though *p53* expression levels were reduced.

An *ERBB2* antisense oligonucleotide used at high concentration inhibited ERBB2 protein expression in a dose-dependent manner and suppressed the proliferation of *ERBB2*-positive breast cancer cell lines *(101)*, and, since the mechanism of *ERBB2* transformation appears to be similar in pancreatic cancer *(102)*, the approach may be suitable for this disease. Expression of *ERBB2* might also be suppressed by treatment of cells with a triple helix-forming agent, since the gene has a purine-rich motif in its promoter, although effects of this approach were disappointing in tumor cells *(103)*.

Antisense reduction of *BCL2* gene expression has been reported to sensitize cells to cytosine arabinoside (ara-C) and methotrexate (MTX), and hence this approach may provide a novel mechanism for improving chemotherapeutic treatment of cancer *(104)*.

Antisense therapeutics are an evolving technology, and there remain several uncertainties about their mechanism of action and potential toxicity. For instance, it has been shown that, although these oligonucleotides activate RNase H activity when bound to mRNA, at high concentration they will bind to and inhibit the catalytic action of the enzyme *(105)*. Some of the inhibitory effects noted may be the result of binding to molecules other than RNA, such as heparin, and this makes it difficult to determine exactly what is causing an inhibitory effect. For instance, studies in smooth muscle cells *(106)* have suggested that the antiproliferative effect of antisense oligonucleotides to c-*myb* and c-*myc* is actually a nonantisense mechanism dependent on a GC-rich sequence, and nonsequence-dependent binding has been noted with basic fibroblast growth factor (bFGF) *(107)*. The motif CpG in a nucleic acid sequence is also thought to be a potential immunomodulator *(108,109)*. Mice injected intraperitoneally with phosphorothioates show a dramatic increase in immunoglobulin secretion, accompanied by increased expression of MHC class II markers, and oligonucleotides containing a CpG motif can induce interferons and augment natural killer cells *(110,111)*.

GENETIC PRODRUG ACTIVATION THERAPY

Genetic prodrug activation therapy (GPAT) exploits selective expression of a metabolic suicide gene within tumor cells, to confer sensitivity to a prodrug, and depends on targeting for specificity *(112)*. The first report of a GPAT system was made by Moolten *(113)*, who described the transduction of a mouse cell line with an HSV-

TK construct, which became sensitive to ganciclovir in vitro, and in vivo studies on tumors in syngeneic animals showed total eradication of neoplastic cells.

Transduction targeting relies on preferential delivery of genes to target cells through selection of a particular phenotype. This may be very simple, as in the targeting of dividing tumor cells in otherwise quiescent brain tissue, which can be achieved using a retroviral vector, or more sophisticated, as in the targeting of tumor cells expressing particular cell-surface receptors using gene transfer systems with ligand moieties.

Transcriptional targeting relies on unique tissue-specific or tumor-specific transcriptional elements to drive expression only in those cells that contain transcription factors capable of activating the promoter elements. As a consequence, for such a system to be effective, the regulatory elements of the promoter/enhancer need to be fully characterized.

These two methods can be combined to provided an improved targeting system, but each system has its own advantages and disadvantages, which are described in more detail in the following sections.

Transduction Targeting

The receptors for the murine leukemia viral envelopes commonly used to package retroviruses for gene therapy applications have been cloned and identified recently as a phosphate receptor (in the case of the amphotropic MLV-A, which infects a variety of species, including human) and a cationic amino acid transporter (in the case of the ecotropic MLV-E, which infects only rodents). The residues in the retroviral envelope proteins determining host range have been identified, which therefore gives the opportunity to engineer novel specificity into the envelope–receptor interaction. Both single-chain antibodies to cell surface antigens and natural ligands to transmembrane receptors have been engineered, either as N-terminal extensions or as replacement cassettes in the envelope protein *(114)*. There has been mixed success with these approaches. Retroviral particles from helper cells expressing a fusion protein between the envelope protein and (as an N-terminal extension) the domain of heregulin β1, which mediates specific interaction with the ERBB3 and ERBB4 receptors, were able to induce tyrosine phosphorylation of the these receptors, on the surface of target cells, but not to produce gene transfer *(115)*. In contrast, when heregulin α or β1 were engineered as replacement cassettes within the envelope, very efficient infection of breast cancer cells expressing the cognate receptors was achieved *(116)*.

Transcriptional Targeting

Transcriptional targeting exploits tumor-specific promoter elements to drive the expression of a toxic protein only in those cells that contain transcription factors able to activate the promoter. The first reported system harnessed one of two promoters, either the hepatoma-associated α-fetoprotein (AFP) or normal liver-associated albumin (ALB), to drive a *VZV-TK* suicide gene. In vitro, it was possible to engineer expression restricted to the malignant hepatoma cells, using the AFP promoter, and expression restricted to normal liver cells, using the ALB promoter *(117)*. Subsequent studies to test the concept in transgenic mice were disappointing because recombinant retrovirus constructs failed to express the suicide gene, attributed to silencing of the retroviral sequences *(18)*.

The author's group has exploited the promoter elements of the proto-oncogene *ERBB2* for this approach *(119–121)*, and, because of the encouraging results of this system in experimental models, a clinical trial to test its safety and efficacy has been approved by the UK regulatory authorities. Others have used the CEA gene promoter *(122–124)* and the *MUC1/DF3* gene promoter *(125,126)* with similar success, and both systems could be suitable for application in pancreatic cancer.

Bystander Effects

One of the phenomena that has been noted by several groups studying the GPAT system is that treatment of mixed populations of transduced and nontransduced cells with prodrug can result in unexpectedly high levels of cell death. This has been termed bystander killing, a feature which is extremely advantageous for GPAT systems, in which the transduction efficiency is poor. In xenografts composed of a mixed population, in which only 10% of cells carried the suicide gene, over half the tumors were eradicated after prodrug treatment *(127)*. It is postulated that the bystander effect is caused by metabolic cooperation between cells, the result of trafficking of small molecules (mol wt < 1000 Daltons) between cells via gap junctions, or that it could result from apoptotic vesicles containing the enzyme (or gene) derived from dying cells being phagocytosed *(127)*; more recent work has suggested that a T-cell-mediated response could contribute. Lung tumors transduced with an HSV-TK gene in immunocompetent mice, and then treated with ganciclovir, showed a 90% reduction in tumor size compared to the saline-treated controls. However, the same study repeated in nude mice (T-cell-deficient) resulted in no change in tumor burden between the ganciclovir-treated and the saline-treated control animals *(128)*.

GENETIC IMMUNOMODULATION

Cytotoxic T-lymphocytes can destroy target cells that present a recognized antigen in the context of the MHC class I presentation machinery. The new understanding of how cellular proteins are processed and presented to the immune system has opened a new avenue of genetic intervention to produce or enhance a cytotoxic response.

Most cytosolic proteins destined for degradation become tagged by attachment of a small protein called ubiquitin, and processed by proteasomes to small peptides, which are transported by a heterodimeric complex of transporters of antigenic peptides (TAP-1 and TAP-2) into the endoplasmic reticulum. Here they may bind within the peptide-binding groove of the MHC class I α-chain to allow it to complex with β2-microglobulin and be transported to the cell surface. There is an enormous amount of allelic variation in class I genes, and each gene product binds only a small repertoire of peptide sequences. Most of the peptides which can be bound in this way are nonapeptides, but a smaller number of octapeptides and decapeptides can also be complexed.

Exposure of a peptide in the MHC class I molecule by an antigen-presenting cell can produce a cytotoxic immune reaction by interaction with a T-lymphocyte with the appropriate specificity of antigen recognition. However, specific T-cell receptor engagement with the MHC class I–peptide complex is insufficient on its own to activate a naive T-lymphocyte; instead, a second signal is required in the form of interaction between the CD28 receptor molecule on the lymphocyte and a co-stimulatory molecule of a family known as B7 on the antigen-presenting cell. One class of T-helper lymphocyte appears to play an important accessory role in the initiation of the immune response by secretion of cytokines, including interleukin-2, which supports the proliferation and activation of the T-cytotoxic lymphocytes.

Tumor cells frequently have defects in the pathway that leads to antigen presentation and potential immune recognition (about 25% of pancreatic cancers have lost class I expression *(129)*, and cancer patients often have a degree of immunodepression, so therapeutic strategies fall into two broad groups: One approach is to restore the missing components and enhance immune recognition, and the other is to engineer vaccines using potential tumor-specific antigens.

Cytokine Gene Therapy

Cytokines are a heterogeneous group of polypeptides that modulate the proliferation, maturation, and function of cells of the immune system. Rosenberg and colleagues *(130)* demonstrated that the systemic administration of interleukin-2 reduced the number of metastases observed in experimental animal tumor models, such as chemically induced sarcomas and mouse melanomas. Encouraging results were also reported in human clinical trials with this and other cytokines *(131,132)* but dose-limiting toxicity experienced with systemic administration led to the approach of genetic engineering to express these molecules locally to stimulate the immune system and reject the tumor. A large number of studies in murine models have now demonstrated that tumor growth can be inhibited and even abrogated by the transfer and expression of various cytokines *(133)*. In general, the most consistent results have come from the modification of tumor cells to express interleukin-2 (IL-2) *(134–151)* and granulocyte–macrophage colony stimulating factor (GM-CSF) *(136,152–154)*, but there are contrasting effects in different tumor types: The most dramatic responses are seem in melanoma and renal cell carcinoma. Encouraging results are now being reported for IL-15 gene transfer into tumor cell deposits, which induces lymphokine-activated killer cells and tumor-infiltrating lymphocytes with increased local levels of interferon-γ (IFN-γ) and GM-CSF secretion *(155–157)*. Coexpression of two cytokine genes in a nonimmunogenic murine pancreatic cancer cell line has recently been engineered, and produced enhanced tumor rejection, compared to expression of either IL-2 or IFN-γ alone *(158)*. In these experiments, mice were inoculated subcutaneously with parental Panc02 tumor cells, and then received a series of four weekly vaccinations with irradiated tumor cells engineered to express IL-2, IFN-γ, or both cytokines together. None of the unvaccinated or control animals survived tumor-free to 100 d, but 30% of those vaccinated with IFN- —expressors, 40% of those vaccinated with IL-2-expressor, and 80% of those vaccinated with the double-expressors were free of disease: These animals were also resistant to subsequent challenge with parental tumor.

Co-Stimulatory Molecule Gene Therapy

Expression of co-stimulatory molecules, such as B7.1, on tumor cells by gene transfer could enable them to activate T-lymphocytes directly, bypassing the requirement for professional antigen-presenting cells, such as dendritic cells or macrophages. This can be achieved either by injection of the gene expression vector into tumor deposits *in situ*, or by transduction of tumor cells extracted from a biopsy specimen and then returned to the patient after irradiation. A major attraction of the approach is that it does not require knowledge of the exact profile of tumor-associated antigens in any particular case, nor even definition of the HLA type of the patient. It has been demonstrated that naive syngeneic mice are able to reject implanted melanoma cells transfected to express B7.1, but the parental cells grew progressively *(159–161)*. The animals were also resistant to subsequent challenge with injection of the parental tumor (not expressing B7).

The costimulatory molecule B7.1 may be more effective than its relative B7.2 in inducing rejection and protective immunity in vivo *(162–164)*, although both appear equally effective at stimulating IL-2 and IFN-γ production. Expression of costimulatory B7 molecules on tumor cells may not make them as effective as professional antigen-presenting cells, but in combination with exogenous IL-10, or IL-6 plus IL-12, this approach has generated cytotoxic T-lymphocytes from naive sygeneic mouse spleen cells in vitro. Allogeneic proliferative and cytotoxic T-lymphocyte responses are also enhanced against primary human tumor cell lines that have been engineered to express B7.1*(165)*.

Tumor Antigen Vaccination

MHC-restricted, tumor-specific cytotoxic T-lymphocytes have been isolated with activity against a number of different tumors. In patients with *ERBB2*-expressing cancers, an HLA-A2-presented peptide derived from the *ERBB2* oncogene was shown to be recognized by tumor-infiltrating lymphocytes *(166)*. Several of the antigens against which they react are candidates for vaccination in the treatment of pancreatic cancer. The tumor-associated antigen carcinoembryonic antigen (CEA) has been used for so-called active adoptive immunotherapy, since it is expressed at much higher levels on tumor cells than on normal cells. Intramuscular injection of a synthetic plasmid expressing human CEA produced a humoral response against the antigen in mice *(167)*, and immunoprotection against challenge with CEA-expressing colon cancer cells *(168,169)*. Similar results have been reported for a recombinant CEA vaccinia vaccine given in combination with systemic interleukin-2 *(170)*.

Both helper CD4+ and cytotoxic CD8+ lymphocytes specific for K-*ras* have been reported in patients with *ras*-positive cancer *(171–173)*, and mutant *p21 ras* can be recognized by human T-cells in vitro *(174–177)*. The tight restriction of mutations to codons 12/13 in this gene makes it perhaps the best candidate for an exclusive tumor-specific antigen. The approach has been explored both in experimental animals and (more recently) in man. Mice were immunized subcutaneously at 2-wk intervals with purified ras oncoproteins mixed with immunologic adjuvants, which enhance the induction of T-cell-mediated immunity. Proliferative and cytolytic T-cell responses directed against the Arg 12 ras protein were generated, resulting in protection against challenge with cells expressing Arg 12 *Ras* and therapeutic benefit in mice bearing established tumors expressing this protein *(178)*. Synthetic *ras* peptides have been tested as a cancer vaccine in patients with advanced pancreatic carcinoma recently *(179)*. Professional antigen-presenting cells (APCs) from peripheral blood were loaded ex vivo with a synthetic ras peptide corresponding to the ras mutation found in tumor tissue from each of five patients. None of the patients showed evidence of a T-cell response against any of the ras peptides before vaccination, but, in two of the patients treated, an immune response against the immunizing ras peptide was identified by laboratory tests (but there was no evident clinical benefit observed in these individuals with advanced, terminal disease). The author's group is presently developing a DNA vaccine consisting of nontransforming fragments of the mutated K-*ras* gene, which is delivered either as an intradermal injection or transfected into purified dendritic cells (professional antigen-presenting cells), and there is some evidence for a specific immune response, both cytotoxic and humoral, in animal models.

Genetic Engineering of Antitumor Lymphocytes

Variants of the CD44 protein family containing sequences encoded by variant exon 6 (v6) are expressed on cancer cells and involved in the metastatic spread of rat and human tumors *(180,181)*. A single-chain antigen-binding fragment of a specific antibody, which recognizes a v6 epitope, was fused to the zeta-chain of the T-cell receptor complex, and the chimeric gene transfected into murine cytotoxic T-lymphocytes (CTL). The resultant CTLs were not MHC-restricted in their CD44v6 recognition, and exhibited lytic activity in vitro toward cells expressing CD44 variants comprising exon v6, and tumor cell xenografts grown in athymic nude mice were suppressed in their growth upon infusion of the genetically manipulated CTLs *(182)*.

Lymphocytes have also been engineered to express a targeted toxin against an oncoprotein expressed on the surface of pancreatic cancer cells, namely the *ERBB2* receptor *(183)*. A chimeric gene was created in which a single-chain antibody against the extracellular domain of the *ERBB2* receptor was fused to a *Pseudomonas* exotoxin and expressed in human lymphocytes. These T-cells were able to kill *ERBB2*+ tumor cells selectively in vitro, and also to inhibit *ERBB2*+ tumor growth after injection in nude mice; there was no evidence of toxicity to cells and tissues not expressing *ERBB2*. It appears that the lymphocytes migrate to the tumor deposits, where they produce and accumulate toxin, which kills the malignant cells expressing the targeted antigen. This could be a very exciting approach to the genetic targeting of cell-mediated immunotherapy.

Gene Therapy Targeted to Tumor Vasculature

Destruction of tumor vasculature may inhibit the primary deposit and its metastases, and the endothelium within the new vessels proliferates much more rapidly than within normal vessels, providing the possibility of differential toxicity to cytokines or antimitotic therapy. Promoters that could be exploited to drive selective gene expression in tumor endothelium include those that are regulated by hypoxia, such as erythropoietin, VEGF, and lactate hydrogenase, and the approach could be combined with hypoxia-selective drug therapy. Genetic modification of endothelial cells may enable the delivery of therapeutic agents to the sites of tumor deposits, since it appears that endothelial cells, injected systemically, collect and proliferate selectively in the neovasculature *(184)*.

GENE THERAPY AS A RATIONAL APPROACH TO CANCER TREATMENT

Genetic intervention for the treatment of cancer is a strategy that is presently attracting a great deal of attention and publicity, not all of which is positive. The hype surrounding the approach (and its exponents) is likely to give way in time to a more conservative view of its place in the care of patients with cancer. Clearly, there are at present major technical challenges to its delivery and there is uncertainty about the most effective gene products, but continued research will resolve these issues. Ultimately, one can expect that genetic intervention therapies will be integrated into the range of options available to the cancer specialist, offered probably in an adjuvant setting combined with surgery, conventional chemotherapy, and radiotherapy. Patients will be selected by the molecular profile of their cancer and their own genetic background for therapies that are more effective and more selective than those available today, and it may even be possible to use genetic intervention to prevent the development of the disease in those predicted to be at high risk. The scientific and technical challenges are not inconsiderable, but there are great potential rewards for patients with pancreatic cancer, and we should look forward to the next decade with optimism.

REFERENCES

1. Lemoine NR. Molecular pathology of pancreatic duct neoplasms. In: Sirica A and Longnecker DS (eds), Biliary and pancreatic ductal epithelium: pathobiology and pathophysiology. Marcel Dekker, New York, 1996; pp. 502–525.
2. McCormick CSF and Lemoine NR. Molecular biology: diagnostic and therapeutic potentials. In: Howard JM (ed), Surgical diseases of the pancreas. Williams and Wilkins, Media, PA 1996; pp. 439–448.
3. Lemoine NR. Genetic intervention for the treatment and prevention of pancreatic cancer. Dig Surg 1995; *11:*170–177.
4. Lynch HT, Smyrk T, Kern SE, Hruban RH, Lightdale CJ, Lemon SJ, et al. Familial pancreatic cancer: a review. Semin Oncol 1996; *23:*251–275.
5. Lynch HT and Fusaro RM. Pancreatic cancer and the familial atypical multiple mole melanoma (FAMMM) syndrome. Pancreas 1991; *6:*127–131.
6. Whelan AJ, Bartsch D, and Goodfellow PJ. Brief report: a familial syndrome of pancreatic cancer and melanoma with a mutation in the CDKN2 tumor-suppressor gene. N Engl J Med 1995; *333:*975–977.
7. Goldstein AM, Fraser MC, Struewing JP, Hussussian CJ, Ranade K, Zametkin DP, et al. Increased risk of pancreatic cancer in melanoma-prone kindreds with p16INK4 mutations. N Engl J Med 1995; *333:*970–974.
8. Bilimoria MM, and Morrow M. The woman at increased risk for breast cancer: evaluation and management strategies. CA Cancer J Clin 1995; *45:*263–278.
9. Gullick WJ, and Handyside AH. Pre-implantation diagnosis of inherited predisposition to cancer. Eur J Cancer 1994; *13:*2030–2032.
10. Whitcomb DC, Gorry MC, Preston RA, Furey W, Sossenheimer MJ, Ulrich CD, et al. Hereditary pancreatitis is caused by a mutation in the cationic trypsinogen gene. Nature Genet 1996; *14:*141–145.
11. Kattwinkel J, Lapey A, Di Sant'Agnese PA, and Edwards WA. Hereditary pancreatitis: three new kindreds and a critical review of the literature. Pediatrics 1973; *51:*55–69.
12. Friend SH. Breast cancer susceptibility testing: realities in the post-genomic era. Nature Genet 1996; *13:*16–17.
13. Goggins M, Schutte M, Lu L, Moskaluk CA, Weinstein CL, Petersen GM, et al. Germline BRCA2 gene mutations in patients with apparently sporadic pancreatic carcinomas. Cancer Res 1996; *56:*5360–5364.
14. Hengge UR, Chan EF, Foster RA, Walker PS, and Vogel JC. Cytokine gene expression in epidermis with biological effects following injection of naked DNA. Nature Genet 1995; *10:*161–166.
15. Gunzburg WH and Salmons B. Retroviral vectors. In: Lemoine NR and Cooper DN, (eds), Gene Therapy, Bios, Oxford, 1996; pp. 33–60.

16. Rosenberg SA, Aebersold P, Cornetta K, Kasid A, Morgan RA, Moen R, et al. Gene transfer into humans—immunotherapy of patients with advanced melanoma, using tumor-infiltrating lymphocytes modified by retroviral gene transduction. N Engl J Med 1990; *323:*570–578.

17. Culver KW, Ram Z, Wallbridge S, Ishii H, Oldfield EH, and Blaese RM. In vivo gene transfer with retroviral vector-producer cells for treatment of experimental brain tumors. Science 1992; *256:*1550–1552.

18. Oldfield EH, Ram Z, Culver KW, Blaese RM, DeVroom HL, and Anderson WF. Gene therapy for the treatment of brain tumors using intra-tumoral transduction with the thymidine kinase gene and intravenous ganciclovir. Hum Gene Ther 1993; *4:*39–69.

19. Culver KW, Van Gilder J, Link CJ, Carlstrom T, Buroker T, Yuh W, et al. Gene therapy for the treatment of malignant brain tumors with in vivo tumor transduction with the herpes simplex thymidine kinase gene/ganciclovir system. Hum Gene Ther 1994; *5:*343–379.

20. Russell SJ and Miller AD. Foamy virus vectors. J Virol 1996; *70:*217–222.

21. Cosset FL, Takeuchi Y, Battini JL, Weiss RA, and Collins MK. High-titer packaging cells producing recombinant retroviruses resistant to human serum. J Virol 1995; *69:*7430–7436.

22. Evans MJ, Rollins SA, Wolff DW, Rother RP, Norin AJ, Therrien DM, et al. In vitro and in vivo inhibition of complement activity by a single-chain Fv fragment recognizing human C5. Mol Immunol 1995; *32:*1183–1195.

23. Rother RP, Squinto SP, Mason JM, and Rollins SA. Protection of retroviral vector particles in human blood through complement inhibition. Hum Gene Ther 1995; *6:*429–435.

24. Ring CJA. Adenovirus vectors. In: Lemoine NR and Cooper DN (eds), Gene Therapy, Bios, Oxford, 1996; pp. 61–76.

25. Crystal RG, Jaffe A, Brody S, Mastrangeli A, McElvaney NG, Rosenfeld M, et al. A phase 1 study, in cystic fibrosis patients, of the safety, toxicity, and biological efficacy of a single administration of a replication deficient, recombinant adenovirus carrying the cDNA of the normal cystic fibrosis transmembrane conductance regulator gene in the lung. Hum Gene Ther 1995; *6:*643–666.

26. Crystal RG, McElvaney NG, Rosenfeld MA, Chu CS, Mastrangeli A, Hay JG, et al. Administration of an adenovirus containing the human CFTR cDNA to the respiratory tract of individuals with cystic fibrosis. Nature Genet 1994; *8:*42–51.

27. Brody SL, Metzger M, Danel C, Rosenfeld MA, and Crystal RG. Acute responses of non-human primates to airway delivery of an adenovirus vector containing the human cystic fibrosis transmembrane conductance regulator cDNA. Hum Gene Ther 1994; *5:*821–836.

28. Yei S, Mittereder N, Wert S, Whitsett JA, Wilmott RW, and Trapnell BC. In vivo evaluation of the safety of adenovirus-mediated transfer of the human cystic fibrosis transmembrane conductance regulator cDNA to the lung. Hum Gene Ther 1994; *5:*731–744.

29. Kochanek S, Clemens PR, Mitani K, Chen H-H, Chan S, and Caskey CT. A new adenoviral vector: replacement of all viral coding sequences with 28 kb of DNA independently expressing both full-length dystrophin and beta-galactosidase. Proc Natl Acad Sci USA 1996; *93:*5731–5736.

30. Bartlett JS, and Samulski RJ. Adeno-associated virus vectors for human gene therapy. In: Lemoine NR and Cooper DN (eds), Gene Therapy, Bios, Oxford, 1996; pp. 77–92.

31. Wolff JA, Malone RW, Williams P, Chong W, Acsadi G, Jani A, and Felgner PL. Direct gene transfer into mouse muscle in vivo. Science 1990; *247:*1465–1468.

32. Danko I and Wolff JA. Direct gene transfer into muscle. Vaccine 1994; *12:*1499–1502.

33. Davis HL, Whalen RG, and Demeneix BA. Direct gene transfer into skeletal muscle in vivo: factors affecting efficiency of transfer and stability of expression. Hum Gene Ther 1993; *4:*151–159.

34. Mahato RI, Kawabata K, Nomura T, Takakura Y, and Hashida M. Physicochemical and pharmacokinetic characteristics of plasmid DNA/cationic liposome complexes. J Pharm Sci 1995; *84:*1267–1271.

35. Mahato RI, Kawabata K, Takakura Y, and Hashida M. In vivo disposition characteristics of plasmid DNA complexed with cationic liposomes. J Drug Target 1995; *3:*149–157.

36. Jiao S, Williams P, Berg RK, Hodgeman BA, Liu L, Repetto G, and Wolff JA. Direct gene transfer into nonhuman primate myofibers in vivo. Hum Gene Ther 1992; *3:*21–33.

37. Scheule RK and Cheng SH. Liposome delivery systems. In: Lemoine NR and Cooper DN, (eds), Gene Therapy, Bios, Oxford, 1996; pp. 93–112.

38. Caplen NJ, Alton EW, Middleton PG, Dorin JR, Stevenson BJ, Gao X, et al. Liposome-mediated CFTR gene transfer to the nasal epithelium of patients with cystic fibrosis. Nature Med 1995; *1:*39–46.

39. Caplen NJ, Gao X, Hayes P, Elaswarapu R, Fisher G, Kinrade E, et al. Gene therapy for cystic fibrosis in humans by liposome-mediated DNA transfer: the production of resources and the regulatory process. Gene Ther 1994; *1:*139–147.

40. Nabel EG, Yang Z, Muller D, Chang AE, Gao X, Huang L, Cho KJ, and Nabel GJ. Safety and toxicity of catheter gene delivery to the pulmonary vasculature in a patient with metastatic melanoma. Hum Gene Ther 1994; *5:*1089–1094.

41. Nabel GJ, Nabel EG, Yang ZY, Fox BA, Plautz GE, Gao X, et al. Direct gene transfer with DNA-liposome complexes in melanoma: expression, biologic activity, and lack of toxicity in humans. Proc Natl Acad Sci USA 1993; *90:*11,307–11,311.

42. Trubetskoy VS, Torchilin VP, Kennel SJ, and Huang L. Use of N-terminal modified poly(L-lysine)-antibody conjugate as a carrier for targeted gene delivery in mouse lung endothelial cells. Bioconjug Chem 1992; *3:*323–327.

43. Trubetskoy VS, Torchilin VP, Kennel S, and Huang L. Cationic liposomes enhance targeted delivery and expression of exogenous DNA mediated by N-terminal modified poly(L-lysine)-antibody conjugate in mouse lung endothelial cells. Biochim Biophys Acta 1992; *1131:*311–313.

44. Remy JS, Kichler A, Mordvinov V, Schuber F, and Behr JP. Targeted gene transfer into hepatoma cells with lipopolyamine-condensed DNA particles presenting galactose ligands: a stage toward artificial viruses. Proc Natl Acad Sci USA 1995; *92:*1744–1748.

45. Cristiano RJ, Smith LC, Kay MA, Brinkley BR, and Woo SL. Hepatic gene therapy: efficient gene delivery and expression in primary hepatocytes utilizing a conjugated adenovirus-DNA complex. Proc Natl Acad Sci USA 1993; *90:*11,548–11,552.

46. Cristiano RJ, Smith LC, and Woo SL. Hepatic gene therapy: adenovirus enhancement of receptor-mediated gene delivery and expression in primary hepatocytes. Proc Natl Acad Sci USA 1993; *90:*2122–2126.

47. Gao L, Wagner E, Cotten M, Agarwal S, Harris C, Romer M, et al. Direct in vivo gene transfer to airway epithelium employing adenovirus-polylysine-DNA complexes. Hum Gene Ther 1993; *4:*17–24.

48. Curiel DT, Agarwal S, Wagner E, and Cotten M. Adenovirus enhancement of transferrin-polylysine-mediated gene delivery. Proc Natl Acad Sci USA 1991; *88:*8850–8854.

49. Wu GY, Zhan P, Sze LL, Rosenberg AR, and Wu CH. Incorporation of adenovirus into a ligand-based DNA carrier system results in retention of original receptor specificity and enhances targeted gene expression. J Biol Chem 1994; *269:*11,542–11,546.

50. Cheng L, Ziegelhoffer PR, and Yang NS. In vivo promoter activity and transgene expression in mammalian somatic tissues evaluated by using particle bombardment. Proc Natl Acad Sci USA 1993; *90:*4455–4459.

51. Yang NS, Burkholder J, Roberts B, Martinell B, and McCabe D. In vivo and in vitro gene transfer to mammalian somatic cells by particle bombardment. Proc Natl Acad Sci USA 1990; *87:*9568–9572.

52. Jiao S, Cheng L, Wolff JA, and Yang NS. Particle bombardment-mediated gene transfer and expression in rat brain tissues. Biotechnol NY 1993; *11:*497–502.

53. Yang NS and Sun WH. Gene gun and other non-viral approaches for cancer gene therapy. Nature Med 1995; *1:*481–483.

54. Sun WH, Burkholder JK, Sun J, Culp J, Turner J, Lu XG, et al. In vivo cytokine gene transfer by gene gun reduces tumor growth in mice. Proc Natl Acad Sci USA 1995; *92:*2889–2893.

55. Nellen W and Lichtenstein C. What makes an mRNA anti-sense-itive? Trends Biochem Sci 1993; *18:*419–423.

56. Carter G and Lemoine NR. Antisense technology for cancer therapy: does it make sense? Br J Cancer 1993; *67:*869–876.

57. Barton CM and Lemoine NR. Antisense oligonucleotides directed against TP53 have antiproliferative effects unrelated to effects on p53 expression. Br J Cancer 1995; *71:*429–437.

58. Bielinska A, Shivdasani RA, Zhang LQ, and Nabel GJ. Regulation of gene expression with double-stranded phosphorothioate oligonucleotides. Science 1990; *250:*997–1000.

59. Sullenger BA, Gallardo HF, Ungers GE, and Gilboa E. Overexpression of TAR sequences renders cells resistant to human immunodeficiency virus replication. Cell 1990; *63:*601–608.

60. Sullenger BA, Gallardo HF, Ungers GE, and Gilboa E. Analysis of trans-acting response decoy RNA-mediated inhibition of human immunodeficiency virus type 1 transactivation. *J Virol* 1991; *65:*6811–6816.

61. Porter A. Gene targeting as an approach to gene therapy. In: Lemoine NR and Cooper DN, (eds), Gene Therapy, Bios, Oxford, 1996; pp. 169–190.

62. Jones PH, Harper S, and Watt FM. Stem cell patterning and fate in human epidermis. Cell 1995; *80:*83–93.

63. Barton CM, Staddon SL, Hughes CM, Hall PA, O'Sullivan C, Kloppel G, et al. Abnormalities of the p53 tumour suppressor gene in human pancreatic cancer. Br J Cancer 1991; *64:*1076–1082.

64. Scarpa A, Capelli P, Mukai K, Zamboni G, Oda T, Iacono C, and Hirohashi S. Pancreatic adenocarcinomas frequently show p53 gene mutations. Am J Pathol 1993; *142:*1534–1543.

65. Simon B, Weinel R, Hohne M, Watz J, Schmidt J, Kortner G, and Arnold R. Frequent alterations of the tumor suppressor genes p53 and DCC in human pancreatic cancer. Gastroenterology 1994; *106:*1645–1651.

66. Ruggeri BA, Klein-Szanto AJP, Huang LY, and Lang D. P53 and RB-1 tumor suppressor gene expression and alterations in human pancreatic cancer. Int J Pancreatol 1994; *16:*193–196.

67. Kalthoff H, Schmiegel W, Roeder C, Kasche D, Schmidt A, Lauer G, et al. p53 and K-RAS alterations in pancreatic epithelial cell lesions. Oncogene 1993; *8:*289–298.

68. Redston MS, Caldas C, Seymour AB, Hruban RH, da Costa L, Yeo CJ, and Kern SE. p53 mutations in pancreatic carcinoma and evidence of common homocopolymer tracts in DNA microdeletions. Cancer Res 1994; *54:*3025–3033.

69. Berrozpe G, Schaeffer J, Peinado MA, Real FX, and Perucho M. Comparative analysis of mutations in the p53 and K-ras genes in pancreas cancer. Int J Cancer 1994; *58:*185–191.

70. Chen PL, Chen YM, Bookstein R, and Lee WH. Genetic mechanisms of tumor suppression by the human p53 gene. Science 1990; *250:*1576–1580.

71. Frebourg T, Sadelain M, Ng YS, Kassel J, and Friend SH. Equal transcription of wild-type and mutant p53 using bicistronic vectors results in the wild-type phenotype. Cancer Res 1994; *54:*878–881.

72. Fujiwara T, Cai DW, Georges RN, Mukhopadhyay T, Grimm EA, and Roth JA. Therapeutic effect of a retroviral wild-type p53 expression vector in an orthotopic lung cancer model [see comments]. J Natl Cancer Inst 1994; *86:*1458–1462.

73. Wills KN, Maneval DC, Menzel P, Harris MP, Sutjipto S, Vaillancourt MT, et al. Development and characterization of recombinant adenoviruses encoding human p53 for gene therapy of cancer. Hum Gene Ther 1994; *5:*1079–1088.

74. Zhang WW, Fang X, Mazur W, French BA, Georges RN, and Roth JA. High-efficiency gene transfer and high-level expression of wild-type p53 in human lung cancer cells mediated by recombinant adenovirus. Cancer Gene Ther 1994; *1:*5–13.

75. Zhang WW and Roth JA. Anti-oncogene and tumor suppressor gene therapy—examples from a lung cancer animal model. In Vivo 1994; *8:*755–769.

76. Liu TJ, Zhang WW, Taylor DL, Roth JA, Goepfert H, and Clayman GL. Growth suppression of human head and neck cancer cells by the introduction of a wild-type p53 gene via a recombinant adenovirus. Cancer Res 1994; *54:*3662–3667.

77. Clayman GL, Trapnell BC, Mittereder N, Liu TJ, Eicher S, Zhang S, and Shillitoe EJ. Transduction of normal and malignant oral epithelium by an adenovirus vector: the effect of dose and treatment time on transduction efficiency and tissue penetration. Cancer Gene Ther 1995; *2:*105–111.

78. Clayman GL, el Naggar AK, Roth JA, Zhang WW, Goepfert H, Taylor DL, and Liu TJ. In vivo molecular therapy with p53 adenovirus for microscopic residual head and neck squamous carcinoma. Cancer Res 1995; *55:*1–6.

79. Liu TJ, el Naggar AK, McDonnell TJ, Steck KD, Wang M, Taylor DL, and Clayman GL. Apoptosis induction mediated by wild-type p53 adenoviral gene transfer in squamous cell carcinoma of the head and neck. Cancer Res 1995; *55:*3117–3122.

80. Clayman GL, Liu TJ, Overholt SM, Mobley SR, Wang M, Janot F, and Goepfert H. Gene therapy for head and neck cancer. Comparing the tumor suppressor gene p53 and a cell cycle regulator WAF1/CIP1 (p21). Arch Otolaryngol Head Neck Surg 1996; *122:*489–493.

81. Yang C, Cirielli C, Capogrossi MC, and Passaniti A. Adenovirus-mediated wild-type p53 expression induces apoptosis and suppresses tumorigenesis of prostatic tumor cells. Cancer Res 1995; *55:*4210–4213.

82. Eastham JA, Hall SJ, Sehgal I, Wang J, Timme TL, Yang G, et al. In vivo gene therapy with p53 or p21 adenovirus for prostate cancer. Cancer Res 1995; *55:*5151–5155.

83. Bookstein R, Demers W, Gregory R, Maneval D, Park J, and Wills K. p53 gene therapy in vivo of hepatocellular and liver metastatic colorectal cancer. Semin Oncol 1996; *23:*66–77.

84. Werthman PE, Drazan KE, Rosenthal JT, Khalili R, and Shaked A. Adenoviral-p53 gene transfer to orthotopic and peritoneal murine bladder cancer. J Urol 1996; *155:*753–756.

85. Hamada K, Alemany R, Zhang WW, Hittelman WN, Lotan R, Roth JA, and Mitchell MF. Adenovirus-mediated transfer of a wild-type p53 gene and induction of apoptosis in cervical cancer. Cancer Res 1996; *56:*3047–3054.

86. Drazan KE, Shen XD, Csete ME, Zhang WW, Roth JA, Busuttil RW, and Shaked A. In vivo adenoviral-mediated human p53 tumor suppressor gene transfer and expression in rat liver after resection. Surgery 1994; *116:*197–203.

87. Fujiwara T, Grimm EA, Mukhopadhyay T, Zhang WW, Owen Schaub LB, and Roth JA. Induction of chemosensitivity in human lung cancer cells in vivo by adenovirus-mediated transfer of the wild-type p53 gene. Cancer Res 1994; *54:*2287–2291.

88. Harper J, Adami G, Wei N, Keyormarsi K, and Elledge S. The p21 Cdk-interacting protein Cip1 is a potent inhibitor of G1 cyclin-dependent kinases. Cell 1993; *75:*805–816.

89. El-Deiry W, Tokino T, Velculescu V, Levy D, Parsons R, Trent J, et al. *WAF1*, a potential mediator of p53 tumor suppression. Cell 1993; *75:*817–825.

90. Caldas C, Hahn SA, da Costa LT, Redston MS, Schutte M, Seymour AB, et al. Frequent somatic mutations and homozygous deletions of the p16 (MTS1) gene in pancreatic adenocarcinoma. Nature Genet 1994; *8:*27–31.

91. Liu Q, Yan Y-X, McClure M, Nakagawa H, Fujimura F, and Rustgi AK. MTS-1 (CDKN2) tumor suppressor gene deletions are a frequent event in esophagus squamous cancer and pancreatic adenocarcinoma cell lines. Oncogene 1995; *10:*619–622.

92. Bartsch D, Shevlin DW, Tung WS, Kisker O, Wells SA, and Goodfellow PJ. Frequent mutations of CDKN2 in primary pancreatic adenocarcinomas. Genes, Chromosomes Cancer 1995; *14:*189–195.

93. Naumann M, Savitskaia N, Eilert C, Schramm A, Kalthoff H, and Schmiegel W. Frequent codeletion of p16/MTS1 and p15/MTS2 and genetic alterations in p16/MTS1 in pancreatic tumors. Gastroenterology 1996; *110:*1215–1224.

94. Mukhopadhyay T, Tainsky M, Cavender AC, and Roth JA. Specific inhibition of K-ras expression and tumorigenicity of lung cancer cells by antisense RNA. Cancer Res 1991; *51:*1744–1748.

95. Georges RN, Mukhopadhyay T, Zhang Y, Yen N, and Roth JA. Prevention of orthotopic human lung cancer growth by intratracheal instillation of a retroviral antisense K-ras construct. Cancer Res 1993; *53:*1743–1746.

96. Yoshida T and Aoki K. Gene therapy for pancreatic cancer. Tanpakushitsu Kakusan Koso 1995; *40:*2727–2731.

97. Aoki K, Yoshida T, Sugimura T, and Terada M. Liposome-mediated in vivo gene transfer of antisense K-ras construct inhibits pancreatic tumor dissemination in the murine peritoneal cavity. Cancer Res 1995; *55:*3810–3816.

98. Bayever E and Iversen P. Oligonucleotides in the treatment of leukemia. Hematol Oncol 1994; *12:*9–14.

99. Bishop MR, Iversen PL, Bayever E, Sharp JG, Greiner TC, Copple BL, et al. Phase I trial of an antisense oligonucleotide OL(1)p53 in hematologic malignancies. J Clin Oncol, 1996; *14:*1320–1326.

100. Cai DW, Mukhopadhyay T, and Roth JA. Suppression of lung cancer cell growth by ribozyme-mediated modification of p53 pre-mRNA. Cancer Gene Ther 1995; *2:*199–205.

101. Colomer R, Lupu R, Bacus SS, and Gelmann EP. erbB-2 antisense oligonucleotides inhibit the proliferation of breast carcinoma cells with erbB-2 oncogene amplification. Br J Cancer 1994; *70:*819–825.

102. Hall PA, Hughes CM, Staddon SL, Richman PI, Gullick WJ, and Lemoine NR. The c-erbB-2 proto-oncogene in human pancreatic cancer. J Pathol 1990; *161:*195–200.

103. Ebbinghaus SW, Gee JE, Rodu B, Mayfield CA, Sanders G, and Miller DM. Triplex formation inhibits HER-2/neu transcription in vitro. J Clin Invest 1993; *92:*2433–2439.

104. Kitada S, Takayama S, De Riel K, Tanaka S, and Reed JC. Reversal of chemoresistance of lymphoma cells by antisense-mediated reduction of bcl-2 gene expression. Antisense Res Dev 1994; *4:*71–79.

105. Gao WY, Han FS, Storm C, Egan W, and Cheng YC. Phosphorothioate oligonucleotides are inhibitors of human DNA polymerases and RNase H: implications for antisense technology. Mol Pharmacol 1992; *41:*223–229.

106. Burgess TL, Fisher EF, Ross SL, Bready JV, Qian YX, Bayewitch LA, et al. The antiproliferative activity of c-myb and c-myc antisense oligonucleotides in smooth muscle cells is caused by a nonantisense mechanism. Proc Natl Acad Sci USA 1995; *92:*4051–4055.

107. Guvakova MA, Yakubov LA, Vlodavsky I, Tonkinson JL, and Stein CA. Phosphorothioate oligodeoxynucleotides bind to basic fibroblast growth factor, inhibit its binding to cell surface receptors, and remove it from low affinity binding sites on extracellular matrix. J Biol Chem 1995; *270:*2620–2627.

108. Krieg AM. CpG DNA: a pathogenic factor in systemic lupus erythematosus? J Clin Immunol 1995; *15:*284–292.

109. Krieg AM, Yi AK, Matson S, Waldschmidt TJ, Bishop GA, Teasdale R, Koretzky GA, and Klinman DM. CpG motifs in bacterial DNA trigger direct B-cell activation. Nature 1995; *374:*546–549.

110. Yamamoto T, Yamamoto S, Kataoka T, and Tokunaga T. Ability of oligonucleotides with certain palindromes to induce interferon production and augment natural killer cell activity is associated with their base length. Antisense Res Dev 1994; *4:*119–122.

111. Yamamoto T, Yamamoto S, Kataoka T, and Tokunaga T. Lipofection of synthetic oligodeoxyribonucleotide having a palindromic sequence of AACGTT to murine splenocytes enhances interferon production and natural killer activity. Microbiol Immunol 1994; *38:*831–836.

112. Harris JD and Lemoine NR. Strategies for targeted gene therapy. Trends Genet 1996; *12:*400–405.

113. Moolten FL. Gene therapy: creating mosaic pattern of drug susceptibility. Mt Sinai J Med 1986; *53:*232.

114. Schnierle BS and Groner B. Retroviral targeted delivery. Gene Ther 1996; *3:*1069–1073.

115. Schnierle BS, Moritz D, Jeschke M, and Groner B. Expression of chimeric envelope proteins in helper cell lines and integration into Moloney murine leukemia virus particles. Gene Ther 1996; *3:*334–342.

116. Han X, Kasahara N, and Kan YW. Ligand-directed retroviral targeting of human breast cancer cells. Proc Natl Acad Sci USA 1995; *92:*9747–9751.

117. Huber BE, Richards CA, and Krenitsky TA. Retroviral-mediated gene therapy for the treatment of hepatocellular carcinoma: an innovative approach for cancer therapy. Proc Natl Acad Sci USA 1991; *88:*8039–8043.

118. Richards CA and Huber BE. Generation of a transgenic model for retrovirus-mediated gene therapy for hepatocellular carcinoma is thwarted by the lack of transgene expression. Hum Gene Ther 1993; *4:*143–150.

119. Harris JD, Gutierrez AA, Hurst HC, Sikora K, and Lemoine NR. Gene therapy for cancer using tumour-specific prodrug activation. Gene Ther 1994; *1:*170–175.

120. Sikora K, Harris J, Hurst H, and Lemoine N. Therapeutic strategies using c-erbB-2 promoter-controlled drug activation. Ann NY Acad Sci 1994; *716:*115–124.

121. Ring CJA, Harris JD, Hurst HC, and Lemoine NR. Suicide gene expression induced in tumour cells treated with recombinant adenoviral, retroviral and plasmid vectors containing the ERBB2 promoter. Gene Therapy 1996; *3:*1094–1103.

122. Osaki T, Tanio Y, Tachibana I, Hosoe S, Kumagai T, Kawase I, Oikawa S, and Kishimoto T. Gene therapy for carcinoembryonic antigen-producing human lung cancer cells by cell type-specific expression of herpes simplex virus thymidine kinase gene. Cancer Res 1994; *54:*5258–5261.

123. Richards CA, Wolberg AS, and Huber BE. The transcriptional control region of the human carcinoembryonic antigen gene: DNA sequence and homology studies. DNA Seq 1993; *4:*185–196.

124. DiMaio JM, Clary BM, Via DF, Coveney E, Pappas TN, and Lyerly HK. Directed enzyme pro-drug gene therapy for pancreatic cancer in vivo. Surgery 1994; *116:*205–213.

125. Manome Y, Abe M, Hagen MF, Fine HA, and Kufe DW. Enhancer sequences of the DF3 gene regulate expression of the herpes simplex virus thymidine kinase gene and confer sensitivity of human breast cancer cells to ganciclovir. Cancer Res 1994; *54:*5408–13.

126. Ring CJA, Martin L-A, Blouin P, Hurst HC, and Lemoine NR. Use of transcriptional regulatory elements of the MUC1 and ERBB2 genes to drive tumor-selective expression of a prodrug-activating enzyme. Gene Therapy 1997; *4:*1045–1052.

127. Freeman SM, Abboud CN, Whartenby KA, Packman CH, Koeplin DS, Moolten FL, and Abraham GN. The "bystander effect": tumor regression when a fraction of the tumor mass is genetically modified. Cancer Res 1993; *53:*5274–5283.

128. Vile RG, Nelson JA, Castleden S, Chong H, and Hart IR. Systemic gene therapy of murine melanoma using tissue specific expression of the HSVtk gene involves an immune component. Cancer Res 1994; *54:*6228–6234.

129. Scupoli MT, Sartoris S, Tosi G, Ennas MG, Nicolis M, Cestari T, et al. Expression of MHC class-i and class-II antigens in pancreatic adenocarcinomas. Tissue Antigens 1996; *48*:301–311.

130. Mazumder A and Rosenberg SA. Successful immunotherapy of natural killer-resistant established pulmonary melanoma metastases by the intravenous adoptive transfer of syngeneic lymphocytes activated in vitro by interleukin 2. J Exp Med 1984; *159*:495–507.

131. Rosenberg SA, Lotze MT, Yang JC, Linehan WM, Seipp C, Calabro S, et al. Combination therapy with interleukin-2 and alpha-interferon for the treatment of patients with advanced cancer. J Clin Oncol 1989; *7*:1863–1874.

132. Rosenberg SA, Lotze MT, Yang JC, Aebersold PM, Linehan WM, Seipp CA, and White DE. Experience with the use of high-dose interleukin-2 in the treatment of 652 cancer patients. Ann Surg 1989; *210*:474–484.

133. Galea-Lauri J and Gaken J. Cancer gene therapy II: immunomodulatory strategies. In: Lemoine NR, and Cooper DN (eds), Gene Therapy Bios, Oxford, 1996; pp. 277–299.

134. Bubenik J, Zeuthen J, Bubenikova D, Simova J, and Jandlova T. Gene therapy of cancer: use of IL-2 gene transfer and kinetics of local T and NK cell subsets. Anticancer Res 1993; *13*:1457–1460.

135. Cordier L, Duffour MT, Sabourin JC, Lee MG, Cabannes J, Ragot T, Perricaudet M, and Haddada H. Complete recovery of mice from a pre-established tumor by direct intratumoral delivery of an adenovirus vector harboring the murine IL-2 gene. Gene Ther 1995; *2*:16–21.

136. Gilboa E, Lyerly HK, Vieweg J, and Saito S. Immunotherapy of cancer using cytokine gene-modified tumor vaccines. Semin Cancer Biol 1994; *5*:409–417.

137. Haddada H, Ragot T, Cordier L, Duffour MT, and Perricaudet M. Adenoviral interleukin-2 gene transfer into P815 tumor cells abrogates tumorigenicity and induces antitumoral immunity in mice. Hum Gene Ther 1993; *4*:703–711.

138. Hathorn RW, Tso CL, Kaboo R, Pang S, Figlin R, Sawyers C, deKernion JB, and Belldegrun A. In vitro modulation of the invasive and metastatic potentials of human renal cell carcinoma by interleukin-2 and/or interferon-alpha-gene transfer. Cancer 1994; *74*:1904–1911.

139. Hurford RK, Jr., Dranoff G, Mulligan RC, and Tepper RI. Gene therapy of metastatic cancer by in vivo retroviral gene targeting. Nature Genet 1995; *10*:430–435.

140. Karp SE, Farber A, Salo JC, Hwu P, Jaffe G, Asher AL, et al. Cytokine secretion by genetically modified nonimmunogenic murine fibrosarcoma. Tumor inhibition by IL-2 but not tumor necrosis factor. J Immunol 1993; *150*:896–908.

141. Kim TS, Russell SJ, Collins MK, and Cohen EP. Immunity to B16 melanoma in mice immunized with IL-2-secreting allogeneic mouse fibroblasts expressing melanoma-associated antigens. Int J Cancer 1992; *51*:283–289.

142. Krauss JC, Strome SE, Chang AE, and Shu S. Enhancement of immune reactivity in the lymph nodes draining a murine melanoma engineered to elaborate interleukin-4. J Immunother Emphasis Tumor Immunol 1994; *16*:77–84.

143. Melani C, Chiodoni C, Arienti F, Maccalli C, Sule Suso J, Anichini A, Colombo MP, and Parmiani G. Cytokine gene transduction in tumor cells: interleukin (IL)-2 or IL-4 gene transfer in human melanoma cells. Nat Immun 1994; *13*:76–84.

144. Musiani P, Modesti A, Brunetti M, Modica A, Vitullo P, Gulino A, et al. Nature and potential of the reactive response to mouse mammary adenocarcinoma cells engineered with interleukin-2, interleukin-4 or interferon-gamma genes. Nat Immun 1994; *13*:93–101.

145. Ohira T, Ohe Y, Heike Y, Podack ER, Olsen KJ, Nishio K, et al. Gene therapy for Lewis lung carcinoma with tumor necrosis factor and interleukin 2 cDNAs co-transfected subline. Gene Ther 1994; *1*:269–275.

146. Patel PM, Flemming CL, Russell SJ, McKay IA, MacLennan KA, Box GM, Eccles SA, and Collins MK. Comparison of the potential therapeutic effects of interleukin 2 or interleukin 4 secretion by a single tumour. Br J Cancer 1993; *68:*295–302.

147. Porgador A, Tzehoval E, Vadai E, Feldman M, and Eisenbach L. Immunotherapy via gene therapy: comparison of the effects of tumor cells transduced with the interleukin-2, interleukin-6, or interferon-gamma genes. J Immunother 1993; *14:*191–201.

148. Roth C, Mir L, Cressent M, Quintin Colonna F, Ley V, Fradelizi D, and Kourilsky P. IL-2 gene transduction in malignant cells: applications in cancer containment. Bone Marrow Transplant 1992; *1:*174–175.

149. Russell SJ, Eccles SA, Flemming CL, Johnson CA, and Collins MK. Decreased tumorigenicity of a transplantable rat sarcoma following transfer and expression of an IL-2 cDNA. Int J Cancer 1991; *47:*244–251.

150. Shawler DL, Dorigo O, Gjerset RA, Royston I, Sobol RE, and Fakhrai H. Comparison of gene therapy with interleukin-2 gene modified fibroblasts and tumor cells in the murine CT-26 model of colorectal carcinoma. J Immunother Emphasis Tumor Immunol 1995; *17:*201–208.

151. Tjuvajev J, Gansbacher B, Desai R, Beattie B, Kaplitt M, Matei C, et al. RG-2 glioma growth attenuation and severe brain edema caused by local production of interleukin-2 and interferon-gamma. Cancer Res 1995; *55:*1902–1910.

152. Rosenthal FM, Cronin K, Bannerji R, Golde DW, and Gansbacher B. Augmentation of antitumor immunity by tumor cells transduced with a retroviral vector carrying the interleukin-2 and interferon-gamma cDNAs. Blood 1994; *83:*1289–1298.

153. Rosenthal FM, Fruh R, Henschler R, Veelken H, Kulmburg P, Mackensen A, et al. Cytokine therapy with gene-transfected cells: single injection of irradiated granulocyte-macrophage colony-stimulating factor-transduced cells accelerates hematopoietic recovery after cytotoxic chemotherapy in mice. Blood 1994; *84:*2960–2965.

154. Wiltrout RH, Gregorio TA, Fenton RG, Longo DL, Ghosh P, Murphy WJ, and Komschlies KL. Cellular and molecular studies in the treatment of murine renal cancer. Semin Oncol 1995; *22:*9–16.

155. Munger W, DeJoy SQ, Jeyaseelan R, Sr., Torley LW, Grabstein KH, Eisenmann J, et al. Studies evaluating the antitumor activity and toxicity of interleukin-15, a new T-cell growth factor: comparison with interleukin-2. Cell Immunol 1995; *165:*289–293.

156. Gamero AM, Ussery D, Reintgen DS, Puleo CA, and Djeu JY. Interleukin 15 induction of lymphokine-activated killer cell function against autologous tumor cells in melanoma patient lymphocytes by a CD18-dependent, perforin-related mechanism. Cancer Res 1995; *55:*4988–4994.

157. Lewko WM, Smith TL, Bowman DJ, Good RW, and Oldham RK. Interleukin-15 and the growth of tumor derived activated T-cells. Cancer Biother 1995; *10:*13–20.

158. Clary BM, Coveney EC, Blazer DGr, Philip R, and Lyerly HK. Active immunotherapy of pancreatic cancer with tumor cells genetically engineered to secrete multiple cytokines. Surgery 1996; *120:*174–181.

159. Townsend SE, Su FW, Atherton JM, and Allison JP. Specificity and longevity of antitumor immune responses induced by B7-transfected tumors. Cancer Res 1994; *54:*6477–6483.

160. Townsend SE and Allison JP. Tumor rejection after direct costimulation of CD8+ T cells by B7-transfected melanoma cells. Science 1993; *259:*368–370.

161. Chen L, Ashe S, Brady WA, Hellstrom I, Hellstrom KE, Ledbetter JA, McGowan P, and Linsley PS. Costimulation of antitumor immunity by the B7 counterreceptor for the T lymphocyte molecules CD28 and CTLA-4. Cell 1992; *71:*1093–1102.

162. Matulonis U, Dosiou C, Freeman G, Lamont C, Mauch P, Nadler LM, and Griffin JD. B7-1 is superior to B7-2 costimulation in the induction and maintenance of T-cell-mediated

antileukemia immunity. Further evidence that B7-1 and B7-2 are functionally distinct. J Immunol 1996; *156:*1126–1131.

163. Yang G, Hellstrom KE, Hellstrom I, and Chen L. Antitumor immunity elicited by tumor cells transfected with B7-2, a second ligand for CD28/CTLA-4 costimulatory molecules. J Immunol 1995; *154:*2794–2800.

164. Hodge JW, Abrams S, Schlom J, and Kantor JA. Induction of antitumor immunity by recombinant vaccinia viruses expressing B7-1 or B7-2 costimulatory molecules. Cancer Res 1994; *54:*5552–5555.

165. Dohring C, Angman L, Spagnoli G, and Lanzavecchia A. T-helper- and accessory-cell-independent cytotoxic responses to human tumor cells transfected with a B7 retroviral vector. Int J Cancer 1994; *57:*754–759.

166. Linehan DC, Goedegebuure PS, Peoples GE, Rogers SO, and Eberlein TJ. Tumor-specific and HLA-A2-restricted cytolysis by tumor-associated lymphocytes in human metastatic breast cancer. J Immunol 1995; *155:*4486–4491.

167. Conry RM, LoBuglio AF, Kantor J, Schlom J, Loechel F, Moore SE, et al. Immune response to a carcinoembryonic antigen polynucleotide vaccine. Cancer Res 1994; *54:*1164–1168.

168. Conry RM, LoBuglio AF, Loechel F, Moore SE, Sumerel LA, Barlow DL, and Curiel DT. A carcinoembryonic antigen polynucleotide vaccine has in vivo antitumor activity. Gene Ther 1995; *2:*59–65.

169. Conry RM, LoBuglio AF, Loechel F, Moore SE, Sumerel LA, Barlow DL, Pike J, and Curiel DT. A carcinoembryonic antigen polynucleotide vaccine for human clinical use. Cancer Gene Ther 1995; *2:*33–38.

170. McLaughlin JP, Schlom J, Kantor JA, and Greiner JW. Improved immunotherapy of a recombinant carcinoembryonic antigen vaccinia vaccine when given in combination with interleukin-2. Cancer Res 1996; *56:*2361–2367.

171. Gedde Dahl Td, Fossum B, Eriksen JA, Thorsby E, and Gaudernack G. T cell clones specific for p21 ras-derived peptides: characterization of their fine specificity and HLA restriction. Eur J Immunol 1993; *23:*754–760.

172. Fossum B, Olsen AC, Thorsby E, and Gaudernack G. CD8+ T cells from a patient with colon carcinoma, specific for a mutant p21 ras-derived peptide (13Gly->Asp), are cytotoxic towards a carcinoma cell line harbouring the same mutation. Cancer Immunol Immunother 1995; *40:*165–172.

173. Qin H, Chen W, Takahashi M, Disis ML, Byrd DR, McCahill L, et al. CD4+ T-cell immunity to mutated ras protein in pancreatic and colon cancer patients. Cancer Res 1995; *55:*2984–2987.

174. Jung S and Schluesener HJ. Human T lymphocytes recognize a peptide of single point-mutated, oncogenic ras proteins. J Exp Med 1991; *173:*273–276.

175. Gedde Dahl Td, Eriksen JA, Thorsby E, and Gaudernack G. T-cell responses against products of oncogenes: generation and characterization of human T-cell clones specific for p21 ras-derived synthetic peptides. Hum Immunol 1992; *33:*266–274.

176. Fossum B, Gedde Dahl Td, Hansen T, Eriksen JA, Thorsby E, and Gaudernack G. Overlapping epitopes encompassing a point mutation (12 Gly—>Arg) in p21 ras can be recognized by HLA-DR, -DP and -DQ restricted T cells. Eur J Immunol 1993; *23:*2687–2691.

177. Fossum B, Breivik J, Meling GI, Gedde Dahl Tr, Hansen T, Knutsen I, et al. A K-ras 13Gly—>Asp mutation is recognized by HLA-DQ7 restricted T-cells in a patient with colorectal cancer. Modifying effect of DQ7 on established cancers harbouring this mutation? Int J Cancer 1994; *58:*506–511.

178. Fenton RG, Keller CJ, Hanna N, and Taub DD. Induction of T-cell immunity against Ras oncoproteins by soluble protein or Ras-expressing *Escherichia coli.* J Natl Cancer Inst 1995; *87:*1853–1861.

179. Gjertsen MK, Bakka A, Breivik J, Saeterdal I, Gedde Dahl Tr, Stokke KT, et al. Ex vivo ras peptide vaccination in patients with advanced pancreatic cancer: results of a phase I/II study. Int J Cancer 1996; *65:*450–453.

180. Rudy W, Hofmann M, Schwartz AR, Zoller M, Heider KH, Ponta H, and Herrlich P. The two major CD44 proteins expressed on a metastatic rat tumor cell line are derived from different splice variants: each one individually suffices to confer metastatic behavior. Cancer Res 1993; *53:*1262–1268.

181. Castella EM, Ariza A, Ojanguren I, Mate JL, Roca X, Fernandezvasalo A, and Navaspalacios JJ. Differential expression of CD44v6 in adenocarcinoma of the pancreas—an immunohistochemical study. Virchows Arch 1996; *429:*191–195.

182. Hekele A, Dall P, Moritz D, Wels W, Groner B, Herrlich P, and Ponta H. Growth retardation of tumors by adoptive transfer of cytotoxic T-lymphocytes reprogrammed by CD44v6-specific scfv-zeta-chimera. Int J Cancer 1996; *68:*232–238.

183. Chen SY, Yang AG, Chen JD, Kute T, King CR, Collier J, et al. Potent antitumour activity of a new class of tumour-specific killer cells. Nature 1997; *385:*78–80.

184. Ojeifo JO, Forough R, Paik S, Maciag T, and Zwiebel JA. Angiogenesis-directed implantation of genetically modified endothelial cells in mice. Cancer Res 1995; *55:*2240–2244.

18

Quality of Life in Pancreatic Cancer

D. Fitzsimmons and C. D. Johnson

INTRODUCTION

Pancreatic cancer is well known to have a short duration of survival after diagnosis, and to be relatively resistant to current therapies. When survival is short, quality of life (QOL) assumes great importance, and clinicians should be concerned not only with the biophysical disease process, but with the consequences of illness on the well-being of their patients. Knowledge of the demands that disease brings, not only in terms of physical threats, but also psychological and social consequences, and how the patient copes with their illness, treatment, and care, can only help greater understanding of disease and illness. Consideration of how to improve the quality as well as quantity of life is of paramount importance. It is recognized that QOL assessment is long overdue in pancreatic cancer *(1)*.

This chapter will review the place of QOL and its assessment in the disease process, and in the interaction of patients with health care professionals, before going on to consider the specific symptoms of pancreatic cancer that can affect QOL. It will describe how advanced cancer affects psychological well-being, and will look in detail at published descriptions of QOL assessments in pancreatic cancer. The authors' own developmental work for a pancreas-cancer-specific module has identified the most relevant issues for patients with this disease and highlights some differences in perception between patients and health care professionals. Finally, the chapter looks at ways in which the various treatments of pancreatic cancer can affect QOL.

QUALITY VS QUANTITY OF LIFE

The principal outcomes of medical and surgical interventions have traditionally been described in terms of mortality and morbidity rates. Despite advances in the treatment of pancreatic cancer, these outcomes remain disappointing. With an increasing incidence, pancreatic cancer is now the fourth leading cause of cancer death in the United States *(2)*. Survival remains poor, and over 90% of patients will die within 1 yr of diagnosis. Predominantly a disease of the elderly, with a majority of cases occurring in those aged 60–80 yr *(3)*, its rising incidence is largely related to a relative increase in the elderly population *(4)*.

The majority of patients present to the clinician with disseminated disease. First symptoms are often nonspecific and may be attributed to other causes, and the patient may simply not realize that something is wrong. Various known risk factors, such as cigarette smoking, excessive alcohol consumption, chronic pancreatitis, and diabetes mellitus, are common and individually rarely increase the index of suspicion *(5,6)*. Strong diagnostic indicators (e.g., jaundice, pain, weight loss) usually indicate that the disease is extensive and consequently incurable. Although diagnostic techniques have improved, detection of the tumor can be difficult, which may result in a delay in reaching a firm diagnosis and referral to the appropriate specialist.

Less than 20% of patients are eligible for resection at the time of diagnosis. For the majority (>80%), medical and surgical intervention will be aimed at control of symptoms. The clinician caring for such patients should aim to maximize QOL within the context of limited survival.

WHAT IS QUALITY OF LIFE?

The term "quality of life" is a key catch-phrase in medicine today *(7)*. However, its definition remains vague, and no gold standard exists. Conceptually, it is an attempt to capture various aspects of subjective health status, such as symptoms, physical performance, and psychosocial well-being, in a comprehensive and standardized assessment. The consensus of opinion is that it is a subjective evaluation of aspects of a person's life, including physical, psychological, occupational (role), social, and cognitive functioning *(8)*. Within health-related QOL, it is an attempt to show how such areas have been influenced by illness and treatment.

The roots of QOL assessment within modern medicine can be linked to the World Health Organization, who, in 1947, considered disease as a biophysical process: "Health is a state of complete physical, mental, and social well-being, and not merely the absence of disease" *(9)*. This was followed by the introduction of the Karnofsky index, which was widely used by physicians as a crude measure of a patient's physical performance *(10)*. The Kennedy administration in the 1960s stated that QOL was a goal for the United States health care system for the year 2000 *(11)*. That decade saw the emergence of specially designed QOL instruments for use within clinical practice.

Since 1980, there has been a proliferation of interest in assessing the patient's QOL in parallel with the emergence of the field of psychosocial oncology. This can be demonstrated by the fact that there are now three times as many publications citing "quality of life" in the literature on the Excerpta Medica database *(12)*. This has been led not only by a need to address QOL for its importance to the patient, but also because QOL evaluation is now obligatory for the evaluation of any new drug or treatment. Accurate QOL assessment is essential in clinical trials. All new MRC and EORTC trials demand intention to measure QOL as part of priority ranking for all research funding proposals.

Quality of life assessment is now widely used in clinical trials to complement the primary end points of survival and cure. Indeed, opinion is increasing that, in palliative and supportive interventions, QOL assessment may well be the primary end point of concern *(13,14)*. Quality of life assessment also has a role in comparing treatments in terms of their cost-effectiveness in the competitive climate of health service resource allocation.

A further application of QOL assessment that is beginning to be addressed is in the individual management of care. Clinicians need to make a well-informed decision with colleagues, patient, and family regarding whether the benefit of treatment in terms of increased survival outweighs the potential risk of toxicity and side effects that may severely compromise the patient's well-being.

There are a number of specially designed QOL instruments that are available. Examples of these are listed in Table 1. These may be loosely grouped into three main categories: generic, disease specific, and dimension specific. A review of clinical studies indicated 75 instruments that had been used in a range of settings *(15)*. In deciding on the type of questionnaire to be used, Streiner and Norman *(16)* advocate the use of generic questionnaires in cross-treatment comparisons or cost-utility analysis (e.g., the Nottingham Health Profile or Short Form 36). However, for a particular disease, a disease-specific instrument would give greater sensitivity. A commonly used cancer-specific questionnaire is the Rotterdam Symptom Checklist. However, an effective compromise is to use both types of measurement.

The resistance observed among many scientific clinicians to the application of QOL instruments, and the frequent failure to generate useful data, rest on several key issues. One is the lack of consideration given to a correct choice of instrument guided by the aim of the study; another is that the researcher has failed to justify the use of a particular instrument with their own operational definition of QOL *(17)*. All too commonly, QOL assessment is an afterthought to the research study, rather than being an integral part of the development of the research protocol.

Quality of life assessment is demanding in terms of time and resources. Many QOL instruments are complex for the patient to complete and are difficult to score. Pitfalls of past research have included a lack of follow-up and missing data *(18)*. Reasons for this cited in the literature include attitudes toward qualitative social research and generation of data that cannot be measured with any degree of accuracy or dependability *(19)*. The reason for the failure of past QOL measurements to yield significant results is considered to be that the instruments used have been global and unidimensional, that is, they concentrate only on the patient's physical functioning *(17)*. These are unable to provide enough information about what is going on in a person's life and about the impact of illness and treatment regimes on that person's usual life activities.

Gill *(20)* believes that the goal for reliable and accurate construction of a QOL instrument centers on balancing the psychometric and clinimetric strategies. The psychometric strategy is usually aimed at finding and combining multiple items that measure a single attribute, e.g., anxiety and depression, thereby achieving internal reliability. This is countered by the clinimetric strategy of measuring multiple attributes with a single index, the goal being face validity. The goal for effective QOL assessment is to use an instrument that is able to capture the specific symptoms, side effects, and psychosocial well-being that affect each patient. Some of these issues are applicable to all cancer patients, and can be measured by generic cancer instruments. Some issues are specific to pancreatic cancer, and their inclusion, which is necessary for a full picture of each patient's QOL, requires construction of a pancreas-cancer-specific instrument. Before an appropriate pancreas-cancer-specific questionnaire can be developed, the clinical and psychosocial features of the disease must be considered.

Table 1
Examples of Quality of Life Assessment Tools

Tool	Ref.
Generic (broad measures)	
Activities of Daily Living (ADL) index	55
Quality of Well Being scale	56
Sickness Impact Profile (SIP)	57
Nottingham Health Profile (NHP)	58
McMaster Health Index questionnaire	59
General Health Questionnaire	60
World Health Organization assessment	61
Short Form 36 (SF-36)	62
Disease-specific (cancer)	
Spitzer's Quality of Life Index	63
European Co-operative Oncology Group (ECOG) scoring system	64
Functional Living Index—Cancer (FLIC)	65
EORTC QLQ-C30	66
Rotterdam Symptom Checklist (RSCL)	67
Linear Analogue Self Assessment (LASA)	68
Functional Assessment of Cancer Therapy (FACT G)	69
Dimension-Specific (e.g., depression, pain)	
Hospital Anxiety and Depression Scale	70
McGill Pain Questionnaire	71
Zung's Self Rating Depression Scale	70
Beck Depression Inventory (BDI)	72
Profile of Mood States (POMS)	73
Psychological Adjustment to Illness Scale (PAIS)	74

SYMPTOMS OF PANCREATIC CANCER

Pancreatic cancer can bring with it many distressing symptoms for the patient. At diagnosis, the chief presenting symptoms reported are pain (radiating to the back in half), bile duct obstruction resulting in jaundice, weight loss, and anorexia *(3,5)*.

One of the central challenges for the clinician is to achieve effective symptom control. Malignant bile duct obstruction brings about not only the clinical symptom of jaundice, but also the distress of pruritis and skin changes. Jaundice may affect the patient's psychological and social well-being. Changes in perceived body image may be of great concern for the patient, as the jaundice emphasizes their illness. Social activities may be curtailed as the patient is aware of the change in physical appearance. Recurrent jaundice after palliative treatment is an ominous sign for many patients, with significant psychological impact.

Nausea and vomiting have been reported in 30–40% of pancreatic cancer patients, although true mechanical obstruction occurs in only 5% of cases *(21)*. Because of the effect of the disease, patients may suffer indigestion and early satiety. The patient may be faced with dietary changes as he or she is unable to consume the same volume of food or the same types of food. For example, some patients are unable to tolerate a high fat/high protein diet, and, after pancreatic resection, diabetes mellitus may necessitate dietary modification. This can have repercussions on the patient and the family as they try to find an adequate diet that is both palatable and tolerated by the patient, and ensures an adequate level of nutrition.

Weight loss and cachexia occur in over 90% of patients with pancreatic cancer *(22)*. As in other advanced cancer patient populations, this can have a significant effect on patient well-being. It can result in changes in body image and also is used by many patients as a marker to assess the stage of their illness. Weight loss is seen as a crucial indication that there is disease progression. Therefore, a goal for the pancreatic cancer patient is to maintain body weight for as long as possible.

Pain is a well-reported problem in pancreatic cancer; up to 85% of patients with advanced disease suffer pain *(23)*. Frequently, the patient presents with dull epigastric pain, and, as disease progresses, pain can radiate to the back *(3)*. The main causes of pain are neoplastic infiltration of nerves and pancreatic duct obstruction, with upstream dilation and ductal hypertension *(24)*. The patient may be faced with pain in the cervical or thoracic spine as a consequence of metastases. Such pain is difficult for the clinician to manage effectively.

Other reported symptoms include steatorrhea and changes in bowel habit, and flatulence, indigestion, fatigue, and muscle weakness *(5)*.

Psychosocial Impact of Pancreatic Cancer

Few studies have examined the impact of pancreatic cancer on the well-being of the patient. One study has investigated the observation of increased depression in these patients *(25)*. Explorations of this link have postulated an association between pain and anxiety and depression, or that the patient has to face the demands that a diagnosis of advanced cancer brings *(26)*.

Pancreatic cancer is less common than colon, breast, lung, and gynecological cancers; therefore, patients may have not heard of the disease before. Alternatively, they may associate it with other cancers, such as colorectal cancer, in which the clinical picture is different and treatment options and prognosis are more favorable. Before reviewing QOL assessment, it will be helpful to consider what is known about QOL in other advanced cancers.

PSYCHOSOCIAL DEMANDS OF ADVANCED CANCER

The diagnosis of cancer can have an overwhelming impact on the patient and his or her family *(8)*. With advanced cancer, not only do they have to face the dilemmas of being labeled as a cancer patient, but also it is usually clear that treatment is limited and survival will be short. Despite changes in public education and in the media, cancer is still associated with thoughts of a painful, long, and undignified death *(8)*. There may well be repercussions of stigma associated with a label of advanced cancer, resulting in isolation of patient and family. They have to enter the health care arena, which, for many, is a new and frightening experience as they cope with the demands of treatment and hospitalization, and with the realization that their advanced cancer may be incurable. There is a potential conflict in the need for truth-telling and optimism. Clinicians are faced with the task of breaking bad news, yet may often have very little preparation for this. A common response of the clinician is distancing from the patient, yet this has the potential to further isolate the patient, and to ensure that psychological morbidity goes unrecognized *(27)*.

Coping with Advanced Cancer

Several studies have investigated how patients and their families cope with the cancer experience and the consequent uncertainty about the future *(28–30)*. One commonly identified coping mechanism is denial or avoidance. Despite attempts to provide the patient with accurate and truthful information, he or she either disregards the news that cancer is present or selectively assimilates only the most optimistic news, resulting in an unrealistic expectation of the illness. Although frustrating for those caring for such patients, it may be a necessary defense mechanism for the patient.

In the face of adversity, some patients cope by finding an acceptable explanation for their illness. This may involve rationalizing their illness through past behavior or life events, such as smoking or blaming the illness on the actions of others *(27)*. Patients commonly ask the question "Why me?", and, in the case of pancreatic cancer, the disease often cannot be attributed to any definite cause. Some patients may be frustrated by this lack of knowledge regarding their illness.

Control

One factor that influences the way that patients cope successfully or otherwise with their illness is their perceived control over their illness and treatment. Patients adapt more easily if they feel that they can contribute to the outcome of their illness. This may be manifest in strategies such as the need for information regarding their illness and treatment, or by direct action to fight against the cancer. Such patients may want surgery or other treatment at any cost, and are willing volunteers for clinical trials. The concept of maintaining hope is crucial for many when faced with such adversity. Helplessness is associated with a strong risk of later depressive illness *(30)*.

Psychosocial support is a crucial element of coping with cancer. This includes not only support from family and friends, and the ability to talk honestly about the illness and future plans, but also support and feedback from the health care team.

QUALITY OF LIFE ASSESSMENT IN PANCREATIC CANCER

Little research has been undertaken to examine QOL in pancreatic cancer. The majority of studies have been undertaken in the past 5 yr and are either cross-sectional or retrospective studies. Many of these studies are subject to methodological flaws in the design and assessment of QOL and most are primarily concerned with assessing a particular treatment. Quality of life assessment is used to this end, but is not reported as an end in itself. Consequently, there are numerous problems with the methods used and the data reported. Key problems center on the definition of QOL regarding its appropriateness and suitability to answer the study research question, the retrospective (rather than prospective) methods used, and the lack of patient responses to QOL assessment.

An extensive literature search on BIDS and Medline for the years 1990–1996 identified only 26 articles using these keywords: quality of life, pancreatic, periampullary, neoplasm, psychological, and social. On examination, only nine were actual research studies, the others being review articles or had mentioned "quality of life" in the article, but had not actually described or assessed it.

A few studies purporting to measure QOL did not use any formal assessment tool, but applied their own criteria to assess QOL. A retrospective analysis of eight patients with potentially curable resections used cytology by ERCP as a prognostic indicator of QOL. No definition or assessment was reported; the authors simply state that in six patients with partial pancreatectomies, postoperative QOL was reported as good *(31)*. An evaluation of pancreatic resection in 158 patients with advanced cancer in one Japanese center used hospital-free survival as an indication of QOL *(32)*. This crude indicator clearly takes no account of functional or psychosocial status of the patients out of the hospital. Although the authors of that study consider that survival and hospital-free survival are the best general means to measure QOL, there is no evidence from professional or patient viewpoints to support such assumptions.

Other studies have taken a similar approach to measuring QOL from retrospectively defined criteria. In a recent study of the role of gemcitabine in advanced pancreatic cancer in phase II clinical trials, an attempt to quantify symptomatic improvement was made by the calculation of a "clinical benefit response" using measures including pain intensity, analgesic consumption, weight loss, and performance status *(33)*. Although the authors state that it is a valid and reliable method, caution should be given to the interpretation of such response regarding patient improvement, when the defined criteria are assessed from an expert viewpoint, and are not validated in independent studies.

A retrospective study audited outcome, between 1975–1986, in 101 patients with pancreatic and periampullary carcinomas *(34)*. Quality of life was assessed using patients' complaints of symptoms and Swiss Group for Clinical Cancer Research (SAKK) score. A comfort index was designed by plotting good palliation (discharge to SAKK score >3) against disease duration. Symptoms impairing QOL were pain, jaundice, and vomiting. However, as discussed earlier, QOL is much more than an expert's observation of clinical symptoms.

Some studies have used unidimensional observer indicators as measures to ascertain QOL. A much-used tool in this context is the Karnofsky index, which is a crude indicator of a patient's physical performance. Ebert et al. *(35)* examined the role of high/low dose octreotide in 10 patients at 3 mo follow-up, using the Karnofsky index, an oncology scoring system, and reports of pain and weight. They concluded that four of 10 patients had QOL similar to healthy controls, but pain was different. Such assumptions should be considered carefully, given the lack of justification to support what actually constitutes "healthy quality of life." Psychological and social well-being will make a substantial impact on such perception. In a later study to compare the outcome of radical resection vs surgical bypass in 128 patients followed-up at 3 mo *(36)*, the use of the Karnofsky index and clinical performance scale indicated that, in the resected group, 82% were mobile and 63% pain free; in the bypass group, 31% were in hospital, 26% pain-free, and 39% had a degree of nausea and vomiting. This study attempts to consider a range of important symptoms, and a basic measure of function, but again does not record these issues from the patient's perspective.

Glimelius et al. *(37)* attempted to measure the cost of pancreatic cancer in terms of QOL using quality of life adjusted years (QALYs) in a study of primary chemotherapy vs best supportive care in 61 inoperable gastrointestinal tumors, 22 of which were pancreatic cancer. This small study indicated a 50% increase in the QALY cost of treatment in pancreatic tumors, but acknowledged that such results need to be interpreted cautiously, with the limited knowledged of QOL assessment in pancreatic cancer.

Other studies have used a variety of QOL assessment tools in their studies. In a randomized placebo controlled trial of tamoxifen in 44 patients with irresectable tumors, the Karnofsky and Hospital Anxiety and Depression Score (HADS) failed to indicate any significant difference in QOL. In an investigation of the effect of pain and depression on QOL in 130 newly diagnosed cancer patients using Memorial pain assessment card, Beck depression inventory, hopelessness scale, functional living index, and weekly activity checklist, only patients with moderate or increased pain showed significantly poorer QOL scores and impaired functional activity *(25)*. This approach is a move in the right direction toward qualitative, patient-centered QOL assessment.

A limited number of cross-sectional studies have compared the outcome of medical and surgical interventions for pancreatic cancer in terms of QOL. In follow-up of 19 patients who had undergone endoscopic insertion of a stent, Ballinger et al. *(38)* used a cancer-specific measure (the Rotterdam Symptom Checklist), the HADS score, and also added two additional questions related to jaundice and pruritis, to assess QOL before ERCP, and then at 1, 4, 8, and 12 wk after stent insertion. After stenting, there was complete relief of jaundice and pruritis, and anorexia was significantly better at 12 wk. Of the 16 patients who complained of indigestion before stenting, relief was significantly better at 1 wk, and there was complete relief at 6–8 wk. Fifteen patients felt that their mood was good/very good before stent insertion, and this was unchanged at 12 wk. In a recent study *(39)*, 31 patients with malignant biliary obstruction completed the EORTC QLQ-C30 and two further questions assessing jaundice and pruritis before insertion of a stent and 1 mo later. Patients reported significant improvement in emotional, cognitive, and global health scores. In addition to the expected improvement in pruritis and jaundice, anorexia, diarrhea, and sleep pattern were also reported to be improved. These studies show how QOL data can be reported in terms of qualitative changes, rather than as the numerical values favored by those usually working with quantitative measurements.

One study has examined QOL following surgical resection. In a cross-sectional survey, 25 patients after Whipple's procedure and age/sex-matched patients after cholecystectomy were followed-up. Six QOL measures were used: the time trade-off technique, direct questioning of objectives, physician global assessment, gastrointestinal QOL index, Visick scale, and sickness impact profile. A clinical assessment of nutritional status was performed using the subjective global assessment, as well as clinical markers of nutritional status (anthropometry, gastrointestinal hormone status). The results indicated that QOL was excellent in the Whipple's group, and not significantly different from the control subjects. Regarding nutritional status, there was no significant difference in gastrointestinal symptoms, although five of the Whipple's patients complained of greasy bowel movements, and one patient complained of difficulty in maintaining weight. Although the purpose of the study was to begin to allow patients to assess their QOL, it was only concerned with the impact of the Whipple's procedure, and did not address the broader issue of QOL in pancreatic cancer. Nevertheless, the use of a broad range of instruments designed to assess a variety of aspects of QOL emphasizes the need to make an all-inclusive assessment. However, in the absence of a disease-specific instrument, the use of many different instruments can be cumbersome.

In summary, then, although the question of QOL in pancreatic cancer is beginning to be addressed in research studies, there is no standardized and comprehensive approach to its assessment. Little consideration has been given to the patient's viewpoint of QOL in pancreatic cancer, with only one study mentioning that patients were able to give supplemental responses to specific issues affecting them. No studies allowed the patient to rate the relevance of each issue regarding their own experience of pancreatic cancer. Some studies, although using well-described QOL assessment tools, had to supplement the chosen tool with additional items that may have influenced the validity and reliability of results obtained *(17)*. What appears obvious is the lack of significant differences between disparate groups, which suggests that the various approaches used have not been specific or sensitive enough to assess QOL in pancreatic cancer. The studies that did obtain significant differences used a number of instruments. Psychometrically, triangulation of measurement approaches increase content and construct validity as a greater proportion of the conceptual domain of QOL will be tapped *(17)*. However, this should be carefully balanced with the realities of clinical practice, in which there is a need for a quick, easy-to-measure assessment tool whose findings can be easily interpreted. This will improve compliance, as the patient may find it difficult to complete lengthy questionnaires. This is particularly pertinent to the pancreatic cancer patient, because these patients may be simply too unwell to complete a long questionnaire. Follow-up of such patients at particularly vulnerable times when their QOL is compromised could be difficult. Consensus of specialist opinion has suggested that there is a need for a pancreatic-cancer specific QOL questionnaire *(40)*.

DEVELOPMENT OF A PANCREATIC CANCER QUALITY OF LIFE QUESTIONNAIRE

At present, no pancreatic-cancer-specific QOL questionnaire exists, and, in the few QOL studies that have been conducted, the instruments used do not include specific symptoms or side effects associated with this disease. Also, there may be psychosocial issues related to the impact of advanced cancer on the patient that have as great or greater importance in assessing QOL in pancreatic cancer.

In developing such a valid and reliable questionnaire for use in cross-sectional clinical trials, attention should focus on the development process itself and the methodology employed. In 1986, the European Organization for Research and Treatment of Cancer (EORTC) established the Quality of Life Study Group to address such issues. A core cancer module, the QLQ-C30, has been developed and refined, and has been demonstrated to have validity and reliability across a range of cancer patient populations and cultures *(41–43)*.

Attention has now focused on the development of add-on disease-specific modules. A lung cancer module has been developed, with breast, colorectal, head and neck, and esophageal modules now undergoing final stages of development. In March 1996, the European Quality of Life in Pancreatic Cancer (EQoLiPA) study group was established. This group is committed to the multilingual development of a pancreatic-cancer-specific module to supplement the EORTC QLQ-C30. The EORTC-published guidelines for module development have been followed. There are essentially four key phases *(44)*:

1. Generation of relevant quality of life issues;
2. Operationalization of a disease-specific questionnaire;

3. Pretesting of questionnaire in a sample patient population, and its refinement; and

4. Large-scale field testing.

All stages are subject to internal peer review by the EORTC Quality of Life Study Group to ensure standardization of the development process. By early 1997, phase 1 and 2 of the pancreatic cancer module had been completed and approved by the EORTC study group. It is anticipated that phase 4 will be completed and the module approved for use by the end of 1998. The following is a description of phase 1 and phase 2 work, highlighting the important issues for patients with pancreatic cancer.

Phase 1: Generation of Quality of Life Issues

There are three key stages in generating a list of disease-specific issues: extensive literature review, interviews with specialists, and interviews with patients. However, the literature review was largely unproductive. In order to ensure that the most relevant and important issues were generated from the patients' perspective, a qualitative study was undertaken to gain an insight into pancreatic cancer patients' views of their illness, treatment, and care, using a social sciences methodology known as grounded theory.

Grounded theory was developed in 1968 as an attempt to bridge the gap between quantitative and qualitative research methods *(45)*. Its main features are that, through a number of open-ended interviews with patients, key themes or categories begin to emerge. These are coded accordingly. As the interviews are conducted, new emerging data is analyzed and compared with the existing interviews. This allows themes to be linked together. Data collection is stopped when such themes can be illustrated at length from the patient interviews. This rich description of data is known as saturation. At this point, other sources of data (for example, literature that has examined the impact of advanced cancer on the patient and family, and also expert views) are examined or sampled to provide the theoretical underpinning to the emerging theory.

A cross-section of 21 patients from the south of England were interviewed about their illness, treatment, and care, and the perceived impact on their QOL. In order to gain an understanding of the specialist's viewpoint on QOL in pancreatic cancer, a review panel of six multidisciplinary health professionals (surgeon, internist, palliative care physician, surgical nurse, palliative care nurse) were individually given a copy of the QLQ-C30, and a list of issues obtained in the literature review, and asked to comment on which issues they thought were most important to the pancreatic cancer patient. These comments were then compared with the completed outcome of the patient interviews, to provide an exhaustive list of relevant issues.

A list of 42 relevant issues was generated. These include specific symptoms of pancreatic cancer, side effects of treatment, and also additional QOL issues related to emotional and social well-being. There was good agreement between health professionals and patients regarding the content of such issues generated (Table 2).

However, a noticeable difference was observed when the context of these issues was examined. The health care professionals described symptoms associated with the disease as having a direct impact on the patient's QOL. The example of pain can illustrate this. Pain as a consequence of malignant bile duct obstruction and/or disseminated disease can affect physical performance, social functioning, and psychological well-being. The professional view is that, as pain becomes more severe, there is a subsequent

Table 2
Issues Relevant to the Pancreatic Cancer Patient

Symptoms/side effects			
Pain	Digestion	Evacuation	Skin/general health
Abdominal pain	Changes in amount of food	Change in bowel habit	Jaundice
Bony pain	Changes in type of food	Color of stool	Itching
Back pain	Feeling full early in meals	Color of urine	Changes in condition of skin
Pain on moving	Pleasure in eating	Excessive wind	Swollen abdomen
Effect of pain medica-tion	Indigestion		Concern about physical appearance
	Taste changes		Hair loss
	Sore/dry mouth		Feeling drowsy during day
	Weight loss		Loss of physical strength
	Infection		Tingling in hands and feet
			Numbness in hands or feet

Additional quality of life issues

Worrying about future health   Ability to talk to others about illness
Worrying about future in general   Receiving information about illness and treatment
Feeling in control of illness   Receiving support
Maintaining hope   Involvement in discussions about treatment and care
Planning future events
Time spent thinking about illness
Family support
Loneliness

effect on these domains, and consequently on QOL. Therefore, the greater the severity of symptoms, the greater the impact on QOL.

However, the pancreatic cancer patient saw the impact of a symptom in terms of the need to embark on, or adapt, coping strategies. As a symptom arose, patients regarded the impact in terms of the perceived threat to their daily life and self-identity. Five main coping strategies were identified, and can be illustrated, using the impact of pain (Table 3). If a symptom was relatively mild, such coping strategies were sufficient to deal with the threat, and impact on their overall perception of QOL was nonexistent or mild. However, if the symptom was severe, these coping strategies were insufficient to deal with the threat, and had a great impact on their QOL. This is in contrast to the relationship described by specialists and also the assumption made by most QOL measures that the presence of a symptom is constant regarding impact on QOL regardless of severity. Such assumptions may be a limitation in these measures, because they neglect the underlying cognitive processes that mediate patients' perceptions of QOL *(14)*.

Portenoy *(46)* in a theoretical model for describing relationships between symptomology and QOL suggests three relationships to explain differences in overall QOL perception in relation to the degree of symptoms (Fig. 1). First, a constant relationship

Table 3
Main Coping Strategies

Strategy	Example
Defending/avoidance	Symptom e.g., pain, is ignored for as long as possible and patient soldiers on regardless
Blaming	Symptom is blamed on external event, e.g., initial onset of pain is blamed on a recent fall, or other disease, such as gallstones
Rationalizing	Symptom is rationalized as a "normal part of the illness," e.g., pain seen in the postoperative patient as expected consequence of surgery
Turning to others	Patient turns to family and/or health professionals to explain symptoms and provide support in tackling symptom
Taking direct action	Patient takes affirmative action against symptom, e.g., takes analgesia or volunteers for participation in clinical trials

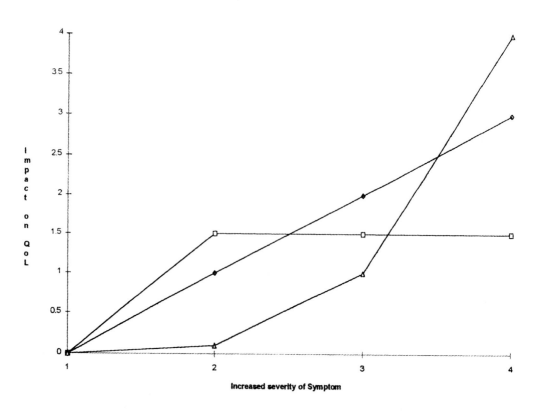

Fig. 1. Symptom intensity and quality of life. Three hypothesized relationships. □: Constant relationship, i.e., each symptom has direct impact on QOL, regardless of severity, ◊: Linear relationship, i.e., impact on QOL of severity of symptom (view observed in clinical practice and view of health professionals in study. △: Curvilinear impact of symptom on QOL—low when mild, potentially overwhelming when high. Related to meaning of symptom on QOL perception. View endorsed by patients in study.

exists, whereby each symptom has a direct impact on QOL, regardless of severity (line □). This view is seen in many QOL measurement tools, in which symptoms or issues are unweighted regarding the effect on overall QOL. Second, a linear relationship is proposed in which severity of symptom is directly proportional to the impact of overall QOL (line ◊). This relationship is assumed in clinical practice, because of the effect of severe symptoms relative to mild and moderate symptoms. Such a viewpoint was endorsed by the healthcare professionals interviewed. Third, Portenoy suggests that a more accurate relationship is shown by a curvilinear line (line △). Here, it is suggested that, when the symptom is mild, impact on overall QOL is low, higher when moderate, and potentially overwhelming when severe. This appears to be the relationship expressed by the patients interviewed.

In addition to enabling the development of a pancreas-cancer-specific module, this study has provided an important insight into how the pancreatic cancer patient copes with his or her illness, treatment, and care. It supports the assumptions that QOL perception is multidimensional and subjective and can only be described accurately by patients themselves. By ensuring that the most relevant and important issues to the patient, rather than to the specialist, are captured in a QOL questionnaire, using both quantitative and qualitative research methods in the developmental process will contribute to the reliability and validity of a pancreatic cancer QOL module.

Phase 2: Operationalization of the Pancreatic Cancer Quality of Life Module

A pancreatic cancer module has now been developed to supplement the EORTC QLQ-C30. It has undergone review by patients and a panel of international specialists to rate the importance of issues generated, and to check for significant omissions. It has undergone refinement following review by the EORTC Quality of Life Study Group guidelines, and has been translated into several European languages for parallel multilingual phase 3 and 4 development by the EQoLiPA study group. At present, it is intended for assessment of QOL in all treatments of pancreatic adenocarcinoma, ductal cell carcinoma and periampullary tumors. Provisionally composed of 26 items, the issues covered are broadly shown in Table 2.

INTERVENTIONS TO IMPROVE QUALITY OF LIFE IN PANCREATIC CANCER

Over the past two decades, there has been considerable advancement in medical and surgical interventions for pancreatic cancer; however, these have failed to have a significant impact on the long-term survival of patients. Although surgical resection is the only intervention that offers a chance of potential cure, only 20% of pancreatic cancer patients may be eligible for such intervention. Consequently, over 80% of patients will receive some form of palliative medical and surgical intervention. The goal of management is to improve symptoms and functioning of patients within the context of a limited survival. Optimizing the patient's QOL should therefore be of prime concern in deciding on choice of treatment intervention.

Surgical Resection

Surgical resection in the form of a pancreatoduodenectomy or Whipple's procedure is the only intervention that can provide patients with long-term survival. These procedures have been refined over past decades, and, with the emergence of specialist pancreatic surgeons, accurate preoperative staging of disease, better anesthetic techniques, intensive care, nutrition, and other supportive care, mortality and morbidity rates have subsequently declined.

However, it is a significant risk to the patient. Patients are still faced with the risk of postoperative complications. Also, there may be a long rehabilitative period for the patient, resulting in a long hospitalization and recuperation at home. The patient may be faced with the clinical onset of diabetes or exocrine sufficiency, and will need to take supplements for the remainder of life. Other long-term problems reported in the literature include nutritional changes, as patients are unable to tolerate their normal diet, delayed gastric emptying, and altered bowel habits, such as dumping syndrome or steatorrhea *(3,47)* Surgery has also been reported to have a negative effect on patients' body image, as they are faced with the mutilating effect of surgery *(8)*. Patients may be faced with a long period in which they are unable to resume their normal daily activities, which compromises their QOL. The demands placed on the family as they cope with the demands of caregiving in the rehabilitative period may also have a significant impact on the patient's well-being.

However, surgery may have a positive impact on patients' QOL. The patient with pancreatic cancer who is eligible for surgery is faced with the hope that he or she is able to undergo such a radical procedure and that this will encourage taking direct action in the fight against the disease. This attitude has been demonstrated in other cancer patient populations. A study examining the psychological morbidity of women undergoing mastectomy or lumpectomy demonstrated that there was greater psychological distress in the lumpectomy group *(48)*. Similarly, in a study of limb-sarcoma patients *(49)* which compared the impact of amputation against limb-sparing surgery and irradiation, the expectation that those undergoing limb-sparing surgery would have a greater QOL was not confirmed, with the surprising observation that amputation had a less negative effect on QOL. In the study by McLeod et al. *(50)*, QOL following a Whipple's procedure was reported as excellent. Although one must be cautious because of very few studies, for the minority of patients who are eligible for resection, the short-term impact on QOL needs to be balanced by the long-term prospect of increasing survival and allowing patients to resume a normal life, albeit for a restricted period. Such decision-making should rest with both clinician and patient, and surgery should be integrated into a total multidisciplinary program for the patient's maximum advantage *(51)*.

Palliative Surgery

Palliative surgery still has an important role in the management of patients, particularly when duodenal obstruction is present. It may also be beneficial to the inoperable patient who is otherwise medically fit *(21)*. This increasing interest in palliative surgery parallels the decline in perioperative mortality and also the emergence of specialist pancreatic surgeons. It is an important option in the management of pancreatic cancer; however, it is imperative that the benefit to the patients in terms of effective palliation for the remainder of their lives is worth the risk that palliative surgery brings. As Watanapa and Williamson *(21)* comment: "It is obviously attractive to avoid a major operation in those with a limited expectation of life, but with two provisos: that the nature and irresectability of the tumor can be established beyond doubt, and that subsequent quality of life is not eroded by the need for further hospital admission."

Surgical palliation carries with it the risks of postoperative complications. In their review *(21)*, Watanapa and Williamson compared the results of endoscopic vs surgical palliation. Although endoscopic palliation was associated with lower mortality rates (9 vs 12%), shorter hospital stay (7 vs 14 d), and lower complications (16 vs 31%), the long-term complications, such as recurrent jaundice and cholangitis, appeared more common (28 vs 16%). This may allow patients to continue to enjoy their life for as long as they remain physically well. If the aim in the surgically fit patient is to relieve symptoms effectively for the remainder of life, allowing the patients the opportunity to adapt to life within the limitations of his or her illness, surgical palliation has an important role in rehabilitating the patient to achieve maximum QOL.

Endoscopic Palliation

For a significant number of patients, on diagnosis, their disease is clearly disseminated, and prognosis is extremely limited. Effective short-term management of symptoms with fewer complications may be the treatment of choice. The advantages of endoscopic palliation are lower procedure-related morbidity and mortality, shorter initial hospitalization, and lower costs *(52)*. Recent cross-sectional studies have demonstrated the benefits of endoscopic stenting on symptoms such as pain, jaundice, and improving appetite, and also on patients' overall QOL *(25,53)*. These factors, in combination with the overall general health and age of the patient, and projected survival, should all be considered when deciding on management of care in the inoperable patient.

Adjuvant Therapies

The benefit of adjuvant therapies in pancreatic cancer continues to be a source of debate in the literature. Because of the biological nature of the tumor, many therapies have proven unsuccessful. Those that have shown benefit need to be addressed in the context of survival, as Jessup, Posner and Huberman *(53)* state: "Since median survival is usually 2–6 mo in patients with advanced disease, a 50% increase in survival, while significant, may not be biologically important, especially if the therapy has toxicity that detracts from the quality of life, and ultimate cure rates remain unchanged." Yet the toxicity of such therapies needs to be balanced with the psychological benefit of chemotherapy. Side effects are often perceived as less important than the feeling that the patient has control of the disease. So the patient may report improved QOL despite moderate or severe side effects. Slevin *(7)* describes this as related to relief of symptoms, increased medical attention, and the hope that something positive is being done against their disease.

The most common chemotherapy agents reported in pancreatic cancer studies have been 5-fluoracil and gemcitabine. Although toxicity of these agents is comparatively low, they may still induce known side effects, such as stomatosis and alopecia. Radiotherapy can cause erythema around the radiation site, and also fatigue. Compliance with treatment regimens may also impact on the patients' daily routine as they attend frequent treatment sessions and follow-up. In a review of 21 hormonal/chemotherapy studies and six radiotherapy and chemotherapy studies between 1983 and 1993, only 26%

of studies gave evidence of the patients' physical performance, and 30% gave no mention of previous treatments. Although toxicities in the studies were minimal, with only one study indicating toxicity, there are methodological drawbacks within the studies, and few trials evaluated the impact of medical treatment on patients' QOL; those that did provided only scant results. An important conclusion drawn from this review was that future studies should focus on phase II screening with new drugs or new combinations, supported by a strong biological rationale and the development of a valid and acceptable tool for evaluating QOL in such patients *(40)*. Such recommendations should be followed with the emergence of novel approaches to controlling this disease, for example, essential fatty acids and matrix metalloproteinase inhibitors, in which the intended therapeutic benefit is control of the disease process rather than cure.

FUTURE DIRECTIONS

Quality of life assessment in pancreatic cancer is still in its infancy, and provides an exciting opportunity for future research and development. Such development should now begin to look at the standardization of QOL assessment and the application of such measurement in research studies, particularly in randomized controlled trials. Only when accurate and comprehensive assessment is obtained can we begin to address the risks and benefits of the disease and treatment in terms of outcome on QOL. A key issue rests on greater understanding in the clinical application of QOL assessment and appreciation of the contribution of other research methodologies that can contribute to our knowledge of all aspects of disease and illness.

Regarding the individual management of care of the pancreatic cancer patient, QOL should be a prime concern when deciding on the best course of action for each patient, especially when faced with the patient whose survival is limited. Caring for such patients and family can be emotionally challenging for all health professionals involved. With the knowledge that prognosis is poor and treatment is limited, the health professional may be reluctant to consider treatment options, as Waegener *(54)* comments:

> "Because of the dismal prognosis, most physicians have a very pessimistic attitude toward patients with pancreatic cancer. This may contribute to the delay in diagnosis. This results in a self-fulfilling prophesy, because patients with a delayed diagnosis are often in a frail medical state and unlikely to benefit from any antineoplastic therapy. Therefore any progress is very slow."

Supportive care interventions have an important role in the management of care of the pancreatic cancer patient. Not only should these be concerned with strategies to relieve symptoms associated with the disease, but also to facilitate the patient and family to adjust to the illness and treatment and optimize their QOL. There is a wealth of literature that examines the management of the cancer patient. Within pancreatic cancer, this should rest in the multidisciplinary management, as Slevin *(7)* suggests: "In addition to having a direct impact on length of survival, the multiplicity of symptoms in individuals with cancer suggests the need for a holistic approach to the psychological and physical symptom management, as well as therapeutic intention."

As clinicians are increasingly aware that the illness is much more than a biological disease process, but impacts on all aspects of a person's life, pancreatic cancer should not be managed in isolation, but should be a process of decision-making among surgeon, oncologist, physician, patient, family, general practitioner, nurse, and other health care professionals, to ensure that our research and clinical endeavors are aimed at maximizing the QOL of the pancreatic cancer patient.

REFERENCES

1. Trede M. Treatment of pancreatic carcinoma—the surgeon's dilemma. Br J Surg 1987; *74:*79,80.
2. Haddock G and Carter DC. Aetiology of pancreatic cancer. Br J Surg 1990; *77:*1159–1165.
3. Carter DC. Clinical features and management of carcinoma of the pancreas. Br J Hosp Med 1995; *54:*459–464.
4. Ashton Key M, Hammersley S, Johnson CD. Incidence and mortality of gastric and pancreatic cancer in England and Wales 1961–1988. Gut 1991; *32:*A580–A581.
5. Krech RL and Walsh D. Symptoms of pancreatic cancer. J Pain Symptom Manage 1991; *6:*360–367.
6. Fontham ETH and Correa P. Epidemiology of pancreatic cancer. Surg Clin North Am, 1989; *69:*551.
7. Slevin ML. Quality of life: philosophical question or clinical reality? Br Med J 1992; *305:*466–469.
8. Fallowfield L. Quality of life: the missing measurement in health care. Souvenir, London, 1990.
9. World Health Organisation Constitution. WHO Chron 1947; *1:*29.
10. Karnofsky DA, Abelman WH, Craver LF, et al. The use of nitrogen mustards in the palliative treatment of carcinoma. Cancer 1948; *1:*634–656.
11. Meeberg GA. Quality of life: a concept analysis. J Adv Nurs 1993; *18:*32–38.
12. Quality of life and clinical trials. Lancet 1995; *346:*1–2 (editorial).
13. Kassa S. Problems in assessing quality of life. J Cancer Care 1993; *2:*100–103.
14. Cella DF. Quality of life: concepts and definitions. J Pain Symptom Manage 1994; *9:*186–192.
15. Gill TM and Feinstein AR. A critical appraisal of the quality of life measurements. JAMA 1994; *272:*619–626.
16. Streiner DL and Norman GR. Health measurement scales: a practical guide to their development and use, 2nd ed., Oxford University Press, Oxford, 1992.
17. Jaloweic A. Issues in using multiple measures of quality of life. Semin Oncol Nurs 1990; *6:*271–277.
18. Hayden KA, et al. Pitfalls in quality of life assessment. Lessons from a Southwest Oncology Group breast cancer clinical trial. Oncol Nurs Forum 1993; *20:*1415–1419.
19. Donovan K, Sanson Fisher RW, and Redman S. Measuring quality of life in cancer patients. J Clin Oncol 1989; *7:*959–968.
20. Gill, TM. Quality of life assessment: values and pitfalls. J Royal Soc Med 1995; *88:*680–682.
21. Watanapa P and Williamson RCN. Surgical palliation for pancreatic cancer: developments during the past two decades. Br J Surg 1992; *79:*8–20.
22. De Wys WD. Weight loss and nutritional abnormalities in cancer patients: incidence, severity and significance. Clin Oncol 1986; *5:*251–261.
23. Kaiser MH, Barkin J, and MacIntyre JM. Pancreatic cancer: assessment of prognosis by clinical presentation. Cancer 1985; *56:*397–402.
24. Lebovits AH and Lefkowitz M. Pain management of pancreatic carcinoma: a review. Pain 1988; *36:*1–11.
25. Kelsen DP. Portenoy RK, Thaler HT, Niedzwiecki D, Passik SD, Tao Y, et al. Pain and depression in patients with newly diagnosed pancreas cancer. J Clin Oncol 1995; *13:*748–755.
26. Passik SD and Breitbart WS. Depression in patients with pancreatic carcinoma. Diagnostic and treatment issues. Cancer 1996; *78:*615–626.

27. Faulkner A and Maguire P. Talking to cancer patients and their families. Oxford: Oxford Medical, Oxford, 1994.

28. Dunkel-Schatter C, Feinstein LG, Taylor SE, and Falke RL. Patterns of coping with Cancer. Health Psych 1992; *11:*79–87.

29. Gammon J. Which way out of the crisis? Coping strategies for dealing with cancer. Professional Nurse 1993; May 488–493.

30. Maguire K. Improving the recognition and treatment of affective disorders in cancer patients. In: Granville-Grasson K (ed), Recent advances in psychiatry, 7th ed. Churchill Livingstone, London, 1992; 15–30.

31. Ishikawa O, Ohigashi H, Nakaizumi A, et al. Surgical resection of potentially curable pancreatic cancer with improved preservation of endocrine function: further evaluation of intraoperative cytodiagnosis. Hepato-gastroenterology 1993; *40:*443–447.

32. Yasue M, Sakamoto J, Morimoto T, et al. Evaluation of the effect of pancreatic resection in advanced pancreatic cancer with special reference using hospital-free survival as a measure of quality-of-life. Jap J Clin Oncol 1995; *25:*37–45.

33. Eypasch E, Williams JI, and Wood-Dauphinee S. Gastrointestinal quality of life index; development, validation and application of a new instrument. Br J Surg 1995; *82:*216–222.

34. Pretre R, Huber O, Robert J, Soravia C, Egeli RA, and Rohner A. Results of surgical palliation for cancer of the head of the pancreas and periampullary region. Br J Surg 1992; *79:*795–798.

35. Ebert M, Friess H, Beger HG, and Büchler MW. Role of octreotide in the treatment of pancreatic cancer. Digestion 1994; *55:*48–51.

36. Bakkevold KE and Kambestad B. Palliation of pancreatic cancer: a prospective multicentre study. Eur J Surg Oncol 1995; *21:*176–182.

37. Glimelius B, Hoffman K, Graf W, et al. Cost-effectiveness of palliative chemotherapy in advanced gastrointestinal cancer. Ann Oncol 1995; *6:*267–274.

38. Ballinger AB, McHugh M, Catnach SM, Alstead EM, and Clark MI. Symptom relief and quality of life after stenting for malignant bile duct obstruction. Gut 1994; *35:*467–470.

39. Luman W, Cull A, Palmer KR. Quality of life following endoscopic stenting for malignant biliary obstruction. Abstract presented at the British Society of Gastroenterology, March, Brighton, 1996.

40. Lionetto R, Pugliese V, Bruzzi P, Rosso R. No standard treatment is available for advanced pancreatic cancer. Eur J Cancer 1995; *31A:*882–887.

41. Niezgoda HE and Pater JL. A validation study of the domains of core EORTC quality of life questionnaire. Qual Life Res 1993; *2:*319–325.

42. Sprangers MA, Cull A, Bjordal K, Groenvold M, and Aaronson NK. The European Organization for Research and Treatment of Cancer. Approach to quality of life assessment: guidelines for developing questionnaire modules. EORTC Study Group on Quality of Life. Qual Life Res 1993; *2:*287–295.

43. Ringdal GI and Ringdal K. Testing the EORTC Quality of Life Questionnaire on cancer patients with heterogeneous diagnoses. Qual Life Res 1993; *2:*129–140.

44. Aaronson NK, Cull A, Kassa S, and Sprangers MG, for the EORTC Study Group on Quality of Life. The EORTC modular approach to quality of life assessment in oncology: an update. In: Spiker B (ed), Quality of life and pharmoeconomics in clinical trials, 2nd ed. Raven, New York, 1995;

45. Strauss A and Corbin J. Basics of qualitative research. Grounded theory procedures and techniques, Sage, London, 1990.

46. Portenoy RK. Pain and quality of life: clinical issues and implications for research. In: Tchekmedyian NS and Cella DF (eds), Quality of life in oncology practice and research, PRR Dominus, New York, 1991.

47. Pitt HA. Curative treatment for pancreatic neoplasms. Standard resection. Surg Clin N Am 1995; *75:*891–904.

48. Maguire P (1985). Barriers to psychological care of the dying. Br Med J 291, 1711–1713.
49. Sugarbaker PH, Barosky I, Rosenberg SA, and Gianola FJ. Quality of life assessment of patients in extremity sarcoma clinical trials. Surgery 1982; *91:*17–23.
50. McLeod RS, Taylor BR, O'Connor BI, Greenberg GR, Jeejeebhoy KN, Royall D, and Langer B. Quality of life, nutritional status, and gastrointestinal hormone profile following the Whipple procedure. Am J Surg 1995; *169:*179–185.
51. Fraser SCA. Quality of life measurement in surgical practice. Br J Surg 1993; *80:*163–168.
52. Lichtenstein DR and Carr-Locke DL Endoscopic palliation for unresectable pancreatic carcinoma. [Review] Surg Clin N Am 1995; *75:*969–988.
53. Palmer KR, Kerr M, Knowles G, Cull A, Carter DC, and Leonard RCF. Chemotherapy prolongs survival in inoperable pancreatic-carcinoma. Br J Surg 1994; *81:*882–885.
54. Jessup JM, Posner M, and Hubeman M. Influence of multi-modality therapy on the management of pancreatic carcinoma. Semin Surg Oncol 1993; *9:*27–32.
54. Waegner DJT, Punt CJA, and Wilke H. Current status and future directions in the perioperative treatment of pancreatic cancer. Ann Oncol 1994; *5(Suppl):*S87–S90.
55. Katz S, Ford AB, Moskowitz RW, et al. Studies of illness in the aged: the index of ADL: a standardised measure of biological and psychosocial function. JAMA 1963; *185:*914–919.
56. Kaplan RM, Bush JW, and Berry CC. Health status types of validity and the index of well being. Health Serv Res 1976; *11:*478–507.
57. Deyo RA, Inui TS, Leninger JD, et al. Physical and psychological functions in rheumatoid arthritis: clinical use of a self-administered instrument. Arch Intern Med 1982; *142:*879–882.
58. Hunt SM, Mckenna SP, McEwan J, et al. A quantitative approach to perceived health status: a validation study. J Epidemiol Community Health 1980; *35:*297–300.
59. Chambers LW, Sackett DL, Goldsmith CH, et al. Development and applications of an index of social function. Health Serv Res 1976; *11:*430–441.
60. Goldberg DP and Williams P. A users guide to the general health questionnaire. Windsor NFER, nelson.
61. Satoris N. A WHO method for the assessment of health related quality of life. In: Walker SR and Rosser RM (eds) Quality of life assessment: key issues for the 1990s, Klewer, London, 1993; pp. 201–207.
62. Ware JE, Gandek B, the IQOLA Project Group. The SF-36 health survey: development and use in mental health research and the IQOLA Project. Int J Ment Health 1994; *23:*49–73.
63. Spitzer WO, Dobson AJ, Hall J, et al. Measuring quality of life of cancer patients: a concise QL index for use by physicians. J Chron Dis 1981; *34:*585–597.
64. Osbond ME, Lavin PT, Babyam RK, et al. Effect of autolymphocyte therapy on survival and quality of life in patients with metastatic cell carcinoma. Lancet 1990; *335:*994–998.
65. Schnipper H, Clinch J, McMurray A, and Levitt M. Measuring the quality of life of cancer patients the functional living index: cancer development and validation. J Clin Oncol 1984; 472–483.
66. Aaronson NK, Ahmedzai S, Bergman B, et al. The European Organisation for Research and Treatment of Cancer QLQ-C30: a quality of life instrument for use in international clinical trials in oncology. J Nat Cancer Inst 1993; *85:*365–376.
67. De Haes JCJM, van Knippenberg FCE, and Neijt JP. Measuring psychological and physical distress in cancer patients: structure and application of the Rotterdam symptom checklist. Br J Cancer 1990; *62:*1034–1038.
68. Priestman TJ and Baum M. Evaluation of quality of life in patients receiving treatment for advanced breast cancer. Linear analogue self assessment (LASA). Lancet 1976; *1:*899–901.
69. Cella DF, Tulskey DS, and Gray G. Functional assessment of cancer therapy (FACT) scale: development and validation of the general measure. J Clin Oncol 1993; *11:*570–579.
70. Zung WWK. Self rating depression scale. Arch Gen Psychiatry 1965; *12:*63–70.
71. Melzack R. The McGill pain questionnaire major properties and scoring methods. Pain 1975; *1:*277.

72. Beck AT, Mendelson M, Mock J, et al. Psychometric properties of the Beck depression inventory: twenty-five years of evaluation. Clin Psych Rev 1988; *8:*77–100.
73. Baker F, Curbow B, and Wingward JR. Role retention and quality of life of bone marrow transplant survivors. Soc Sci Med 1991; *32:*697–704.
74. Morrow GR, Chiarello RJ, and Derogatis LR. A new scale for assessing patients psychological adjustment to medical illness (PAIS). Psych Med 1978; *8:*605–610.

INDEX

A

Abdominal pain
 palliation, 247
Acidic fibroblast growth factors (FGF1), 25–27, 39–42
Acinar cell adenocarcinoma
 Lewis rats, 53, 54
Adeno-associated virus (AAV), 298
Adenomatoid ductal hyperplasia, 56, 57
Adenomatous hyperplasia, 56, 57
Adenoviral vectors, 297, 298
Adjuvant therapy
 QOL, 333, 334
Adriamycin, 271
Advanced cancer
 coping, 324
AIN-76A diet, 63, 64
AKT2, 4
Allele-specific oligodeoxynucleotides (ASOH)
 K-ras mutations, 116, 117, 121
American Joint Committee (AJCC) staging classification, 160
American Society for Gastrointestinal Endoscopy (ASGE) recommendations, 243
Amphiregulin, 22–24, 35
Androgen-induced growth factor (FGF-8), 25
Angiography, 162
 cost, 162
 tumor resectability assessment, 186
Animal models, 53–66
 carcinogen distribution and metabolism, 54–56
 carcinogenic mechanisms, 56
 dietary additives, 64, 65
 diet modulation, 63, 64
 gene abnormalities, 57–62
 hormones, 65
 neoplastic phenotypes, 62, 63
 precursor lesions, 56, 57
 species differences, 63
Antioxidant micronutrients, 64, 65
Antisense technology, 299, 300

 dominant gene expression blockade, 301, 302
Antrectomy, 219, 220, 229
Azaserine-induced carcinoma
 rat, 61, 62
Azaserine-rat model
 dietary additives, 64, 65

B

B7.1, 305, 306
Basic fibroblast growth factor (FGF2), 25–27, 39–42, 302
BCL2, 302
Betacellulin, 22–24, 35
Biliary bypass with antrectomy, 219, 220, 229
Biliary obstruction, 235
Biliary sepsis
 ERCP, 243
Biolioenteric anastomosis, 236
Bladder cancer
 p53 mutations, 124
Blood samples
 K-ras mutations, 120, 121
Body image, 323
Bombesin, 65
BRCA2
 homozygous deletions, 9
 mutations, 12, 126
Breast cancer
 TGF-B, 89–94
*Bst*NI, 116, 117

C

CA 19-9, 137–144
 false-positive rates, 140
 predictive value, 140
 prognosis, 143, 144
 sensitivity, 141
 specificity, 140
 tumor resectability, 142, 143
 vs.imaging, 142, 143
 vs.tumor antigens, 144–148
CA 50, 144
 vs CA 19-9, 144, 145

CA 242, 147
  vs CA 19-9, 147
CA 494, 148
  vs Ca 19-9, 148
Cachexia, 323
CAn, 11
Carcinoembryonic antigen (CEA), 306
Carcinogen metabolism
  pancreas, 56
CD4+, 306
CD8+, 306
CD44, 307
CDK4 mutations, 7
Cell cycle control
  pancreatic cancer, 10, 11
  TGF-B, 77–96
Cell growth
  TGF-B, 77–80
c-erbB-2, 36, 37
c-erbB-3, 37
Chemoradiation, 286–288
  M. D. Anderson Cancer Center, 287, 290
  pancreaticoduodenectomy, 196
  postoperative, 288, 289
  preoperative, 289, 290
  Radiation Therapy Oncology Group
      (RTOG), 289
Chemotherapy
  endpoints, 266
  QOL, 266
  radiation, 273, 274
  recent developments, 266, 267
Cholangitis, 243
Cholecystojejunostomy, 250, 254
Cholecystokinin (CCK), 64, 65
Chronic pancreatitis
  CA 19-9, 140
  c-erbB-2, 36, 37
  c-erbB-3, 37
  EGF, 25
  growth factors, 33–47
  maldigestion, 33, 34
  pain pathogenesis, 33
  pathophysiology, 33, 34
Cirrhosis, 140
Cisplatiin, 273
c-K-ras mutations, 56–58
Classification of pancreatic cancer
  Japanese Pancreas Society, 214
Clinical trials
  QOL assessment, 320

c-MET, 29
c-myb, 302
c-myc, 78, 302
Colon cancer
  p53 mutations, 124
  TGF-B, 82–84
Computed tomography (CT), 159–162,236,
      282, 283
  cost, 162
  jaundice, 157
  pancreatic cancer, 157, 158
  tumor resectability assessment, 183, 184
  tumor resectability prediction, 150
Computed tomography (CT) angiography,
      158, 159
Computed tomography (CT)-guided
      percutaneous biopsy, 165
  cost, 165
Cost
  CT vs angiography, 162
  FDG-PET, 165
  image-guided percutaneous biopsy, 165
  malignant obstructive jaundice, 246
  MRI, 163
  scintigraphy, 165
Co-stimulatory molecule gene therapy, 305, 306
Cripto, 29
  chronic pancreatitis, 37–39
Cyclin-dependent protein kinase (CDK), 10
Cyclin D1 protein, 91
Cyclin E, 91
Cyclins, 10
Cyclophosphamide, 273
Cytokine gene therapy, 305

D

3-D CT arteriography, 162
Diet, 323
Dietary additives
  animal models, 64, 65
Dietary fat, 64
Diet modulation
  animal models, 63, 64
Distal pancreatectomy (DP)
  resection rate, 216
  survival rate, 216–220
DPC4, 7, 8, 11, 81
  inactivation, 9, 10
  mutations, 12, 25
Ductal adenocarcinoma
  molecular genetics, 14

Duodenal fluid
K-ras mutations, 120, 121
Duodenal obstruction, 254
DUPAN-2, 145, 146
vs CA 19-9, 146

E

E2f, 78
EGF receptor type 1 (HER-1), 35–37
EGF receptor type 2 (HER-2), 24
EGF receptor type 3 (HER-3), 24
EGF receptor type 4 (HER-4), 24
Elastase-1-myc transgenic mouse model, 60
Endoglin, 75
Endometrial carcinoma, 86–89
Endoscopic palliation
QOL, 333
Endoscopic retrograde cholangio-
pancreatography (ERCP), 236
biliary sepsis, 243
tumor resectability assessment, 183–185
Endoscopic retrograde
cholangiopancreatography (ERCP)
brushings
K-ras mutations, 120, 121
Endoscopic stents, 235–249
abdominal pain palliation, 247
complications, 243, 244
malignant obstructive jaundice, 244–246
morbidity, 235
mortality, 236
patient selection, 236
QOL, 326
Endoscopic ultrasound (EUS), 158, 164
EORTC QLQ-C30, 326, 327
EORTC Quality of Life Study Group, 327
Epidermal growth factor (EGF), 22, 23
Epidermal growth factor (EGF) receptor, 24,
25, 35–37
ERB2, 302
ERBB2, 307
Erythropoietin, 307
Estrogen, 65
European Quality of Life in Pancreatic
Cancer (EQoLiPA), 327
Ewings sarcoma, 95
Experimental models, 53–66
Extended pancreatic resection, 222, 223
Japanese experience, 213–229
methods, 213, 214
morbidity, 216

mortality, 216
outcome, 216–218
pancreatic cancer, 213–229
QOL, 228, 229
resection rate, 216
results, 216–220
subjects, 213, 214
vs pancreatectomy, 216–218
Extended radical Whipple resection
morbidity and mortality, 206, 207, 210
pancreatic adenocarcinoma, 201–211
quality of life, 326, 331, 332
resectability, 204–206
results, 204–208
survival rate, 207, 208
technique, 201–204
External beam intraoperative radiotherapy
(EB-IORT), 285, 288, 291
External beam irradiation (ExBRT), 282,
283, 287, 291
Extrapancreatic extension
CT detection, 160
Extrapancreatic tumor hypoglycemia
syndrome, 27

F

Familial atypical multiple-mole melanoma
(FAMMM) syndrome, 12
Familial pancreatic cancer
definition, 12
screening, 126, 127
Familial pancreatic carcinoma
molecular genetics, 12, 13
Fat
dietary, 64
F-18 fluorodeoxyglucose positron emission
tomography (FDG-PET), 164, 165
cost, 165
Fibroblast growth factors (FGF), 25–27, 39–42
Fibroblast growth factors receptor 1 (FGFR-1),
26, 41, 42
Fibroblast growth factors receptor 2 (FGFR-2),
26, 41, 42
Fibroblast growth factors receptor 3 (FGFR-3),
25, 26, 41
Fibroblast growth factors receptor 4 (FGFR-4),
26, 41
Fibroblast growth factors receptor 5 (FGFR-5),
26, 41
Fibroblast growth factors receptor 6 (FGFR-6),
26

Fibroblast growth factors receptor 7 (FGFR-7), 26

Fibroblast growth factors receptors (FGFR), 25–27, 39–42

Fine needle aspirations (FNAs)
    K-ras mutations, 120, 121

Flat hyperplasia, 56, 57

5-fluoracil, 189, 269, 270
    ExBRT, 287
    radiation, 273, 274

5-fluoracil + adriamycin + mitomycin-C, 271

5-fluoracil + adriamycin + mitomycin-C + streptozocin, 271

5-fluoracil (5-FU)
    QOL, 333

5-fluoracil + mitomycin-C+ methotrexate + vincristine + cyclophosphamide, 273

5-fluoracil + mitomycin-C- + streptozocin, 271

5-fluoracil + streptozotocin + cisplatin + ExBRT (RT-FSP), 287

G

Gastric cancer
    TGF-B, 84–86

Gastric outlet obstruction
    metallic stents, 247, 248

Gastrin, 65

Gastroenterostomy
    morbidity, 247

Gastrojejunostomy, 236, 254, 256, 257, 261

Gemcitabine, 288
    pancreatic adenocarcinoma, 267
    QOL, 333

General Rules for Cancer of the Pancreas, 214, 215, 226

Gene targeting, 300

Gene therapy
    pancreatic cancer, 295–308
    tumor vasculature, 307

Genetic immunomodulation, 304–307

Genetic prodrug activation therapy (GPAT), 302–304
    bystander effects, 304
    transcriptional targeting, 303, 304
    transduction targeting, 303

Genetic therapy
    antitumor lymphocytes, 307

Germ-line therapy, 295

Gianturco Z stent, 239

Glia-activating factor (FGF-9), 25

Gliomas, 92–94

Goserelin, 270, 271

Granulocyte-macrophage colony stimulating factor (GM-CSF), 305

Growth factor receptors
    chronic pancreatitis, 33–47

Growth factor-related binding protein 2 (GRB2), 24

Growth factors
    chronic pancreatitis, 33–47

H

Hamsters, 53–66

Helical CT, 158, 159, 161, 162, 176, 186, 191, 282, 283

Heparin-binding EGF-like growth factor (HB-EGF), 22–24, 35

Hepatocyte growth factor, 29

Hereditary nonpolyposis colorectal carcinoma (HNPCC) syndrome
    etiology, 11
    RER+, 84

Hereditary predisposition syndromes
    prevention, 295, 296

Homologous recombination, 300

Homozygous deletions
    pancreatic cancer, 9, 10

Hormones
    animal models, 65

Hospital Anxiety and Depression Score (HADS), 326

Human pancreatic cancer
    PGFs, 21–29

Human pancreatic ductal adenocarcinoma, 24, 25

Human pancreatic tumors
    histological classification, 58, 62

Hyperplasias, 114

Hyperthermia, 286

I

IL-2, 305, 306

IL-15, 305

Image-guided percutaneous biopsy, 165
    cost, 165

Insulin, 27–29

Insulin-like growth factor I (IGF-I), 27–29

Insulin-like growth factor II (IGF-II), 27–29

Insulin-like growth factor (IGF) receptors, 27–29

Insulin receptor substrate-1 (IRS-1), 27
Intraoperative radiotherapy, 283–286
Invasive ductal adenocarcinoma
    extended radical Whipple resection, 201–211
Iodinated intravenous contrast media, 159
Islet amyloid polyptide (IAPP), 149, 150
Islet cell cancer
    radiation therapy, 290, 291

J

Japanese experience
    extended pancreatic resection, 213–229
Japanese N factor classification, 214
Japanese staging classification, 204
    vs UICC, 204
Jaundice, 254, 322
    CT vs transabdominal ultrasound, 157
Johns Hopkins Hospital National Familial
        Pancreatic Tumor Registry, 12, 127
JV18-1, 9

K

Karnofsky index, 320, 325
Keratinocyte growth factor (FGF-7), 25
Kocher maneuver, 187–189
K-ras, 11, 307
    mutations, 4, 25, 115–122, 301, 302

L

Lactate hydrogenase, 307
Laparoscopic biliary bypass, 253–262
    animal studies, 255–259
    clinical experience, 259–262
    rationale, 254
Laparoscopic cholecysojejunostomy, 259, 260
Laparoscopic gastric bypass, 253–262
    animal studies, 255–259
    clinical experience, 259–262
    rationale, 254
Laparoscopic gastroenterostomy
    malignant duodenal obstruction, 250
Laparoscopic ultrasound (LUS), 164, 175, 176
Laparoscopic ultrasound (LUS) probes, 175, 176
Laparoscopy
    pancreatic cancer diagnosis and staging,
        171–177
    pancreatic cancer staging
        rationale, 171–174
        technique, 174, 175
    peritoneal cytology, 174
    tumor resectability assessment, 185, 186

Laparotomy, 177
    vs laparoscopy, 186
Latent TGF-B-binding protein (LTBP), 74
Latent TGF-B (LTGF-B), 74
Lewis antigens
    biochemical structure, 137, 138
Lewis rats
    acinar cell adenocarcinoma, 53, 54
Liposomes, 298
Lithostatin, 34
Loss of heterozygosity (LOH), 9, 81
Lymphadenectomy, 222
Lymph nodes metastasis, 210,226

M

M. D. Anderson Cancer Center
    chemoradiation, 280, 287
MAD/Smad, 77, 81
Magnetic resonance imaging (MRI), 159,
        160, 162, 163
    cost, 163
Malignant duodenal obstruction
    laparoscopic gastroenterostomy, 250
Malignant obstructive jaundice
    endoscopic vs surgical palliation, 244–246
MAP kinase, 24
mdm-2, 25
Memorial Sloan-Kettering Cancer Center
        (MSKCC)
    cholecystojejunostomy, 250
    staging laparoscopy, 185, 186
Metallic expandable endoprostheses, 239–241
Metallic stents
    gastric outlet obstruction, 247, 248
Methotrexate, 273
Methylthioadenosine phosphorylase
        (MTAP), 10
Microsatellites, 11, 84
    molecular detection, 125
Mismatch repair genes, 11, 12
Mismatch repair (MMR) enzymes, 11
Mitomycin-C, 271, 273
Molecular genetics, 3–15
Moloney murine leukemia virus (MMLV),
        297
Morbidity
    endoscopic stents, 235
    extended pancreatic resection, 216
    extended radical Whipple resection, 206,
        207, 210
    gastroenterostomy, 247

Mortality
  endoscopic stents, 236
  extended pancreatic resection, 216
  extended radical Whipple resection, 206,
      207, 210
MR angiography (MRA), 163
Mucous cell hyperplasia, 56, 57
Mucous cell hypertrophy, 56, 57
Multihit tumorigenesis, 3
Multistep tumorigenesis, 3
Mutator phenotype, 125
MYC mutation, 4

N

Naked DNA, 298
National Familial Pancreatic Tumor Registry
  Johns Hopkins Hospital, 12, 127
Nausea, 322
N-ethyl-*N*-nitrosoguanidine, 55
Nitrosamine,4-(methylnitrosamino)-1-(3-
      pyridyl)-1-butanone (NNK), 55
N-nitrosobis(2-oxopropyl)amine (BOP), 53,
      55, 63
Nodal metastases
  CT detection, 160
Nonpapillary ductal hyperplasia, 56, 57
Nonverbal vectors, 298, 299
Nottingham Health Profile, 321

O

Obstruction
  biliary, 235
  gastric outlet, 247, 248
Obstructive jaundice, 254
Oltipraz, 64
Oncogenes, 4, 5
  activation, 5
Oncogenesis, 71, 72
Osteosarcomas, 94, 95

P

p15, 81
  gliomas, 94
  mutations, 79
p16, 6, 7, 81
  gliomas, 94
  inactivation, 9, 10
  mutations, 12, 79, 91, 126
p21, 11
p27, 79, 80
  endometrial carcinoma, 88, 89

p53, 5, 6, 11, 300, 301
  activities, 6
  inactivation, 9, 10
  mutations, 6, 25, 59, 60
    molecular detection, 122–125
Paclitaxel, 288
Pain, 33, 247, 323
Palliative pancreaticoduodenectomy, 219,
    220
Palliative surgery
  QOL, 332, 333
PANC-I cells, 25
Pancreas
  carcinogen metabolism, 56
Pancreatectomy
  vs extended pancreatic resection, 216–218
Pancreatic adenocarcinoma
  antigens, 148, 149
  extended radical Whipple resection, 201–211
  gemcitabine, 267
  pancreaticoduodenectomy
    results, 195
  prognosis, 171
  regional pancreatectomy vs standard
      pancreaticoduodenectomy, 186, 187
  survival, 171
Pancreatic cancer
  cell cycle control, 10, 11
  chemotherapy, 265–274
  combination chemotherapy, 271–274
  CT vs ultrasound, 157, 158
  definition, 12
  development, 114, 115
  diagnosis
    laparoscopy, 171–177
    radiologic techniques, 157–166
  etiopathogenesis, 95, 96
  extended pancreatic resection, 213–229
  gene therapy, 295–308
  homozygous deletions, 9, 10
  incidence, 113
  molecular genetics, 3–15
  PGFs, 21–29
  psychosocial impact, 323
  quality of life, 319–335
  radiation therapy, 281–292
  screening, 113–130
  sporadic, 12
  staging
    laparoscopy, 171–177
    radiologic techniques, 157–166

survival, 21, 113, 265
symptoms, 235, 322, 323
TGF-B, 80–82
tumor antigens, 137–150
tumor markers, 137, 138
Pancreatic cancer quality of life
        questionnaire
    development, 327–331
Pancreatic Cancer Registry, 221, 222, 226, 227
Pancreatic cancer resection
    Japanese vs Western survival, 224
    prognostic factors, 226
Pancreatic demoplasia, 266
Pancreatic ductal adenocarcinoma
    CT, 159
    human, 24, 25
Pancreatic fistula, 221
Pancreatic imaging
    patient outcome, 166
    principles, 157–159
Pancreatic intraepithelial neoplasias, 114
Pancreaticoduodenectomy, 187–195
    chemoradiation, 196
    Kocher maneuver, 187–190
    pancreatic adenocarcinoma, 195
    pylorus preservation, 193–195
    resectability rates, 171
    retroperitoneal vascular dissection, 190–
        193
    Western experience, 195, 196
Pancreatic resection
    extent, 186–195
    standard forms, 181–196
Pancreatic tumors
    histological classification, 58, 62
Pancreatoduodenectomy
    Japanese history, 208, 209
    QOL, 331
    resection rate, 216
    residual cancer, 209
    survival rate, 216–220
Papillary ductal hyperplasia, 56, 57
Paracaval soft-tissue resection, 187–189
Particle bombardment, 299
p16/CDK4/RB pathway, 11
PCR
    K-ras mutations, 116, 117, 121
    microsatellites, 125
    p53 mutations, 122–124
PCR-RFLP
    K-ras mutations, 116, 117, 121

Percutaneous biopsy
    CT-guided, 165
    ultrasound-guided, 165
Peritoneal cytology
    laparoscopy, 174
Pigs
    laparoscopic bypass, 255–259
p27^{kip1}, 83, 84, 91
Plastic endoprosthesis, 236–239
    stent occlusion, 238
Plastic stent migration, 244
Platelet-derived growth factor (PDGF), 29
Polypeptide growth factors (PGFs)
    human pancreatic cancer, 21–29
Polypeptide growth factors (PGFs)
    receptors, 21–29
Portal vein resection, 223
Postoperative chemoradiation, 288, 289
Preoperative chemoradiation, 289, 290
Primitive neuroectodermal tumors (PNETs),
        92, 93
Psychosocial demands
    advanced cancer, 323, 324
Psychosocial impact
    pancreatic cancer, 323
Psychosocial oncology, 320
Pure pancreatic juice (PPJ)
    CA 19-9, 140
    K-ras mutations, 120, 121
Pylorus preservation
    pancreaticoduodenectomy, 193–195

Q

QOL
    extended pancreatic resection, 228, 229
Qualitiy of life(QOL) assessment
    tools, 321, 322
Quality of life adjusted years (QALYs), 325,
        326
Quality of life assessment, 324–327
    resistance, 321
Quality of life (QOL)
    chemotherapy, 266
    defined, 320–321
    improvement, 331–334
    pancreatic cancer, 319–335
    surgical resection, 326
    TP, 223
    vs quantity, 319, 320
Quality of life (QOL) assessment, 320
    clinical trials, 320

R

Radiation sensitivity
  etiologic factors, 281
Radiation therapy, 281–292
  adjuvant treatment, 288–290
  altered fractionation schedules, 286
  chemotherapy, 273, 274
  intraoperative, 283–286
  islet cell cancer, 290, 291
  QOL, 333, 334
Radiation Therapy Oncology Group (RTOG)
  chemoradiation, 289
Radiology Diagnostic Oncology Group
    study
  CT vs MRI, 163
RAF-1, 24
Raf-1/MAP kinase pathway, 11
ras-GTP, 24
Rats
  azaserine-induced carcinoma, 61, 62
Regional pancreatectomy, 221
  vs standard pancreaticoduodenectomy,
    186, 187
Replication error phenotype (RER), 11, 12
Replication errors (RER+), 84
Resectable pancreatic tumor
  defined, 159, 160
Residual cancer
  pancreaticoduodenectomy, 209
Retroperitoneal vascular dissection, 190–193
Retroviral vectors, 297, 298
Rhabdomyosarcoma, 95
Rotterdam Symptom Checklist, 321, 326
Roux-en-Y jejunostomy, 254

S

Scintigraphy, 159, 164, 165
  cost, 165
Serial analysis of gene expression (SAGE),
    127–129
Short Form 36, 321
Single-strand conformation polymorphism
    (SSCP)
  p53 mutations, 122–124
Somatic genetic therapy, 295
  technology, 296–300
Somatostatin, 65
Son-of-sevenless (SOS), 24
SPAN-1, 145
vs CA 19-9, 145, 146

Spiral CT, 158, 159, 161, 162, 176, 186, 191
Sporadic pancreatic cancer
  definition, 12
Standard pancreaticoduodenectomy
  vs regional pancreatectomy, 186, 187
Stent occlusion, 244
  plastic endoprosthesis, 238
Stool samples
  K-ras mutations, 120, 121
  p53 mutations, 124
Strecker stent, 239
Streptozocin, 271, 287
Superior mesenteric artery (SMA), 182,
    185–190, 192, 193
Superior mesenteric-portal vein (SMPV),
    182, 185–187, 190, 191
Surgical resection, 181–196
  malignant obstructive jaundice, 244–246
  QOL, 331, 332
  quality of life, 326
Swiss Group for Clinical Cancer Research
    (SAKK), 325
Syrian golden hamsters, 53

T

Tamoxifen (Tam), 86, 89, 90, 271
T cell suppressor factor (TcSF), 92
Testosterone, 65
Testosterone:dihydrotestosterone ratio
    (T:DHT), 148, 149
TGF-a, 35
TGF-B
  cancer etiopathogenesis, 95, 96
  cancer growth regulation, 80–96
  growth inhibition, 79, 80
TGF-B1
  breast cancer, 89–94
  colon cancer, 82, 83
  endometrial carcinoma, 86–89
  gastric cancer, 84–86
  gliomas, 92–94
  osteosarcomas, 94, 95
TGF-B2
  breast cancer, 89–94
  endometrial carcinoma, 86–89
  gastric cancer, 84–86
  gliomas, 92–94
  osteosarcomas, 94, 95
TGF-B3
  breast cancer, 89–94
  endometrial carcinoma, 86–89

gastric cancer, 84–86
osteosarcomas, 94, 95
TGF-B antisense, 93, 94
TGF-B receptors (TBR), 45
TGF-B receptor type I, 45, 75, 80, 81, 90, 91
TGF-B receptor type II, 45, 75, 80, 90, 91
TGF-B receptor type III, 45, 75, 81
Tissue polypeptide antigen (TPA), 148, 149
Tissue polypeptide specific antigen (TPS), 148, 149
Total pancreatectomy (TP), 223
    resection rate, 216
    survival rate, 216–220
TP53, 300, 301
Transabdominal ultrasound, 157, 163, 164
Transforming growth factor alpha (TGF-a), 22–24
Transforming growth factor-B (TGF-B), 71–96
    activation, 74
    cell growth, 77–80
    chronic pancreatitis, 42–46
    functions, 73, 74
    oncogenesis, 71, 72
    receptor binding, 75–77
    regulation, 75–77
    structure, 73, 74
Transgenic mouse model, 60
Trypsin inhibitors, 64, 65
Tumor-associated antigens (TAAs), 137–150
Tumorigenesis, 3
Tumor markers
    pancreatic cancer, 137, 138
Tumor resectability
    assessment, 181–185
    extended radical Whipple resection, 204–206

Tumor-suppressor gene function
    replacement, 300, 301
Tumor-supressor genes, 5–9

U

Ubiquitin-proteasome pathway, 80
Ultrasound, 157, 158, 163, 164, 236
Ultrasound-guided percutaneous biopsy, 165
    cost, 165
Union Internationale Contre Le Cancer (UICC) staging classification, 204
    vs Japanese classification, 226
Urine
    p53 mutations, 124

V

Vaccina virus, 298
Vascular involvement
    CT vs angiographic detection, 160, 161
Vincristine, 273
Viral vectors, 297, 298
Vomiting, 322

W

WAF1, 123, 124, 301
Wallstent, 241, 248
Weight loss, 323
Western experience
    pancreaticoduodenectomy, 195, 196
Whipple resection, 201–211, 326, 331, 332
Wide-field irradiation, 287
World Wide Web
    National Familial Pancreatic Tumor Registry, 127

Lightning Source UK Ltd.
Milton Keynes UK
UKOW01f1533290813

216184UK00004B/44/P